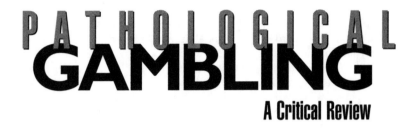

PATHOLOGICAL GAMBLING
A Critical Review

Committee on the Social and Economic Impact
of Pathological Gambling

Committee on Law and Justice

Commission on Behavioral and Social Sciences and Education

National Research Council

NATIONAL ACADEMY PRESS
Washington, D.C.

NATIONAL ACADEMY PRESS • 2101 Constitution Avenue, N.W. • Washington, D.C. 20418

This study was supported by the National Gambling Impact Study Commission. Any opinions, findings, conclusions, or recommendations expressed in this publication are those of the author(s) and do not necessarily reflect the views of the organizations or agencies that provided support for the project.

Library of Congress Cataloging-in-Publication Data

Pathological gambling : a critical review / Committee on the Social
and Economic Impact of Pathological Gambling [and] Committee on Law
and Justice, Commission on Behavioral and Social Sciences and
Education, National Research Council.
    p. cm.
    Includes bibliographical references and index.
    ISBN 0-309-06571-2 (hardcover)
    1. Compulsive gambling—United States. I. National Research
Council (U.S.). Committee on the Social and Economic Impact of
Pathological Gambling. II. National Research Council (U.S.).
Committee on Law and Justice.
    RC569.5.G35 P38 1999
    616.85′841—dc21   99-06598

Additional copies of this report are available from the National Academy Press, 2101 Constitution Avenue, N.W., Lock Box 285, Washington, D.C. 20005. (800) 624-6242 or (202) 334-313 (in the Washington Metropolitan Area).

This report is also available online at http://www.nap.edu

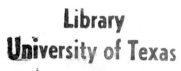

iii

Acknowledgments

The following persons, many who prepared papers or presentations for the committee, are acknowledged and thanked for sharing their expertise on pathological gambling, and for giving of their time to participate in and support the public workshops hosted by the National Research Council:

Curtis L. Barrett, University of Louisville
Alex Blaszczynski, The Liverpool Hospital, Sydney, Australia
Carl Braunlich, Purdue University
David Comings, City of Hope Medical Center, Duarte, California
Sue Cox, Texas Council on Problem and Compulsive Gambling, Richardson
Renee Cunningham-Williams, Washington University School of Medicine
Jeff Derevensky, McGill University, Montreal, Canada
Carlo C. DiClemente, University of Maryland, Baltimore County
William Eadington, University of Nevada
Richard Evans, University of Houston
Don Feeney, Minnesota State Lottery, Roseville
Joanna Franklin, National Council on Problem Gambling, Washington, DC
Peter Goyer, Cleveland Medical Center, Ohio

Mark Griffiths, The Nottingham Trent University, Nottingham,
    Australia
Rina Gupta, McGill University, Montreal, Canada
Matthew A. Hall, Harvard Medical School
Erik Hollander, Mt. Sinai School of Medicine, New York
Durand F. Jacobs, American Board of Professional Psychology,
    California
Norm Kruedelbach, Veterans Administration Medical Center,
    Ohio
Robert Ladouceur, Université Laval, Quebec, Canada
Henry Lesieur, Institute for Problem Gambling, Middletown,
    Connecticut
Scott Lukas, McClean Hospital, Cambridge, Massachusetts
Janet Mann, American Academy of Health Care Providers in the
    Addictive Disorders, Cambridge, Massachusetts
Richard McCleary, University of California at Irvine
Lia Nower, Washington University
Judy Patterson, American Gaming Association, Washington, DC
Marcus D. Patterson, American Academy of Health Care
    Providers in the Addictive Disorders, Cambridge,
    Massachusetts
William Rhodes, Abt Associates Inc., Cambridge, Massachusetts
I. Nelson Rose, Whittier Law School
Lori Rugle, Trimeridian Inc., Carmel, Indiana
William Semple, Cleveland Medical Center, Ohio
Randy Stinchfield, University of Minnesota Medical School
Bradley Stoner, Washington University
Rodger Svendson, Minnesota Institute of Public Health, Anoka
Jack Thar, Indiana Gaming Commission, Indianapolis
Tony Toneatto, Addiction Research Foundation, Calgary, Canada
Joni Vander Bilt, Harvard Medical School
Rachel Volberg, Gemini Research, Northhampton,
    Massachusetts
Lynn Wallisch, Texas Commission on Alcohol and Drug Abuse,
    Austin
Robert Wildman, Dickson, O'Bryan, Dugan and Associates,
    Nevada
Harold Wynne, Wynne Resources, Edmonton, Alberta, Canada
Kurt Zorn, Indiana University

This report has been reviewed in draft form by individuals chosen for their diverse perspectives and technical expertise, in accordance with procedures approved by the Report Review Committee of the National Research Council. The purpose of this independent review is to provide candid and critical comments that will assist the institution in making the published report as sound as possible and to ensure that the report meets institutional standards for objectivity, evidence, and responsiveness to the study charge. The review comments and draft manuscript remain confidential to protect the integrity of the deliberative process.

We thank the following individuals for their participation in the review of this report: John Bailar, Irving B. Harris Graduate School of Public Policy Studies, University of Chicago; Robert Boruch, Graduate School of Education and Wharton School, University of Pennsylvania; Philip J. Cook, Sanford Institute of Public Policy, Duke University; Stephen Cornell, Udall Center for Studies in Public Policy, University of Arizona; John Dombrink, Department of Criminology, Law, and Society, University of California, Irvine; Reid Hastie, Center for Research on Judgment and Policy and Department of Psychology, University of Colorado; John Kihlstrom, Department of Psychology, University of California, Berkeley; Robert S. Lawrence, School of Medicine and School of Hygiene and Public Health, Johns Hopkins University; Scott O. Lilienfeld, Department of Psychology, Emory University; John Monahan, Professor of Law, Psychology, and Legal Medicine, University of Virginia School of Law; Eric J. Nestler, Professor of Psychiatry and Neurobiology, Yale University School of Medicine; Henry W. Riecken, Professor of Behavioral Sciences, University of Pennsylvania School of Medicine (emeritus); and Lee N. Robins, Department of Psychiatry, Washington University of School of Medicine.

Although the individuals listed above have provided constructive comments and suggestions, it must be emphasized that responsibility for the final content of this report rests entirely with the authoring committee and the institution.

The National Academy of Sciences is a private, nonprofit, self-perpetuating society of distinguished scholars engaged in scientific and engineering research, dedicated to the furtherance of science and technology and to their use for the general welfare. Upon the authority of the charter granted to it by the Congress in 1863, the Academy has a mandate that requires it to advise the federal government on scientific and technical matters. Dr. Bruce Alberts is president of the National Academy of Sciences.

The National Academy of Engineering was established in 1964, under the charter of the National Academy of Sciences, as a parallel organization of outstanding engineers. It is autonomous in its administration and in the selection of its members, sharing with the National Academy of Sciences the responsibility for advising the federal government. The National Academy of Engineering also sponsors engineering programs aimed at meeting national needs, encourages education and research, and recognizes the superior achievements of engineers. Dr. William A. Wulf is president of the National Academy of Engineering.

The Institute of Medicine was established in 1970 by the National Academy of Sciences to secure the services of eminent members of appropriate professions in the examination of policy matters pertaining to the health of the public. The Institute acts under the responsibility given to the National Academy of Sciences by its congressional charter to be an adviser to the federal government and, upon its own initiative, to identify issues of medical care, research, and education. Dr. Kenneth I. Shine is president of the Institute of Medicine.

The National Research Council was organized by the National Academy of Sciences in 1916 to associate the broad community of science and technology with the Academy's purposes of furthering knowledge and advising the federal government. Functioning in accordance with general policies determined by the Academy, the Council has become the principal operating agency of both the National Academy of Sciences and the National Academy of Engineering in providing services to the government, the public, and the scientific and engineering communities. The Council is administered jointly by both Academies and the Institute of Medicine. Dr. Bruce Alberts and Dr. William A. Wulf are chairman and vice chairman, respectively, of the National Research Council.

Contents

PATHOLOGICAL GAMBLING

Executive Summary

Gambling in America has deep cultural roots and exists today as a widely available and socially accepted recreational activity. Over 80 percent of American adults now report having gambled sometime during their lifetime—on casino games, lotteries, sports betting, horse racing and off-track betting, and other gambling activities. It is estimated that in 1997 they collectively wagered more than $551 billion. This market has increased the intensity of competition for gambling dollars among state-sponsored lotteries and commercial gambling enterprises, leading to legalization in some states in which gambling had previously been voted down. Presently, gambling in some form is legal in all but 3 states, casinos or casino-style games are available in 21 states, and 37 states have lotteries. Resistance by many state legislatures to casino gambling and state-sanctioned sports betting continues, but state and tribal governments are increasingly relying on gambling revenues.

Although the recent institutionalization of gambling appears to have benefited economically depressed communities in which it is offered, gambling has social and economic costs. Two major concerns of public health and other policy officials are whether, in the currently expanding gambling environment, the number or proportion of pathological gamblers in the United States is increasing and the possible effects of pathological gambling on individuals, families, and communities.

The charge to the Committee on the Social and Economic Impact of Pathological Gambling was to identify and analyze the full range of research studies that bear upon the nature of pathological and problem gambling, highlighting key issues and data sources that can provide hard evidence of their effects.

Pathological gambling differs from the recreational or social gambling of most adults, who view it as a form of entertainment and wager only small amounts. In 1975, the Commission on the Review of the National Policy Toward Gambling estimated that less than 1 percent of the U.S. population were "probable compulsive" gamblers. Pathological gambling was first included as a mental health diagnosis in 1980 in the *Diagnostic and Statistical Manual of Mental Disorders* (DSM), the official publication of the American Psychiatric Association, classified in the section on disorders of impulse control. It was described as a chronic and progressive failure to resist impulses to gamble, characterized by undesirable outcomes ranging from borrowing money from family or friends and losing time at work, to being arrested for offenses committed to support gambling. Much of the literature examined by the committee on pathological gambling also reflects the American Psychiatric Association's conceptualization of pathological gambling as a disorder characterized by people's continuous or periodic loss of control over their gambling behavior, a preoccupation with gambling and with obtaining money with which to gamble, irrational thinking, and a continuation of the behavior despite adverse consequences.

The current description of pathological gambling in DSM-IV characterizes pathological gambling in relatively precise operational terms; provides the basis for measures that are reliable, replicable, and sensitive to regional and local variation; distinguishes gambling behavior from other impulse disorders; and suggests the utility of applying specific types of clinical treatments. Moreover, the DSM-IV criteria appear to have worked well for clinicians for the past five years. However, because it is a clinical description with little empirical support beyond treatment populations, there still are problems with its use to define the nature and etiology of pathological gambling and when trying to esti-mate prevalence.

The Committee on the Social and Economic Impact of Patho-logical Gambling has conducted an extensive review of the rel-evant scientific literature. The committee concludes that patho-logical gambling is a significant enough problem to warrant funding support for a more sustained, comprehensive, and scien-tific set of research activities than currently exists.

The availability of legal gambling has increased sharply in the past 20 years. More people are gambling, and they are wager-ing more. As a result, there is increased concern about pathologi-cal gambling. Clinical evidence suggests that pathological gam-blers engage in destructive behaviors: they commit crimes, they run up large debts, they damage relationships with family and friends, and they kill themselves. With the increased availability of gambling and new gambling technologies, pathological gam-bling has the potential to become even more widespread. A greater understanding of this problem through scientific research is critical. Recent methodological and theoretical advances in epi-demiology, medicine, and the social and behavioral sciences should aid this understanding.

The committee estimates that 1.5 percent of adults in the United States, at some time in their lives, have been pathological gamblers. We estimate that, in a given year, 0.9 percent of adults in the United States, or 1.8 million, are pathological gamblers. Men are more likely than women to be pathological gamblers, and the proportion of pathological gamblers among adolescents is higher than it is among adults. The committee estimates that, in a given year, as many as 1.1 million adolescents between the ages of 12 and 18 are pathological gamblers. However, the com-mittee recognizes that adolescent measures of pathological gam-bling are not always comparable to adult measures and that dif-ferent thresholds for adolescent gambling problems may exist. Given various ways in which pathological gambling has been operationalized in prevalence studies among adolescents, this estimate should be viewed with caution.

Because the existing research on other subgroups in the population is less well developed, the committee was unable to determine the degree to which other groups, such as elderly people and poor people, have disproportionately high rates of pathological gambling.

To understand changes in gambling and pathological gambling over time, as well as the nature and origins of pathological gambling, both cross-sectional and longitudinal studies of gambling will be necessary. The committee recommends that the Centers for Disease Control and Prevention and the National Institutes of Health should routinely include measures of pathological gambling in their annual surveys, and that measures of gambling and related leisure activities and outcomes (e.g., debts) should be added to other prospective, longitudinal studies on health or mental health. Doing so not only would add valuable information about gambling over time, but would also provide important information about baseline measures and other disorders that tend to cooccur with pathological gambling.

Research is beginning to elucidate the onset and course of pathological gambling. For example:

• Pathological gambling often occurs with other behavioral problems, including substance abuse, mood disorders, and personality disorders.
• Recent research suggests that the earlier one starts to gamble, the more likely one is to become a pathological gambler.
• Pathological gamblers are more likely than nonpathological gamblers to report that their parents were pathological gamblers. These findings, in conjunction with twin studies and recent neuroscience studies, suggest that pathological gambling may be influenced by familial factors and the social environment.

An accurate examination of the costs of pathological gambling requires an assessment of the costs and benefits of gambling generally. Gambling appears to have net economic benefits for economically depressed communities, but the available data are insufficient to determine with accuracy the overall costs and benefits of gambling. Pervasive methodological problems prevent firm conclusions about the social and economic effects of gambling or pathological gambling on communities, nor can the committee say whether pathological gamblers contribute disproportionately to overall gambling revenues. Similarly, the committee could not determine how legalized gambling affects community or national rates of suicide and crime. Additional studies are required to advance understanding of these important matters.

Current, but limited, research indicates that pathological gamblers who seek treatment generally improve. This research is inadequate to determine whether any particular treatment approach is more effective than any other or the extent to which people recover on their own. The effectiveness of promising treatments that are emerging in the mental health field (for example, cognitive-behavioral and pharmacotherapy treatments) should be carefully evaluated. The unmet need for treatment of pathological gambling is unknown. Future research should evaluate the extent of unmet need and what barriers contribute to it, such as lack of insurance coverage, stigmatization, or the unavailability of treatment. Because pathological gambling often occurs with other disorders, such as substance abuse and antisocial personality disorder, the committee recommends that those undergoing treatment for those disorders be assessed routinely for pathological gambling.

Advances in computer and telecommunications technology have increased the availability of gambling. New technology holds the potential to change the subjective experience of gambling and to increase how often, how much, and how long people gamble. Research should be conducted to assess the effects on pathological gambling of remote access to gambling (e.g., Internet gambling), new gambling machines, and gambling while alone.

Overall, the committee found that much of the available research on all aspects of pathological gambling is of limited scientific value. Our conclusions are greatly influenced by a relatively small body of newer, better research that meets or exceeds contemporary standards for social and behavioral research. The future research recommended by the committee should be held to those standards.

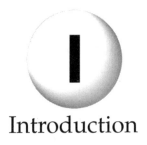

Introduction

Gambling is deeply rooted in American culture (Findlay, 1986). In precolonial times, the proceeds from lotteries authorized by the ruling English monarchy were used to subsidize explorations to, and settlements within, the New World (Ezell, 1960). As colonial America matured, government and private lotteries, as well as social gambling, were common. The colonial era of gambling ended with the spread of Jacksonian morality, aided by numerous well-publicized scandals. Civil War reconstruction introduced a second era of gambling, as lotteries were employed as a form of voluntary taxation to rebuild the war-torn South (Rose, 1998; Ezell, 1977). Gambling continued to spread until 1890, when a scandal involving the Louisiana lottery resulted in federal legislation that effectively banned state lotteries and prohibited other forms of gambling for nearly 70 years (Rose, 1998; Ezell, 1977).

The United States is now in the midst of a third era of widespread legalized gambling, which began in 1931 when Nevada relegalized casinos (Rose, 1986, 1995). Initially, Americans in this era limited legal gambling opportunities to the Nevada casinos, charitable bingo, and pari-mutuel gambling, such as horse and dog track racing. Popular forms of illegal gambling, such as offtrack betting, back room casino games, and numbers, were associated with organized crime and were treated as vice crimes by law enforcement institutions. Then, beginning in 1964, gambling expanded greatly after New Hampshire initiated the first modern state lottery, signifying a change in traditional social and moral barriers. As of this writing, some form of gambling is legal in all but 3 states, casino or casino-style gambling is available in 21 states, and 37 states have lotteries (National Opinion Research Center, 1999). In 1988, Congress passed the Indian Gaming Regulatory Act, which allows tribes to operate any form of gambling currently legalized in the state in which the tribe resides. Resistance by many state legislatures to casino gambling and state-sanctioned sports betting continues, but in numerous jurisdictions other forms of gambling have become institutionalized, with state budgets increasingly dependent on gambling revenues.

The advent of state-sponsored lotteries marked a significant policy shift in which the states moved from tolerance to active sponsorship and aggressive marketing of their own games. Public support of this shift is beyond question, with over 80 percent of adults in the United States participating in various forms of commercial or state-sponsored gambling sometime during their lives. Collectively Americans wagered over $551 billion in 1997 in legal gambling activities (*International Gaming and Wagering Business*, 1998). Although gambling is popular and has social and economic benefits, there are also costs involved for individuals, families, and communities stemming from pathological and problem gambling.

COMMITTEE CHARGE

In August 1996, President Clinton signed P.L. 104-169, establishing the National Gambling Impact Study Commission, whose purpose is to conduct a comprehensive study of the social and economic impacts of gambling in the United States. Section 4(a), (2)(C) of the new law called for "an assessment of pathological or problem gambling, including its impact on individuals, families, businesses, social institutions, and the economy." The act further states under Section (b)(1): "In carrying out its duties under section 4, the Commission shall contract with the National Research Council of the National Academy of Sciences for assistance in conducting the studies required by the Commission under section 4(a), and in particular the assessment required under subparagraph (C) of paragraph (2) of such section." In response to a subsequent request from the National Gambling Impact Study Commission, the National Research Council established the Committee on the Social and Economic Impact of Pathological Gambling.

The committee's charge was to identify and analyze the full range of research studies that bear upon the nature of pathological and problem gambling, highlighting key issues and data sources that may provide scientific evidence of prevalence and multiple effects.

In its review and assessment of the contemporary research on pathological and problem gambling, the committee examined the diverse and frequently debated issues regarding the conceptualization of pathological gambling, its prevalence and effects on individuals and society, its causes and cooccurrences with other psychiatric disorders and substance abuse, what we know about preventing and treating it, and the role of technology in the development of gambling. This review included consideration of over 4,000 gambling-related references, of which approximately 1,600 were determined to be related to pathological or problem gambling. Of these, about 300 were found to be empirical research studies. It was this relatively narrow subset of studies, primarily published in peer-reviewed journals, that the committee concentrated on in determining the strength of the available literature in all key areas.

BRIEF HISTORY OF PATHOLOGICAL AND PROBLEM GAMBLING

For as long as humans have gambled, there has been apprehension about excessive risk-taking and intemperate gambling. Histories of gamblers who lose control recur through the centuries, and from early times their behavior was labeled an addiction (France, 1902, cited by Wildman, 1997). In early Roman law, the original addict was a debtor (Rosenthal, 1992) who, because he could not pay what he owed, was brought into court and enslaved (Glare, 1982; Wissowa, 1984). Hence, judges pronouncing sentence could make the addict the slave of his creditor. These early "addicts" were not limited to gamblers, although in early Roman times gambling was rampant (France, 1902, cited by Wildman, 1997).

Descriptions of many features of what is now clinically described as pathological gambling have appeared in historical accounts of many world cultures, as well as in American literature since the early colonial period. Some famous Roman emperors were avid gamblers, and there is some evidence that Claudius and Nero would meet a modern definition of a pathological gambler (Wildman, 1997). Fear of a loss of control by his soldiers due to gambling caused King Richard the Lion-Hearted to restrict dice playing during the crusades (Fleming, 1978). In the 17th century, gambling was regarded as a vice that ranged from the making of small wagers to the staking of all the gambler's earthly property, and in some instances the person's title (Wildman, 1997; Rose, 1988). Dostoyevsky in *The Gambler* (1866), a fictionalized account of his own experiences, writes of the cognitive distortions, loss of control and self-esteem, and hopelessness currently associated with clinical definitions of severe gambling problems.

Many historians and other writers have noted patterns of behaviors that resemble current descriptions of clinical symptoms of gambling problems (e.g., Cotton, 1674; Stith, 1752; Dostoyevsky, 1866; France, 1902, Wildman, 1997; Rosenthal, 1998). Landon Carter (cited by Findlay, 1986) spoke for the southern gentry when he compared a man with a passion for gambling to a slave. In 1791 an article in *The Western County Magazine* refers to gambling as an addiction, and describes the preoccupation and distraction, citing many cases of individuals who lost everything and committed suicide (see Steinmetz, 1869). Admonitions against gambling were also prominent during the 1820s and 1830s, as part of the temperance movement. In 1834, Charles Caldwell, a physician and prominent medical educator, labeled gambling an addictive vice that would render men mad (Caldwell, 1834). Another physician, J.T. Taylor, also described gambling as an addiction and, like Cotton almost 200 years before him, describes most of the criteria and associated features of gambling problems that comprise the current clinical description of pathological gambling as determined by the American Psychiatric Association (1994). He describes the shame, guilt, and secrecy of the gambler; preoccupation with gambling; neglect of wife and home; neglect of employment; extravagant spending; turning to theft and other illegal activities to support gambling and other expenses; and, finally, suicide (see Taylor, 1838). During the 1840s and 1850s, clergymen and reformers such as Henry Ward Beecher and William Alcott described the gambler's descent through addiction and madness into crime (see Fabian, 1990:55-56).

In the first half of the 20th century, psychoanalysts became interested in gambling (Rosenthal, 1987). Starting in 1914 with Von Hattingberg, they contributed case reports and speculative essays in which patients were often identified as gambling addicts. Freud was particularly interested in why people would deliberately seek out and repeat self-destructive behaviors. He believed that it was not for money that the gambler gambled, but for the gambling itself, what psychoanalysts would refer to today as "the action." Freud thought gambling was an addiction; he placed it in a triad with alcoholism and drug dependence (Freud, 1928).

During the 1930s, legalized gambling became widely available in the United States. With 21 states opening racetracks with pari-mutuel betting and the relegalization of casino gambling in Nevada, gambling problems began to gain attention. The first meeting of Gamblers Anonymous took place in Los Angeles in December 1957. The self-help fellowship was founded on the belief that character changes within gamblers themselves were necessary to ameliorate problematic gambling and its effects, and that changes could be made by adopting spiritual principles used by those recovering from addictions (Gamblers Anonymous, 1997). As the fellowship expanded, its now famous 20 questions became the de facto standard used to gauge whether or not gambling behaviors were compulsive (see Appendix A). The questions became the basis for modern classification systems that determine the chronicity and seriousness of gambling problems in part by the consequences of gambling behavior. Subsequently, explanations of the cause of gambling problems began to focus on the gambler's personal attributes rather than solely on social and economic consequences. People with gambling problems were conceptually transformed into problem gamblers. And if the gambling problems were chronic, the problem gambler was considered a "compulsive gambler," an early term for pathological gambler.

ORGANIZATION OF THE REPORT

The purpose of this report is to describe the current scientific knowledge about the definition, extent, nature, effects, and treatment of pathological gambling, as well as emerging technologies that may affect them in the future.

Chapter 2 considers the concept of gambling and describes contemporary patterns of excessive or pathological gambling. It considers gambling from two distinct perspectives: (1) how clinicians and researchers understand gamblers and the ranges of their behaviors and (2) how such behaviors, particularly pathological gambling, can be understood in terms of the harmful consequences associated with these actions. In the course of this discussion, a nomenclature unfolds and is offered for future use. The chapter also lays a foundation for our review of the scholarly literature pertaining to the extent and nature of pathological gambling, its social and economic effects, and its treatment. Finally, this chapter suggests ways of improving understanding of pathological and problem gambling. Inherent throughout is a critical scientific consideration of pathological gambling as both a psychological and a social construct, and an analysis of its definition as a psychiatric disorder.

Chapter 3 describes the prevalence of pathological gambling in the United States, making note of complications and limitations in the existing research. Chapter 4 assesses our understanding of the origins of pathological gambling. Chapter 5 discusses the social and economic benefits of gambling and assesses the literature about the effects of pathological gambling on individuals, families, communities, and society. In it we discuss the few available studies of socioeconomic effects as examples of how knowledge in this area can be advanced. Chapter 6 reviews characteristics of treatment seekers, treatment approaches and effectiveness, and health care and prevention issues. Chapter 7 considers how advances in the organization and technology of gambling have affected pathological gambling and may increasingly do so in the future.

REFERENCES

American Psychiatric Association
1994   *DSM-IV: Diagnostic and Statistical Manual of Mental Disorders* (4th ed.). Washington, DC: American Psychiatric Association.
Caldwell, C.
1834   *An Address on the Vice of Gambling Delivered to the Medical Pupils of Transylvania University. November 4.* Lexington, KY: J. Clark and Co.
Cotton, C.
1674   *Games and Gamesters of the Restoration. The Compleat Gamester.* Reprinted in 1971 by Kennikat Press, Port Washington, NY.
Dostoyevsky, F.
1866   The gambler. In *The Gambler and Other Stories,* C. Garnett, ed. New York: Macmillan.
Ezell, J.S.
1960   *Fortune's Merry Wheel.* Cambridge, MA: Harvard University Press.
Fabian, A.
1990   *Card Sharps, Dream Books, and Bucket Shops: Gambling in 19th-Century America.* Ithaca, NY: Cornell University Press.
Findlay, J.M.
1986   *People of Chance: Gambling in American Society from Jamestown to Las Vegas.* New York: Oxford University Press.
Fleming, A.M.
1978   *Something for Nothing: A History of Gambling.* New York: Delacorte.
France, C.
1902   The gambling impulse. *American Journal of Psychology* 13:364-407.
Freud, S.
1928   Dostoevsky and parricide. Pp. 175-196 in *Standard Edition of the Complete Psychological Works of Sigmund Freud,* Vol XXI, J. Strachey, trans. ed. London: Hogarth, 1961.
Gamblers Anonymous
1997   *Gamblers Anonymous: Sharing Recovery Through Gamblers Anonymous.* Los Angeles: Gamblers Anonymous.
Glare, P.G.W.
1982   *Oxford Latin Dictionary.* Oxford, England: Clarendon Press.
International Gaming and Wagering Business
1998   The United States gross annual wager. *International Gaming and Wagering Business* (supplement) 19(8):3.
National Opinion Research Center
1999   *Gambling Impact and Behavior Study: Final Report to the National Gambling Impact Study Commission.* March 18. Chicago: University of Chicago Press.

Rose, I.N.
1986   *Gambling and the Law* (1st ed.). Hollywood, CA: Gambling Times.
1988   Gambling and the law. *Journal of Gambling Behavior* 4:240-260.
1995   Gambling and the law: Endless fields of dreams. *Journal of Gambling Studies* 11:15-33.
1998   Technology and the Future of Gambling. Unpublished manuscript. Whittier Law School, Costa Mesa, CA.

Rosenthal, R.J.
1987   The psychodynamics of pathological gambling: A review of the literature. In *The Handbook of Pathological Gambling*, T. Galski, ed. Springfield, IL: Thomas.
1992   Pathological gambling. *Psychiatric Annals* 22:72-78.
1998   The Medicalization of Gambling: Its History as Addiction, Compulsion, and Disease. Unpublished manuscript. Department of Psychiatry, University of California, Los Angeles.

Steinmetz, A.
1869   *The Gaming Table: Its Votaries and Victims, in All Times and Countries, Especially in England and France.* Montclair, NJ: Patterson Smith, 1969.

Stith, W.
1752   *The Sinfulness and Pernicious Nature of Gaming: A Sermon Preached Before the General Assembly of Virginia.* March 1, 1752. Williamsburg, VA: William Hunter.

Taylor, J.S.
1838   *The Victims of Gambling: Being Extracts from the Diary of an American Physician.* New York: Boston, Weeks, Jordon and Co.

Von Hattingberg, H.
1914   Analerotik, angstlust und eigesinn. *Internationale Zeitschrift fur Psychoanalyse* 2:244-258.

Wildman, R.W. II
1997   *Gambling: An Attempt at an Integration.* Edmonton, Alberta, Canada: Wynne Resources.

Wissowa, G.
1984   *Paulys Real-Encyclopadie der Classischen Altertumswissenschaft.* Stuttgart, Germany: Metzler.

2

Gambling Concepts and Nomenclature

Terms used to describe behaviors in similar contexts or venues have an influence on how those behaviors are defined and viewed. Understanding the extent and nature of pathological gambling, as well as its social and economic impact, requires as clear a definition as possible. A discrete, acceptable, and useful definition of pathological gambling would be based on a nomenclature applicable in a wide diversity of contexts (American Psychiatric Association, 1994). Nomenclature refers to a system of names used in an art or science and is critical in conceptualizing, discussing, and making judgments about pathological gambling and related behaviors. A nomenclature inclusive of pathological gambling must be suitable for use in scholarly research, clinical diagnosis and treatment, and community and other social contexts. The nomenclature must also reflect a variety of perspectives because research scientists, psychiatrists, other treatment care clinicians, and public policy makers tend to frame questions about gambling differently, depending on their disciplinary training, experience, and special interests. In the absence of an agreed-upon nomenclature, these and other groups interested in gambling and gambling problems have developed different paradigms or world views from which to consider these matters. Consequently, the act of gambling has been considered by various observers to provide evidence of recreational interest, diminished mathematical skills, poor judgment, cognitive distortions, mental illness, and moral turpitude. These varied views have stimulated debate and controversy.

Historically, the word "gambling" referred to playing unfairly or cheating at play. A gambler was defined as a fraudulent gamester, sharper, or rook who habitually plays for money, especially extravagantly high stakes (*Oxford English Dictionary*, second edition, 1989). In modern times, gambling has come to mean wagering money or other belongings on chance activities or events with random or uncertain outcomes (Devereux, 1979). Gambling in this sense implies an act whereby the participant pursues a monetary gain without using his or her skills (Brenner and Brenner, 1990). This is the dictionary definition of gambling as well (*Oxford English Dictionary*, second edition, 1989). Throughout history, however, gambling also has involved activities requiring skill. For example, a bettor's knowledge of playing strategies can improve his or her chances of winning in certain card games; knowledge of horses and jockeys may improve predictions of probable outcomes in a horse race (Bruce and Johnson, 1996). The use of such skills may reduce the randomness of the outcome but, because of other factors that cannot be predicted or analyzed, the outcome remains uncertain. As used in this report, the term "gambling" refers both to games of chance that are truly random and involve little or no skill that can improve the odds of winning, and to activities that require the use of skills that can improve the chance of winning. By its very nature, gambling involves a voluntary, deliberate assumption of risk, often with a negative expectable value. For example, in casino gambling the odds are against the gambler because the house takes its cut; thus, the more people gamble, the more likely they are to lose.

ROLE OF RISK-TAKING IN
THE GAMBLING EXPERIENCE

Throughout history, scholars and writers have theorized about why human beings gamble. These explanations have encompassed evolutionary, cultural, religious, financial, recreational, psychological, and sociological perspectives (Wildman,

1998). A current and widely disseminated theory is that people engage in gambling because it has the capacity to create excitement (Boyd, 1976; Steiner, 1970). People seek stimulation and try to optimize their subjective experience by shifting sensations. Sensation-seeking and shifting these experiences, as a basic and enduring human drive, can be compared to a child's exploration of his or her environment to develop fundamental mastery of skills and satisfy curiosity. The experiences that humans regularly seek include novelty, recreation, and adventure (Zuckerman, 1979; Ebstein et al., 1996; Benjamin et al., 1996). To paraphrase William Arthur Ward, a 20th century American philosopher, the person who risks nothing, has nothing. Indeed, it is common for individuals to take risks in life. Risk-taking underlies many human traits that have high significance for evolutionary survival, such as wanting and seeking food (Neese and Berridge, 1997). Moreover, risk-taking is reinforced by the emotional experiences that follow, such as relief from boredom, feelings of accomplishment, and the "rush" associated with seeking excitement. Individuals vary considerably in the extent to which they take risks. Some limit their risk-taking to driving a few miles over the posted speed limit, whereas others actively pursue mountain climbing, skydiving, or other exciting sports with a high risk of harm.

Gambling is neither a financially nor a psychologically risk-free experience. In addition to the possibility that gamblers will lose their money, they also risk experiencing a variety of adverse biological, psychological, and social consequences from gambling (American Psychiatric Association, 1994). Personal aspirations and the social setting, however, can affect the likelihood of an individual's engaging in risky behavior, since aspirations will influence the perceived benefits and constraints of the risky situation. The potential payoff of betting stimulates innate risk-taking tendencies. Although exceptions exist, games with the highest "action," such as high-stakes poker and dice games, serve as more powerful stimuli to accelerate a player's risk-taking by increasing the payoff if the bet is won. Even those not normally inclined to buy a lottery ticket, for example, often may do so when several million dollars in winnings are at stake (Clotfelter and Cook, 1989). The simple association between gambling and action, including the prospects of "winning big," which characterizes most popular gambling activities, can maintain stable gambling behaviors despite incredible odds against winning (Lopes, 1987).

MEDICALIZATION OF PATHOLOGICAL GAMBLING

Understanding of the adverse consequences of excessive gambling has undergone profound change. For most of history, individuals who experienced adverse consequences from gambling were viewed as gamblers with problems; today, we consider them to have psychological problems. This change is analogous to the change in the understanding of alcoholics and alcoholism, and it has been reflected in, or stimulated by, the evolving clinical classification and description of pathological gambling in the various editions, between 1980 and 1994, of the *Diagnostic and Statistical Manual of Mental Disorders* (called DSM) published by the American Psychiatric Association. Changes over time in the DSM reflect a desire to be more scientific in determining appropriate criteria for pathological gambling by accounting for its similarities to other addictions, especially substance dependence (American Psychiatric Association, 1980, 1987, 1994; Lesieur, 1988; Rosenthal, 1989; Lesieur and Rosenthal, 1991). Today pathological gambling is understood to be a disorder characterized by a continuous or periodic loss of control over gambling, a preoccupation with gambling and with obtaining money with which to gamble, irrational thinking, and a continuation of the behavior despite adverse consequences.

The official medicalization of excessive gambling is marked by its inclusion in the DSM (American Psychiatric Association, 1980, 1987, 1994). It is not surprising, however, that some scholars (e.g., Szasz, 1970, 1987, 1991) have objected to medicalizing certain socially or culturally offensive behaviors in general, and gambling intemperance in particular (Rosecrance, 1985).[1] Never-

---

[1] For a discussion of nonmedical models for understanding excessive gambling, see the section on other theories and conceptualizations of pathological gambling later in this chapter.

theless, in the United States and elsewhere, although not in all nations or cultures, people with serious gambling problems are now described as suffering from a disorder that reflects a psychiatric illness or disease state. And despite significant gaps in research and a generally deficient state of scholarly literature, pathological gambling is known to be a robust phenomenon (Shaffer et al., 1997) that also is complex in its origins and accompanying disorders, and in its negative social and economic effects. Moreover, all these factors can be affected by traditional, contemporary, and constantly emerging gambling-related technologies.

Conceptualizing gambling behavior on a simple continuum ranging from no gambling to pathological gambling may provide a useful model for developing a public health system of treatment, but it is insufficiently detailed to provide a scientific explanation of the emergence of pathological gambling. The list of important terms used in this report for gambling behaviors suggests that they cover a wide range (see Box 2-1). These terms are important to the discussion of prevalence in Chapter 3.

When considering the range of gambling involvement, it is important to note that today about 20 percent of Americans do not gamble at all; that most gamblers do so for social or recreational reasons without experiencing any negative consequences; and that cooccurrences with other types of problems, as well as negative social and economic effects experienced by individual gamblers and their families, theoretically increase with the level, chronicity, and severity of gambling problems. In other words, once gamblers cross the threshold and enter into the range of problem gambling (described as Level 2 in Box 2-1) they begin to manifest adverse effects; since there are far more problem gamblers than pathological gamblers, most adverse affects are believed to be experienced or caused by problem gamblers. Although this increasing relationship is often asserted or implied in the literature, neither an increasing association nor a progressive gambling behavior continuum is supported by available research. Moreover, the range of different gambling behaviors is believed to be dynamic: for example, social or recreational gamblers can become problem gamblers; problem gamblers can become pathological gamblers, return to a level of social or recreational gam-

---

Box 2-1
Important Gambling Terms Used by the Committee

Compulsive gambling: The original lay term for pathological gambling, it is still used by Gamblers Anonymous and throughout much of the self-help treatment community.

Disordered gambling: Inspired by language in DSM pertaining to Disorders of Impulse Control and used by Shaffer et al. (1997) in their meta-analysis to serve as a conceptual container for the panoply of terms associated with gambling-related problems and pathology. The term is used occasionally in this report to describe the combination of problem and pathological gambling.

Excessive gambling: Reference to an amount of time or money spent gambling that exceeds an arbitrarily defined acceptable level.

Intemperate gambling: Synonymous with excessive gambling.

Level 0 gambling: No gambling at all.

Level 1 gambling: Social and/or recreational gambling (see below) with no appreciable harmful effects.

Level 2 gambling: Synonymous with problem gambling.

---

bling, or even discontinue gambling.[2] In addition, the time involved in shifting from one level to another is commonly believed to be subject to extreme variance, although this has not been empirically demonstrated.

---

[2]There is no direct empirical evidence supporting either the possibility that pathological gamblers can or cannot return to and remain in a state of social or recreational gambling. This pattern has been observed, however, among people with alcohol, heroin, cocaine, and other addictions (e.g., Shaffer and Jones, 1989). Nevertheless, the percentage of those who seek treatment and do return successfully to social or recreational gambling is likely to be so small that clinicians generally and accurately believe that it is not likely. Therefore, they are reluctant to consider this possibility as part of treatment efforts. In practice, pathological gamblers attending Gamblers Anonymous or undergoing forms of treatment other than self-help usually consider themselves as "recovering" from, but not ever cured of, their gambling disorder.

Level 3 gambling: Synonymous with pathological gambling as defined in DSM-IV in which 5 or more criteria out of 10 are present.

Pathological gambling: A mental disorder characterized by a continuous or periodic loss of control over gambling, a preoccupation with gambling and with obtaining money with which to gamble, irrational thinking, and a continuation of the behavior despite adverse consequences.

Probable pathological gambler: A common reference in prevalence research studies and other gambling literature to a person who is suspected of being a pathological gambler on the basis of some criteria, but who has not been clinically evaluated as such.

Problematic gambling: Synonymous with either disordered gambling or excessive gambling.

Problem gambling: Gambling behavior that results in any harmful effects to the gambler, his or her family, significant others, friends, coworkers, etc. Some problem gamblers would not necessarily meet criteria for pathological gambling.

Recreational gambling: Gambling for entertainment or social purposes, with no harmful effects.

Social gambling: Synonymous with recreational gambling.

CONTEMPORARY PATHOLOGICAL GAMBLING

The assumption underlying the existing research is that gambling problems exist and can be measured (Volberg, 1998). Despite agreement among researchers at this fundamental level and a widely recognized and accepted definition of Level 3 (pathological gambling) as described in Box 2-1, there is widespread disagreement about the conceptualization, definition, and measurement of Level 2 (problem gambling). Conceptual and methodological confusion is common in emerging scientific fields (Shaffer, 1986, 1997b), but debate about problem gambling creates public confusion and uncertainty about gambling problems and their effects on society (Volberg, 1998).

For example, in considering excessive gambling behavior, clinicians and the majority of researchers in the United States and abroad rely on well-established psychiatric classifications (nosologies) and descriptions (nosographies) of pathological gambling that have evolved over the past 20 years (American Psychiatric Association, 1980, 1987, 1994). However, debate is ongoing as to their validity, as well as about broader conceptualizations of excessive gambling ranging from problem to pathological (Rosenthal, 1989; Shaffer et al., 1997; Rosecrance, 1985). A number of competing conceptual models and definitions have arisen to explain the origins of these behaviors. Compounding this classification difficulty is the wide variety of labels or terms found in the literature to describe people with gambling problems. For these reasons it can be useful to conceptualize progressively harmful gambling behaviors on a continuum similar to the progressive stages and harmful effects of alcoholism, including: abstinence, social or controlled drinking, problem drinking with loss of control (disruption of work and social functions but minimal organ damage), and severe problem drinking with organ damage. To ensure clarity and consistency in our use of such labels and terms in this report, they are defined in Box 2-1. The following section focuses on the medical conceptualization of pathological gambling, beginning with a discussion of how it differs from problem gambling.

Pathological Gambling Versus Problem Gambling

Although clinicians and researchers concur that understanding the nature, scope, and severity of gambling-related problems is important, there is much variation in the language used to designate various levels of gambling involvement and their consequences. For example, investigators often use the terms "problem gambling," "at-risk gambling," "potential pathological gambling," "probable pathological gambling," "disordered gambling," and "pathological gambling." Some authors have used terms for adolescents that are different from the terms generally used for adults (e.g., Volberg, 1993; Winters et al., 1993). The labeling difficulty arises in part because epidemiologists and clinical researchers do not use the same terminology. Also, various terms arise when investigators characterize broadly defined samples of extreme gamblers. Nevertheless, the frequency and intensity of problems associated with gambling can range from none to a lot. Thus, in the absence of rigorously achieved and convincing validity data, any classification label is inherently arbitrary to some degree and may be too simple to describe such a complex and multidimensional concept as gambling severity (Walker and Dickerson, 1996). This issue, however, is encountered in all psychiatric classifications, not just pathological gambling. The challenge is to establish agreed-on terminology so that researchers, clinicians, and others in the field can communicate precisely.

Imprecise terms, such as "potential pathological gamblers" or "probable pathological gamblers," among other terms, have been promulgated by research relying on a variety of instruments. Use of various terms has contributed substantially to confusion about what constitutes Level 2 problem gambling. Some people have criticized the fact that the American Psychiatric Association's DSM-IV designates only one term to connote a gambling disorder (pathological gambling), because it does not adequately serve investigations that need to describe individuals who are experiencing less extreme difficulties. Since people who meet at least one but less than five of the DSM-IV criteria suggested for a diagnosis of pathological gambling have experienced some level of difficulty, they also warrant attention. However, their problems are extremely variable and range from trivial to serious. Furthermore, these individuals may be progressing toward a pathological state, or they may be pathological gamblers in remission who are recovering (i.e., they met DSM-IV criteria for having been a pathological gambler sometime during their lifetime, but they do not currently meet the criteria suggested for such a diagnosis).

The term "pathological" is defined in the *Oxford English Dictionary* as "caused by or evidencing a mentally disturbed condition." In 1980, the American Psychiatric Association adopted the term "pathological gambling" as the official nomenclature in the DSM-III to describe excessive gambling as an impulse disorder (the DSM criteria are discussed in the next section). Sometimes the terms "pathological" and "compulsive" are used interchangeably; however, "compulsive" is the historical and lay term and the one used by Gamblers Anonymous (1997). But for most researchers and many clinicians, the notion of compulsive gambling as a description of pathological gamblers is a technical misnomer (Lesieur and Rosenthal, 1991). In the psychiatric lexicon, a compulsive behavior is involuntary and "ego-dystonic"—that is, external or foreign to the self. The DSM-IV defines compulsions as "repetitive behaviors or mental acts, the goal of which is to prevent or reduce anxiety or stress, not to provide pleasure or gratification" (American Psychiatric Association, 1994:418). It is an "unwilling" attempt to rid oneself of discomfort and pain. In some cases, individuals perform rigid, stereotyped acts according to idiosyncratically elaborated rules without being able to indicate why they are doing them. Examples of a compulsion would include repetitive hand washing or the irresistible urge to shout an obscenity (see American Psychiatric Association, 1980, 1987, 1994). Pathological gamblers, in contrast, typically experience gambling as ego-syntonic and pleasurable until late in the disorder.

The DSM-IV provides a widely accepted definition of and diagnostic criteria for pathological gambling, but the term "problem gambling" is somewhat more difficult to conceptualize and define. In much of the research literature, problem gambling is used as an overlay to include pathological gambling (Shaffer et al., 1997). In fact, the concepts are inextricable, because on the continuum of gambling behaviors pathological gambling encompasses problem gambling (i.e., all pathological gamblers have been problem gamblers). Moreover, pathological and problem gamblers can experience varying levels of problem chronicity over time. However, problem gambling is most commonly characterized as describing those individuals who meet less than five DSM-IV criteria for a diagnosis of pathological gambling (Lesieur and Rosenthal, 1998). Shaffer and his colleagues considered these as cases that could be "in transition" and described in-transition gamblers as moving either toward or away from pathological states; however, they also noted that in-transition gamblers may not necessarily be in an earlier stage of the disorder. It is important to note that these authors observed that in-transition gamblers may never develop the attributes of pathological gambling; in-transition gamblers may languish in this state or begin to move toward recovery.

The concept of a continuum of problem severity implies that

people can be located at a point on a continuum. They can move from that point, developing more or less serious difficulties. This analysis suggests that gambling problems reflect an underlying unidimensional construct. Although individuals can theoretically move across a continuum of problem severity and some scholars believe that gambling problems may best be conceptualized as a developmental continuum of gambling behaviors with respect to frequency and intensity, there is no empirical evidence that actual progression of the illness is linear (Shaffer et al., 1997). Moreover, clinicians and the self-help treatment community believe that pathological gamblers cannot successfully return to a level of social or recreational gambling.

Development of the DSM Criteria

Largely through the efforts of Robert Custer, pathological gambling was first included in the DSM in 1980 (see DSM-III in Appendix B). Custer had treated pathological gamblers and written about their illness for several years (Custer, 1980; Custer and Custer, 1978). For the first inclusion in DSM-III, there was no testing of criteria beforehand. Instead, inclusion was based on his clinical experience and those of other treatment professionals. The original DSM-III criteria started with a statement about progressive loss of control and then listed seven items. Three or more had to be met for a diagnosis of pathological gambling. The emphasis was on damage and disruption to the individual's family, personal, or vocational pursuits and issues that had to do with money (five of the seven original criteria fell into this latter category). There also was added an exclusion criterion: "not caused by antisocial personality disorder."

The DSM-III criteria were criticized for their unidimensionality, emphasis on external consequences, and middle-class bias (Lesieur, 1984). With the revision of the diagnostic manual in 1987 (DSM-III-R), it was decided to emphasize the similarity to substance dependence, literally by copying the criteria, substituting "gambling" for "use of a substance." This can be clearly seen from an earlier published draft of DSM-III-R when the two sets of criteria are placed side by side (Rosenthal, 1989:103). The only item that appears different, item 5 in the finalized version, seems less so if one considers the symptom of "chasing" one's losses as an attempt to negate or reverse the progressive dysphoria—the shame and guilt—consequent to the gambling (see Appendix B). Thus it resembles the taking of a substance to relieve or avoid painful symptoms (e.g., Weider and Kaplan, 1969; Khantzian, 1975, 1985).

A year after the publication of the new criteria, a group of treatment professionals found considerable dissatisfaction with them, with some preference expressed for a compromise between the old DSM-III and the newer DSM-III-R criteria (Rosenthal, 1989). On the basis of these complaints, a questionnaire was constructed and administered to 222 self-identified compulsive gamblers and 104 substance-abusing controls who gambled at least socially (Lesieur and Rosenthal, 1991; Bradford et al., 1996). The results were analyzed to determine which items best discriminated between the two groups. A new set of nine criteria emerged that combined DSM-III and DSM-III-R, with the addition of one new item: "gambles as a way of escaping from problems or intolerable feeling states." With the exception of "illegal acts," all items were selected by at least 85 percent of the compulsive gamblers. For example, the item pertaining to being preoccupied with gambling was selected by 97 percent of the compulsive gamblers and just 3 percent of the social gamblers (Bradford et al., 1996).

Following a presentation of these findings to gambling research and treatment professionals at several national and international conferences, it was decided that one additional item—"repeated unsuccessful attempts to control, cut back or stop gambling"—should be added. The final phase was a field trial using 453 subjects (Lesieur and Rosenthal, 1998) to test this additional item (representing loss of control). The analysis found that adding or deleting it did not affect the threshold for diagnosis, and that it was highly correlated with other criteria. Based on these findings and the preference of clinicians in the United States and abroad that it be included, "loss of control" was reinstated as a diagnostic criterion, but with the wording improved from DSM-III-R.

The resulting definition of pathological gambling was published in 1994 in the *Diagnostic and Statistical Manual of Mental Disorders* (DSM-IV). This is the latest in an evolving effort by the

American Psychiatric Association to operationally define the disorder. The definition includes 10 criteria, which describe both the individual attributes of sufferers and the social consequences that result from their behavior. Also described are associated features and disorders, specific culture and gender features, prevalence, course, familial pattern, differential diagnosis, and exclusion criteria. As such, the criteria are intended to provide guidance for clinically diagnosing pathological gambling as a disorder of impulse control. To be diagnosed as a pathological gambler, an individual must meet at least five criteria (Bradford et al., 1996; Lesieur and Rosenthal, 1998). For the criteria and full text of the DSM-IV definition, see Appendix B.

The 10 criteria that resulted from this process represent three clusters or dimensions: damage or disruption, loss of control, and dependence. In the category of dependence are tolerance (needs to gamble with increasing amounts of money in order to achieve desired excitement), withdrawal (restless or irritable when attempting to cut down or stop), preoccupation with gambling, and gambling as a way to escape from problems. The wording and selection of items and the diagnostic cut-off point of five or more were based on clinical data; a partial exclusion criterion was then added: "The gambling behavior is not better accounted for by a Manic Episode." Although somewhat controversial, this exclusion was added because excessive gambling may result when a patient is experiencing acute mania, without the disorder itself being present (American Psychiatric Association, 1994).

The current description of pathological gambling in DSM-IV has been found to characterize pathological gambling in relatively precise operational terms; to provide the basis for measures that are reliable, replicable, and sensitive to regional and local variation; to distinguish gambling behavior from other impulse disorders; and to suggest the utility of applying specific types of clinical treatments (Shaffer et al., 1994). Moreover, the DSM-IV criteria appear to have worked well for clinicians for the past five years. However, because it is a clinical description with little empirical support beyond treatment populations, there still are problems with its use to define the nature and origins of pathological gambling, and when trying to estimate prevalence.

The Clinical Picture

Descriptions of the clinical course of pathological gambling date back to 1892 (Quinn, 1892). The traditional description of the disorder has included four phases: the reaction to winning, losing, desperation, and hopelessness (Custer, 1982; Custer and Milt, 1985; Lesieur and Rosenthal, 1991). Recent research has suggested an alternative model, with as many as six phases of development into and out of a gambling addiction: initiation, positive consequences, negative consequences, turning points, active quitting, and relapse prevention (Shaffer and Jones, 1989; Shaffer, 1997; Prochaska et al., 1992; Marlatt et al., 1988). Clinical studies suggest that, as gambling progresses toward a pathological state, there is frequently an increase in the amounts wagered and the time devoted to gambling and a corresponding increase in depression, shame, and guilt (Rosenthal, 1992). Studies primarily of gamblers seeking help suggest that as many as 20 percent will attempt suicide (Moran, 1969; Livingston, 1974; Custer and Custer, 1978; McCormick et al., 1984; Lesieur and Blume, 1991; Thompson et al., 1996), and two out of three help seekers have turned to criminal activities to support their gambling (Lesieur et al., 1986; Brown, 1987; Lesieur, 1989). Pathological gambling can exacerbate other mental disorders, and stress-related physical illnesses are common (Lorenz and Yaffee, 1986). Chapters 4 and 5 discuss these issues in more detail.

Pathological gambling differs from the social and recreational gambling of most adults. Social or recreational gamblers are those who gamble for entertainment and typically do not risk more than they can afford (Custer and Milt, 1985; Shaffer et al., 1997). If they should chase their losses, they do so only briefly and have little preoccupation with gambling. In pathological gambling, however, players generate adverse consequences for themselves and others involved in their life. Clinicians report that, although money is important, male pathological gamblers often say they are seeking action, an aroused euphoric state that may be similar to the high from cocaine or other stimulating drugs. Pathological gamblers report a "rush" characterized by sweaty palms, rapid heartbeat, and nausea or queasiness. This can be experienced while gambling, in anticipation of gambling, or in response to any situation or feeling that reminds them of gambling (Rosenthal and Lesieur, 1992). Pathological gamblers may go for days without sleep, and for extended periods without eating or taking care of other bodily needs. Clinicians have described the presence of cravings, tolerance—the need to make increasingly larger bets or take greater risks to produce the desired level of excitement (Lesieur, 1994)—and withdrawal symptoms (Wray and Dickerson, 1981; Meyer, 1989; Rosenthal and Lesieur, 1992).

Although there are other kinds of intense physiological reactions, clinicians also report that some pathological gamblers are less interested in the excitement or action and more interested in escape. They are seeking to numb themselves and report a quest for oblivion. This motivation for escape may be understood as a quest to reduce psychological discomfort and as an attempt to attain a more normal state—a self-medication (Khantzian, 1975, 1977). These reactions are reported by many women gamblers (Lesieur and Blume, 1991), as well as many slot and video poker machine players. Many pathological gamblers, both male and female, report experiencing amnesic episodes, trances, and dissociative states (Jacobs, 1988; Kuley and Jacobs, 1988; Lesieur and Rosenthal, 1994; Brown, 1996; O'Donnell and Rugle, 1996).

Pathological gamblers also evidence distortions in their thinking (Gaboury and Ladouceur, 1989; Walker, 1992). These cognitive distortions include denial, fixed beliefs, superstition and other kinds of magical thinking, and notably omnipotence. Pathological gamblers experiencing cognitive distortions deny the reality of their gambling situation, including their odds of winning or losing (e.g., Langer, 1975; Langer and Roth, 1975; Ladouceur and Mayrand, 1984; Coulombe et al., 1992; Ladouceur et al., 1995). They may fixate on particular numbers, days of the week, colors of clothing, or a particular slot machine or may possess other magical objects that for them signify or enhance luck (Toneatto, personal communication to the committee, June 2, 1998). Rosenthal (1986) contends that such feelings of omnipotence are born out of desperation: the more helpless the situation, the greater their sense of certainty that they know what will happen next, and that they will achieve a positive outcome.

Bad luck, greed, or poor money management are not sufficient for someone to be a pathological gambler—although these factors do exert influence on the mental state of a gambler. For example, some individuals seek help during the early phase of their gambling career, even while they are still winning. They are astute enough to become concerned about their intense physical or psychological reactions, or about the effect their preoccupation with gambling is having on other aspects of their lives (Rosenthal, 1992; Rosenthal and Lorenz, 1992). One need not lose everything to be a pathological gambler, nor is it necessary to think about gambling every day. Some sufferers are binge gamblers, who sporadically experience consequences or cause damage in their lives or the lives of others. And some pathological gamblers may gamble excessively only at one type of game and are not interested in other types of gambling, whereas other pathological gamblers may play other games in order to support their game of choice (Lesieur, 1984).

Pathological Gambling as an Exculpatory Condition

As noted by Rachlin et al. (1984), the DSM-III created a new category of impulse control disorders, and this class of mental disorders was continued in the DSM-IV (American Psychiatric Association, 1980, 1994). With this new class of disorders came the opportunity for lawyers to use this kind of disorder as the foundation for the application of the insanity defense for criminal offenses. The insanity defense, however, rests in part on the distinction between an overwhelming uncontrollable impulse and the inability or unwillingness to control an impulse. The National Council on Compulsive Gambling has stated that the "APA diagnostic criteria [have] taken compulsive gambling out of the criminal, antisocial department and redefined this behavior as a neurosis, as are all compulsions" (cited in Rachlin et al., 1984:145). Rachlin et al. suggest that, despite their support for efforts to secure help for troubled people, the inclusion of pathological gambling in the DSM-IV should not encourage exculpation or exonoration for criminal offenses that are gambling related (p. 145). They observe that impulse disorders consist of the failure to resist impulses rather than an overwhelming uncontrollable impulse. In a cautionary note, the DSM-IV states that "[I]nclusion here, for clinical and research purposes, of a diagnostic category such as Pathological Gambling or Pedophilia does not imply that the condition meets legal or other non-medical criteria for what constitutes mental disease, mental disorder, or mental disability. The clinical and scientific considerations involved in categorization of these conditions as mental disorders may not be wholly relevant to legal judgments, for example, that take into account such issues as individual responsibility, disability determination, and competency" (American Psychiatric Association, 1994:xxvii). For additional information and examples of legal case rulings, see Morse (1994, 1998); U.S. v. Scholl, 959 F. Supp. 1189 (D. Ariz. 1997); People v. Lowitzki, 674 N.E.2d 859 (111.App. 1996); People v. Kindlon, 629 N.Y.S.2d 827 (App. Div. 1995); and Venezia v. U.S., 884 F. Supp. 919 (D.N.J. 1995).

CLASSIFICATIONS AND CONTROVERSIES

The American Psychiatric Association (1994) classifies pathological gambling as one of five different impulse disorders under a category called "Impulse-Control Disorders Not Elsewhere Classified." The other impulse disorders in this classification are intermittent explosive disorder (discrete episodes of aggressive behavior), kleptomania (stealing objects not needed or of value), pyromania (fire setting), and trichotillomania (hair pulling with noticeable loss). There are many other psychiatric disorders that involve problems of impulse control (e.g., substance use disorders, antisocial personality disorders, conduct disorders, schizophrenia). However, these other disorders have other features, beyond difficulty regulating impulses, that better classify them.

This cluster of impulse disorders suggests that there may be an important relationship between pathological gambling and the other impulse control disorders (e.g., pyromania, kleptomania). For example, these phenotypically different conditions could represent alternative manifestations of a shared predisposition toward impulsivity. Since there is no agreement in the field on the precise meaning of mental disorder, Wakefield (1992) suggests that a disorder is better thought of as a "harmful dysfunction," an idea that integrates social values (harmful) and scientific concepts (dysfunction): "dysfunction is a scientific term referring to the failure of a mental mechanism to perform a natural function for which it was designed by evolution" (Wakefield, 1992:373). The class of impulse disorders in which pathological gambling has been placed represents a set of behaviors that are violations of social mores and customs and therefore considered harmful. The dysfunctional nature of these disorders in general and pathological gambling in particular, however, remains to be determined. As we have previously indicated, mental disorders with impulsive features often have failed to satisfy the legal system's need for exculpatory conditions. These disorders have not been considered as "causal" in the scientific sense and have therefore not withstood courtroom challenges.

This matter becomes even more complicated when considering the matter of comorbidity from the perspective of DSM-IV classification. Comorbidity is the medical term used to describe the cooccurrence of two or more disorders in a single individual; comorbidity is extremely common among pathological gamblers (Crockford and el-Guebaly, 1998). The problem of conceptually distinct multiple diagnoses can be taken to suggest that pathological gamblers suffer from a variety of interactive disorders. However, there is an alternative possibility that has gained considerable support among clinicians: multiple diagnoses reflect an underlying problem with the constructs of mental disorders. The frequency of cooccurring disorders as described in the DSM suggests that these categorical distinctions exhibit "extraordinary and obstinate heterogeneity" (Carson, 1991, cited in Blatt and Levy, 1998: 83-84). Given this conceptual difficulty, although we describe comorbidity issues and pathological gambling more in Chapter 4, we do not emphasize this aspect of the disorder in the report. Nevertheless the reader is encouraged to keep comorbidity issues in mind when reading the discussions that follow of pathological gambling as an impulse disorder, as an addiction, and as considered by other theories and conceptualizations.

Pathological Gambling as an Impulse Disorder

An impulse refers to incitement to action arising from a state of mind or some external stimulus; or a sudden inclination to act, without conscious thought; or a motive or tendency coming from within (*Oxford English Dictionary*, 2nd edition, 1989). The essential feature of an impulse control disorder, as defined by DSM-IV, is "the failure to resist an impulse, drive, or temptation to perform an act that is harmful to the person or to others" (American Psychiatric Association, 1994:609). This implies a loss of control over behavior. There may be a sense of tension prior to committing the act, in which case committing it brings relief. The act is often pleasurable, though it may be followed by guilt and regret.

Existing literature on pathological and problem gambling uses many terms to describe impulsive behaviors from a variety of important perspectives, including "sensation-seeking," "behavioral disinhibition," and "risk-taking" (Lopes, 1987; Monroe, 1970; Zuckerman, 1979, 1983; Zuckerman et al., 1972). There is substantial literature suggesting that the descriptions are correct and contribute to both the origins and the maintenance of gambling involvement and problem gambling (Davis and Brisset, 1995). For example, indicators of behavioral disinhibition—the inability or unwillingness to inhibit behavioral impulses—have been associated with gambling involvement (Ciarrochi et al., 1991; Condas, 1990; Graham and Lowenfeld, 1986; Moravec and Munley, 1983; Templer et al., 1993; Castellani and Rugle, 1995).

In a study of cocaine treatment-seekers (Steinberg et al., 1992), the only measure that differentiated those with gambling problems from those without problems was a measure of disinhibition. In a study comparing a group of pathological gamblers in treatment to controls from the community, Specker and colleagues (1996) found that a significantly higher proportion of pathological gamblers had at least one other impulse control disorder (35 versus 3 percent). Similarly, the findings of increased antisocial behaviors and a history of criminal offenses among pathological gamblers also suggest disinhibitory tendencies (Cunningham-Williams et al., 1998; Blaszczynski and McConaghy, 1989; Busch, 1983; Hickey et al., 1986; Roy et al., 1989). Also, elevated rates of childhood attention-deficit hyperactivity disorder (ADHD) (Carlton et al., 1987; Carlton and Manowitz, 1994) and adult ADHD (Castellani and Rugle, 1995; Rugle, 1998) have been observed among pathological and problem gamblers.

Despite this evidence, this body of research may be misleading. The very few prospective studies of these addictions (e.g., Vaillant, 1983) require us to consider an alternative hypothesis: that involvement with gambling or other addictive behavior patterns can change the personality (Zinberg, 1975). The experience of alcoholism or pathological gambling may shift personality attributes so that, when researchers examine subjects who already have experienced alcoholism or pathological gambling patterns, they seem to have personality traits that are different from nondrinkers or nonpathological gamblers. Thus, it is possible that pathological gambling causes the development of these abnormal personality attributes, rather than that these attributes lead to pathological gambling.

Research suggests that the construct of behavioral disinhibition also relates to the risk for alcoholism (McGue et al., 1997). The presence of this trait may contribute to the high rate of alcoholism, estimated to be 33 percent, among pathological gamblers (Stinchfield and Winters, 1996). Moreover, relatively high levels of behavioral disinhibition differentiate the offspring of alcoholics from the offspring of nonalcoholics (Sher et al., 1991), suggesting that deviations in behavioral disinhibition are familial and may be a contributing cause, rather than merely a consequence of the development of alcoholism. By inference, the development of pathological gambling may be similarly affected by this behavioral trait.

Other dimensions of impulse control that have been examined in the gambling literature are sensation-seeking, novelty-seeking, and arousal. Zuckerman's theory of sensation-seeking as applied to gambling suggests that "individuals entertain the risk of monetary loss for the positive reinforcement produced by states of high arousal during periods of uncertainty, as well as the positive arousal produced by winning" (Zuckerman, 1979). Cloninger (1987) suggests a relationship between a desire for diverse sensations and alcohol consumption. Both Zuckerman and Cloninger's theories are relevant to gambling, in that they imply that gambling behaviors reflect tendencies to take risks and enjoy complex or varied stimulation.

The empirical literature in this area of gambling is inconclusive. Some investigations have found that pathological gamblers score higher on sensation-seeking scales than controls (Kuley and Jacobs, 1988; Stoltz, 1989); others have not found strong associations (Blaszczynski et al., 1990; Dickerson et al., 1990); and still others have found that gamblers scored within the average range on a measure of excitement-seeking (Castellani and Rugle, 1995). Similarly, researchers have not found elevated heart rates among gamblers in the laboratory setting (Anderson and Brown, 1984; Rule and Fischer, 1970; Rule et al., 1971), yet they have found elevated rates during play at various casino and video terminal games (Anderson and Brown, 1984; Leary and Dickerson, 1985). The lack of elevated heart rate in the laboratory may reflect a real difference in reaction—that simulated action is different from the real action of gambling. It also could mean a poor simulation, other characteristics of the laboratory setting, or a variety of other influences that remain difficult to identify.

Coventry and Norman (1997) summarized several problems specifically with studies of arousal and gambling. One example is heart rate fluctuation as a function of relaxation, frequent movement, or being in a simulated environment. The inherent unreliability of averaging heart rate measures, since gambling activity for certain games like slot machines is intermittent, is also a problem with such studies. Coventry and Norman also attempted to account for some of these methodological problems in their study of offtrack horse bettors and found significant increases in heart rate compared to baseline nongambling conditions, as bettors placed their bets. Unfortunately, as the authors point out, in order to be unobtrusive, this study used a less than ideal measure of heart rate (photo-plethysmography) and measured bettors' heart rate for only one race.

Gambling problems also may originate from attempts to relieve or change subjective states (e.g., Kuley and Jacobs, 1988; Rosenthal, 1989; Shaffer, 1996, 1997b). It is therefore not surprising that negative emotionality, that is, the tendency to experience psychological distress and a negative mood state, is a personality construct frequently associated with gambling severity. Supporting evidence includes high rates of depressive-like thinking patterns among frequent gamblers (McCormick et al., 1987) and significantly elevated rates of lifetime and current affective disorders among pathological gamblers (Specker et al., 1996). Whereas gambling involvement may serve to manage or attenuate highly uncomfortable emotions, alternatively, gambling may also reflect attempts to regulate or shift emotions from one state to another to satisfy a need for novel experiences or entertainment. The experience of altered emotional states may not predate the onset of gambling problems. It is possible that people shift their emotional states using gambling, and then fall into a gambling pattern that stimulates problems.

There is considerable consensus that gambling involves impulsiveness. In some studies, data do not systematically address the extent to which risk-taking and other dimensions of impulse control (i.e., sensation- and novelty-seeking, arousal, negative emotionality) are interrelated, or how they interact to affect initiation into and progression of gambling behavior. The established relationship between behavioral disinhibition and gambling may be the result of the correlation of each variable with sensation-seeking. Increased heart rates may be more attributable to other causes, like the anticipated outcome of a future event, not the response to an immediate event, such as the excitement of a race (Coventry and Norman, 1997), or verbalizations made by the gambler during gambling (Coulombe et al., 1992; Gaboury and Ladouceur, 1989; Gaboury et al., 1988; Griffiths, 1994; Ladouceur et al., 1988). And although the retrospective study by Rugle and Rosenthal (1993) suggests that, at least in a subgroup of pathological gamblers with high impulsivity, the impulsivity preceded the onset of gambling problems, longitudinal studies have not been conducted to establish that differences in impulse control characteristics predate the onset of gambling disorders, a necessary condition to establish a causal relationship. Interestingly, however, prospective studies are beginning to emerge suggesting that these traits may be transmitted genetically (Comings, 1998).

Pathological Gambling as an Addiction

Preoccupation, tolerance, and other DSM-IV criteria for pathological gambling, such as repeated unsuccessful efforts to stop gambling and becoming restless or irritable when attempting to stop, are indicative of physiological dependence (Wray and

Dickerson, 1981; Meyer, 1989; Rosenthal and Lesieur, 1992). In addition, the self-help community has thought of what it terms compulsive gambling as an uncontrollable emotional illness (Gamblers Anonymous, 1997). As such, many researchers have turned their attention to the extensive body of literature on addictions to explain pathological and problem gambling behavior. For example, research has begun to explore the possible biochemical basis of excessive gambling and its effects on the brains of pathological gamblers (Hickey et al., 1986; Koepp et al., 1998; Comings, 1998; Lukas, 1998). Although intriguing, these studies are primarily of persons in treatment with no control groups. Moreover, the basis for believing that pathological gambling should be classified as an addiction is almost entirely theoretical. As indicated above, DSM nomenclature has highlighted the similarity of pathological gambling to substance abuse since its third edition in 1987 (American Psychiatric Association, 1980, 1987, 1994), but it uses only the terms "abuse" or "dependence," not addiction.

To test the hypothesis that pathological gambling is a dependent state, studies such as those recently reviewed by Comings (1998) must further address associated genetic, molecular, and environmental factors taking into account other cooccurring conditions and an array of risk factors—all among a diverse population (i.e., men and women, old and young, ethnically representative, rural and urban) of gamblers and nongamblers, problem gamblers and those without problems, and treated and untreated gamblers.[3] Research also should explore the possibility that pathological gambling is a spectrum disorder, which means it shares the underlying genes and observable behavior with other psychiatric disorders. Finally, research in, this area should also consider the possibility of gambling as an addiction with respect to: (1) behavioral signs, (2) psychophysiological signs (e.g., toler-

---

[3]Under a grant from the National Institute for Responsible Gaming, Peter Goyer and William Semple of the Cleveland Medical Center in Brecksville, Ohio, are using positron-emission tomography brain imaging (i.e., PET scanning technology) to study regional cerebral blood flow, and dopamine-2 receptor indices in pathological gamblers. Preliminary findings were presented to the committee on June 2, 1998, in Irvine, California.

ance, withdrawal), and (3) consequences to the person and his or her social functioning or surroundings.

Other Theories and Conceptualizations of Pathological Gambling

The committee was charged to review excessive gambling as "pathological" as determined by the American Psychiatric Association. We were not charged with the task of determining the impact of excessive gambling caused by poor judgment untainted by illness. Although this report focuses on a medical model of gambling problems, readers should note that other models can also illuminate gambling-related excesses. For example, gambling can be understood as one aspect of a much larger problem, namely that a large and increasing number of households have trouble living within their means. For some households, the array of temptations to spend more than they can afford and the pressures to do so from advertising and a culture of conspicuous consumption may overwhelm self-control and skill in managing money. Those who cannot resist the temptation to spend beyond their means tend to be constantly in debt and constantly dealing with the consequences of their improvidence through legal and even illegal means. For some, the problem is credit cards and the Home Shopping Channel. For others, it's gambling or speculating in investments. At-risk people may differ with respect to which type of temptation is most alluring, but the consequences and the social costs to themselves and their friends, family, employers, and creditors are the same regardless. The primary strategy for dealing with the problem of temptation has usually been to limit the availability of stimulants and opportunities. Excessive gamblers may be intemperate because they fail to resist temptation or fail to regulate impulses to act.

Besides the medical model, several other conceptual models and theories have been advanced to explain pathological gambling. These include a general theory of addictions, the reward deficiency syndrome, behavioral-environmental reasons, the biopsychosocial model, and the moral model, among others. Although these models are not directly comparable, according to

Rugle (1998), "the importance of such models is their potential for determining intervention and research strategies, public opinion and policy decisions, and the self-perceptions of pathological gamblers themselves." The discussion below briefly describes three models for which there is some empirical support in the literature: behavioral-environmental reasons, a general theory of addictions, and the reward deficiency syndrome. (For detailed discussion of biogenetic and medical explanations of pathological gambling, see Chapter 4).

Behavioral-Environmental Reasons

Gambling may be viewed as a behavior that has been shaped in part by the environment, that is, pathological gamblers are people who have been susceptible to conditioning. The sequence of outcomes in some forms of gambling (e.g., slot machines) is quite similar to a partial reinforcement schedule (Knapp, 1976; Skinner, 1953, 1969). Winning, for example, represents a positive reinforcement. With partial reinforcement, rewards occur with some wagers, but not all. Gamblers are uncertain about which bets will produce rewards. In some forms of partial reinforcement, rewards come only after a certain number of responses (bets), but the number of responses is always changing. This is called a variable ratio schedule of reinforcement (Skinner, 1969). Variable ratio schedules of reinforcement do not produce learning as quickly as fixed ratio schedules of positive reinforcement (e.g., winning every bet), but after learning has occurred, extinction of behaviors acquired via variable ratio schedules of reinforcement is more difficult than with any other type of reinforcement schedule. This phenomenon may explain people's persistence in gambling despite large losses (Skinner, 1969).

Furthermore, the greater the size of the rewards, the more resistant the behavior is to extinction, a result that suggests gamblers who experience large wins early in their gambling careers may be most susceptible to addiction. Some theorists have pointed out that gambling can provide reinforcement even in the absence of a win. Reid (1986) noted that near misses or losses that were "close" to being wins also encouraged gambling. For example, when two same-type fruits appear in a slot machine, there is a brief period of excitement and thrill as one hopes for the third needed to win the jackpot. Even if the third fruit does not quite line up with the other two, there is still some thrill from the thought of nearly winning. Not surprisingly, some slot machines are designed to ensure a higher than chance frequency of near misses. Such reinforcement can occur at no expense to the casino.

Finally, the casino environment itself provides reinforcing effects, such as flashing lights, ringing bells, bright lighting and color schemes, and the clanging of coins as they fall into the winning collection bins of slot machines (Knapp, 1976). People are often "primed" when casinos give away rolls of free coins, or allow people to gamble without charge for limited periods of time. For all of these reasons, excessive gambling may be viewed as a conditioned response to powerful reinforcers.

General Theory of Addictions

In response to the conceptual confusion affecting understanding of addictive and impulse disorders generally, Jacobs and others have emphasized the need for an overriding conceptual framework—a credible and testable theory, supported by an empirically derived database—that could clearly address the causes and the course of addictive behaviors (Jacobs, 1987, 1988; Shaffer et al., 1989). Jacobs has proposed an interactive model of addiction, defining it as a dependent state that is acquired over time by a predisposed person in an attempt to relieve a chronic stress condition. Using pathological gambling as the prototype addiction, he posited that two interacting sets of factors (an abnormal physiological arousal state and childhood experiences resulting in a deep sense of personal inadequacy and rejection) in a conducive environment may produce addiction to any activity or substance that possesses three attributes: (1) it blurs reality by temporarily diverting the person's attention from the chronic aversive arousal state, (2) it lowers self-criticism and self-consciousness through an internal cognitive shift that deflects preoccupation from one's perceived inadequacies, and (3) it permits complimentary daydreams about oneself through a self-induced dissociative process.

The general theory holds that a given individual's addictive pattern of behavior represents that person's deliberately chosen means for entering and maintaining a dissociative-like state while indulging. Jacobs also characterizes this feature as a type of self-management or self-medicating strategy (Khantzian, 1985); that is, the person's addictive behavior represents the best solution to the stresses generated by longstanding underlying problems. Testing this theory on pathological gamblers, persons with other kinds of addictions, and normal control subjects, Jacobs and others have found principally through self-report research, that similar dissociative states are reported by pathological gamblers, alcoholics, and compulsive overeaters (Kuley and Jacobs, 1988; Marston et al., 1988). However, others have found that, although his work represents an important step toward the development of multidimensional models, Jacobs has largely ignored the importance of the social setting factors (Lesieur and Klein, 1987; Rosecrance, 1988; Zinberg, 1984) that influence the development, maintenance, and recovery from addictive behaviors (Shaffer et al., 1989).

Reward Deficiency Syndrome

Kenneth Blum and his colleagues adopted the concept of a reward deficiency syndrome to refer to alterations in brain chemistry that can interfere with the brain's reward process. This theory holds that genetic commonalties in a spectrum of behavioral disorders (including alcoholism, substance abuse, smoking, compulsive overeating and obesity, attention-deficit disorder, and pathological gambling) may be the underlying cause of a chemical imbalance that alters the signaling in the brain's reward process. The chemical imbalance appears to supplant normal feelings of well-being with negative feelings. A recent study found that the genetic anomaly that interferes with the brain's reward process was present in more than 50 percent of a sample of white pathological gamblers (Comings et al., 1996). This research and related issues are discussed in Chapter 4 in the section on biology-based studies of pathological gambling.

MEASURING PATHOLOGICAL GAMBLING[4]

As interest in pathological gambling increased during the 1990s, researchers have conducted an increasing number of epidemiological surveys and, to a lesser extent, clinical investigations. Accordingly, scientists developed several screening and diagnostic instruments for this research. The committee identified 25 different such assessment instruments that have been used to measure pathological and problem gambling (Shaffer et al., 1997). Of these, 12 were primarily used with adults and 3 were primarily used as adolescent measures. These instruments were used principally as screening tools. As part of the Survey of American Gambling Attitudes and Behavior commissioned by the U.S. Commission on a National Policy Toward Gambling, Kallick and her colleagues at the University of Michigan Survey Research Center developed the first instrument reported in the literature in 1975: the ISR (Institute for Social Research) Test (Kallick et al., 1979). Many of the recently developed tests are based on the DSM-III or subsequent DSM-based definitions to assess and measure pathological gambling.

Table 2-1 lists the primary gambling screening and diagnostic tools used in survey or clinical research cited in the literature. As indicated in the table, many of the measures have not been evaluated and the others have received minimal psychometric evaluation. The exception is the South Oaks Gambling Screen (SOGS), which has been widely used in numerous epidemiological studies (see Shaffer et al., 1997) and has been applied to samples derived from treatment, Gambler's Anonymous, help-line, and several general population settings (e.g., Lesieur and Blume, 1987; Stinchfield, 1998). The widespread use of the SOGS in population surveys did not occur without criticism. The concern is that the use of screening instruments that were developed principally for use in clinical settings requires caution in studies of the general population. In contrast to diagnostic interviews, the aim of screening tools is to identify the *possible* presence of the target

---

[4]The committee acknowledges Rachel Volberg's written contribution pertaining to the history and development of diagnostic and screening instruments.

TABLE 2-1 Measures of Pathological and Problem Gambling

Tool	Type	Number of Items	Psychometrics
For Adults			
ISR (1974)	Screening	18	Not evaluated
CCSM (1984)	Screening	28	Not evaluated
SOGS (1987)	Screening	20	Evaluated with clinic-referred, Gamblers Anonymous, help-line callers, general population
MOGS (1990)	Screening	12	Not evaluated
SOGS-R (1991)	Screening	20	Evaluated with general population
DSM-IV screen (1996)	Screening	10	Evaluated with general population
DIS (1995)	Diagnostic	5	Not evaluated
SGC (1996)	Screening	18	Evaluated with general population
PG-YBOCS (1998)	Screening	10	Not evaluated
DIGS (1997)	Diagnostic interview	20	Evaluated with clinic-referred, help-line, general population
EDJP (1997)	Distorted cognitions	12 per game	Not evaluated
SIR (1998)	Treatment planning	135	Not evaluated
For Adolescents			
SOGS-RA (1993)	Screening	11	Evaluated with general population
DSM-IV-J (1992)	Screening	10	Evaluated with general population
MAGS (1994)	Screening	7–12	Evaluated with general population

problem. Clinical screening measures typically yield conservative scoring decisions (such as the SOGS designation of "probable pathological gambler") that are designed to guard against false negatives—the mistake of claiming that there is no problem when in fact one exists.[5]

A screening tool is most valuable when it is used to determine the need for conducting a more definitive assessment. When screening measures are used in population surveys, they necessarily yield liberal estimates of the disorder. Culleton (1989) has raised the question of the appropriateness of applying a screening test, such as the SOGS, to establish a prevalence rate in a general population. He criticizes this method on the basis of the low predictive value of a test that screens for a disorder with a low base rate among the general population. These concerns remind us that, even when an instrument has high sensitivity and specificity, "the actual predictive value of the instrument could be much more limited, depending on the prevalence of the disorder of interest" (Goldstein and Simpson, 1995:236). This argument suggests that the use of any measure will result in an overestimation of the prevalence of pathological gambling in the general population, given the likelihood that the disorder is a relatively infrequent phenomenon (Volberg and Boles, 1995).

However, future research cannot address whether the SOGS, or any other instrument, provides an overestimate or an underestimate of pathological gambling until the instrument's statistical association with independent and valid standards of the disorder is determined. In this view, the use of screening instruments to estimate a "true" prevalence of a disorder is one of several important methods in the process of acquiring prevalence estimates. Of course, all efforts to establish a prevalence estimate of pathological gambling rest on the assumption that a valid standard of the disorder exists. However, it is not clear whether, in the field of psychiatry in general and for pathological gambling in particular,

---

[5]In fact, screening instruments can be designed to guard against false positives too. The emphasis shifts depending on the objectives of the screen. Conservative screening implies that the true rate of the phenomenon being screened is known, which is often not the case.

such standards exist (Shaffer et al., 1997). The process of establishing construct validity for disorders such as pathological gambling is complex and difficult; we take a brief but important digression into a more technical examination of this process in the next section.

The Process of Determining Construct Validity

Scientific research inevitably involves measuring things. The study of psychopathology involves measuring things that are not readily visible either to the naked eye or with contemporary technological instruments (such as microscopes or neuroimaging equipment). Even if we measure something consistently—that is, with reliability—scientists may remain uncertain of the thing that they are measuring. The concept of validity refers to "the veracity or accuracy of some measurement of a construct" (Malagady et al., 1992:61). Construct validity refers to the idea that scientific instruments are measuring precisely what they claim to be measuring.

It is traditional to establish the construct validity of a clinical disorder by integrating evidence from many different sources (e.g., clinical descriptive studies and etiological investigations) and establishing that the evidence is consistent with the theory that underlies the conceptualization of the disorder. "The problem of construct validation becomes especially acute in the clinical field since for many of the constructs dealt with, it is not a question of finding an imperfect criterion, but of finding any criterion at all" (*Psychological Bulletin Supplement*, 1954:4-15; as cited in Cronbach and Meehl, 1955:285). To establish the construct validity of pathological gambling, scientists will have to work through a rigorous and systematic process.

Malgady and colleagues (1992) suggest a classic three-part framework for validating a psychiatric diagnosis such as pathological gambling. First, clinicians and scientists must establish content validity for the disorder, then conduct research on criterion-related validity, and finally arrive at construct validity. Malagady and colleagues note that "the question of validity is whether or not the quantitative or qualitative values assigned to units under observation accurately depict the units' variations in the construct or entity that is the intention of measurement" (Malagady et al., 1992:61). "Symbolically, validity of some measure (X) is estimated by its correlation, or concordance, with another measure (Y) of the criterion or of a criterion-related indicator that is external to X. When two X measurements are rendered by different interviewers at the same time or at different times or even by different interviewers at different times, the correlation between the measurements is an estimate of reliability. To qualify as a bona fide validity paradigm, the criterion-related indicator (Y) must be external to X, meaning that it was obtained by a different assessment technique, and must have relevance to the construct that is the target of measurement" (p. 61). To date, this paradigm has not been employed by any gambling researchers.

Thus, the scientific work plan to develop measures of pathological gambling would begin with identifying measurable behaviors and attitudes that theoretically reflect the underlying construct of pathological gambling. For example, is pathological gambling best understood as an addictive disorder, an impulse disorder, or one of many problems associated with a more fundamental disorder, such as depression? Individual and environmental factors that influence gambling onset and the development of an excessive gambling pattern would be identified. These factors could include player attributes (e.g., poor judgment and decision making, heightened motivation to seek stimulating sensations), social setting, some special characteristic of the games, or combinations of these elements. The measure would reflect the views of the onset, escalation, and maintenance of pathological gambling and be subjected to the rigors of validity testing so that, as evidence accumulates regarding the measure's validity, the underlying construct—that it is actually measuring pathological gambling—is affirmed.

Ultimately, establishing construct validity is an unending process. Given the problems inherent in any discussion of the construct validity of pathological gambling, Bland et al. (1993:60) have suggested: "In the absence of a validating criterion, or 'gold standard,' it could be argued that perhaps the most that can be hoped for, as with unstructured clinical assessment, is social consensus on diagnostic classification" (e.g., concordance among SOGS interviews or convergence of multiple methods of classification). "The standardization of the diagnostic process is a useful way of increasing to respectable levels low concordance coefficients" (p. 61). In other words, although scientists and clinicians now may be able to measure and assess gambling-related problems reliably, this does not mean, nor should it imply, that either group knows exactly what it is that they are evaluating.

Validity as a Theory-Driven Construct

Given the array of instruments that purport to identify gambling-related problems and pathology, and the potential pitfalls in their design and use among the general population in particular, it is essential to sort through the psychometric characteristics of these screening devices. The two most commonly examined psychometric attributes are reliability and validity. Reliability refers to the capacity of an instrument to measure a relatively enduring trait with some level of consistency over time, across social settings, and between raters. If a given instrument consistently measures a phenomenon, it is said to be reliable. Validity pertains to actually measuring that which is sought to be measured, as opposed to something else. As Goldstein and Simpson (1995) suggest, "Validity refers to the questions 'for what purpose is the indicator being used?' and 'how accurate is it for that purpose?'" (pp. 229-230). If an instrument distinguishes between pathological or problem gambling and another cooccurring condition—alcoholism, for example—it is said to be valid in that regard. Validity also relates to sensitivity and specificity: if a net is thrown out, it must have mesh small enough to catch the cases of interest, but large enough to let escape those cases that do not have the attribute being sought. Sensitivity represents how small the openings are to catch cases and specificity represents how large the openings are to let noncases escape. Reliability and validity, although related concepts, are sometimes confused; reliability is often mistaken for a measure of validity.

Screening Instrument Validation

The problems associated with determining an instrument's validity begin with its very definition. Validity is neither static nor an inherent characteristic of a screening instrument. As indicated in the previous section, determining the validity of an instrument or a construct is an unending and dynamic investigative process. For example, we cannot simply conclude that an instrument has been shown to be valid for all purposes and all settings. "An indicator (e.g., an instrument, such as a test, a rating, or an interview) can be valid for one purpose, but not for another" (Goldstein and Simpson, 1995:230). Directed by theoretical and ultimately practical purposes, validity is the dynamic consequence of applying an instrument to a specific measurement task. However, in the field of gambling studies, there is a paucity of theory-driven research in general and prevalence research in particular (Shaffer, 1997a). When conventional wisdom and theory shift or change, the validity of a measurement instrument can be terminated abruptly. The history of the SOGS provides an instance of the relative nature of validity. Although for some time researchers considered that the SOGS lifetime measure had been found valid and reliable (Volberg, 1994:238), the same investigators now suggest that the SOGS lifetime measures "over-state the actual prevalence of pathological gambling" (Volberg, 1997:41) because it combines those with a history of a gambling problem and those who currently have a problem.

CONCLUSIONS

Gambling behavior inherently involves risk-taking, may involve limited skill, and may best be conceptualized on a continuum ranging from no gambling, to social and recreational gambling, to problem gambling, and to pathological gambling. Pathological gambling often cooccurs with other disorders, and its social and economic effects theoretically increase once the threshold of problem gambling is crossed, although this dynamic relationship has not yet been demonstrated empirically. In addition, little is known about the dynamics of gamblers as they move from one level of gambling behavior to another.

Clinical evidence suggests that pathological gamblers engage in destructive behaviors: they commit crime, they run up large debts, they damage relationships with family and friends, and some kill themselves. Since 1980, pathological gambling has been categorized as a "Disorder of Impulse Control Not Elsewhere Classified" in three versions of the *Diagnostic and Statistical Manual of Mental Disorders* published by the American Psychiatric Association. The effort by the American Psychiatric Association to operationalize pathological gambling has been evolving and today DSM-IV provides a useful definition and diagnostic criteria that is relied on heavily by both clinicians and researchers. As a diagnostic guide, DSM-IV suggests that persons meeting 5 or more of the 10 criteria should be classified and treated as pathological gamblers. Even though the DSM-IV definition of pathological gambling is now widely accepted, there remains debate over the precise classification and construct validity of pathological gambling, and also over the conceptualization and definition of less severe problem gambling, which is not addressed in the DSM-IV. The debate includes the issue of whether or not pathological gambling should be viewed as a dependent state or an addiction rather than as a disorder of impulse control.

The history of pathological and problem gambling research reflects the developmental process of shifting scientific attempts to measure a singular phenomenon. The field is still relatively immature compared with many others and, as a result, does not demonstrate a coherent program of scientific inquiry.

The committee recognizes that, although the term pathological gambling and its accepted definition adequately represent severe cases of excessive gamblers, there is a need for more research to validly define other levels of gambling severity. Not all gamblers experience an excessive relationship with the games they play; not all excessive gamblers experience compulsive or pathological behaviors; not all pathological gamblers experience impairment in every aspect of their activities. A multilevel system with agreed-on terminology, such as that proposed by Shaffer and Hall (1996) should be considered by experts in the field. Such consideration could lead to integration of diverse research findings and to a more accurate reflection of the clinical picture.

Scholars of pathological and problem gambling are still struggling with how to demonstrate the validity of pathological gambling as a primary disorder independent of other mental illness, even as scholars in psychiatry in general continue to encounter many of these same validity problems across the full range of mental disorders (e.g., Cronbach and Meehl, 1955; Dohrenwend, 1995; Malagady et al., 1992). A high priority for future research is to further advance the validity of pathological gambling constructs. In order to establish coherent theories and models of pathological gambling, a rigorous scientific work plan is required. This effort will put the concept of pathological gambling to the test by generating the empirical evidence necessary to fully evaluate its construct validity. Simply entering the psychiatric nomenclature is not a proxy for validity. Many psychiatric diagnoses have come and gone over the years.[6]

Although various instruments are available to assess the prevalence of pathological and problem gambling, each instrument is best understood by viewing it through an evaluative lens that can focus on its origin, driving motivation, relationship to funding, and inherent strengths and weaknesses. Notwithstanding improved diagnostic criteria provided by DSM-IV, until the field develops standardized tools with demonstrated psychometric properties, the ability of an instrument to successfully determine whether an individual is a pathological gambler remains dependent on the method of validation, interviewing technique, sampling design, and other methodological factors. Consequently, in the absence of a well-formulated model or theory and the subsequent construct validity that results from a program of empirical research, scientifically based knowledge and understanding cannot be advanced.

Contemporary scientists stand on the shoulders of those who came before. The efforts of pioneers who undertook the early research on pathological gambling, usually without institutional support, provide the platform on which current investigators stand. The current conceptualization, definition, and diagnostic criteria for pathological gambling must be carefully studied. The

---

[6]For example, the symptom cluster called "post-traumatic stress disorder" first appeared in the DSM-III in 1980, replacing diagnoses such as "shell shock" and "combat fatigue" (Breslau and Davis, 1987). Conversely, in 1973, "homosexuality" was removed from the second edition of the DSM (American Psychiatric Association, 1973), reflecting the medical profession's shift toward viewing sexual orientation as something other than a disorder that needed to be treated (Bayer, 1981).

French biologist Jean Rostand reminds us "nothing leads the scientist so astray as a premature truth" (Rostand, 1939). The field of gambling studies is in its early days. It is therefore timely to encourage those who study gambling and its effects, as well as those in positions to support such research, to pursue empirical studies for further validation and understanding of this public health problem. Future research that measures the incidence of related psychiatric disorders along with pathological gambling, interactive processes, and genetic predispositions will provide important insight into these questions.

REFERENCES

American Psychiatric Association
  1973   *DSM-II: Diagnostic and Statistical Manual of Mental Disorders* (2nd ed.). Washington, DC: American Psychiatric Association.
  1980   *DSM-III: Diagnostic and Statistical Manual of Mental Disorders* (3rd ed.). Washington, DC: American Psychiatric Association.
  1987   *DSM-III-R: Diagnostic and Statistical Manual of Mental Disorders* (3rd ed., revised). Washington, DC: American Psychiatric Association.
  1994   *DSM-IV: Diagnostic and Statistical Manual of Mental Disorders* (4th ed.). Washington, DC: American Psychiatric Association.
Anderson, G., and R. Brown
  1984   Real and laboratory gambling, sensation-seeking and arousal. *British Journal of Addiction* 75:401-410.
Bayer, R.
  1981   *Homosexuality and American Psychiatry: The Politics of Diagnosis.* New York: Basic Books, Inc.
Benjamin, J., L. Lin, C. Patterson, B.D. Greenberg, D.L. Murphy, and D.H. Hamer
  1996   Population and familial association between the D4 dopamine receptor gene and measures of novelty seeking. *Nature Genetics* 12(January):81-83.
Bland, R.C., S.C. Newman, H. Orn, and G. Stebelsky
  1993   Epidemiology of pathological gambling in Edmonton. *Canadian Journal of Psychiatry* 38:108-112.
Blaszcyznski, A.P., and N. McConaghy
  1989   Anxiety and/or depression in the pathogenesis of addictive gambling. *International Journal of the Addictions* 24:337-350.
Blaszczynski, A.P., N. McConaghy, and A. Frankova
  1990   Boredom proneness in pathological gambling. *Psychological Reports* 67:35-42.
Blatt, S.J., and K.N. Levy
  1998. A psychodynamic approach to the diagnosis of psychopathology. Pp

73-109 in *Making Diagnosis Meaningful: Enhancing Evaluation and Treatment of Psychological Disorders*, J.W. Barron et al., eds. Washington, DC: American Psychiatric Association.

Blum, K., J.G. Cull, E.R. Braverman, T.J.H. Chen, and D.E. Comings
1997   Reward deficiency syndrome: Neurobiological and genetic aspects. Pp 311-327 in *Handbook of Psychiatric Genetics*, K. Blum, E.P. Noble et al., eds. Boca Raton, FL: CRC Press Inc.

Boyd, W.H.
1976   Excitement: The gambler's drug. In *Gambling and Society*, W.R. Eadington, ed. Springfield, IL: Thomas.

Bradford, J., J. Geller, H.R. Lesieur, R.J. Rosenthal, and M. Wise
1996   Impulse control disorders. Pp. 1007-1031 in *DSM-IV Sourcebook: Volume 2*, T.A. Widiger, A.J. Frances, H.A. Pincus, et al., eds. Washington, DC: American Psychiatric Association.

Brenner, R., and B.A. Brenner
1990   *Gambling and Speculation: A Theory, a History, and a Future of Some Human Decisions*. Cambridge, England: Cambridge University Press.

Breslau, N., and G.C. Davis
1987   Posttraumatic stress disorder: The stress or criterion. *Journal of Nervous and Mental Disease* 175(5):255-264.

Brown, R.I.F.
1987   Pathological gambling and related patterns of crime: Comparisons with alcohol and other drug addictions. *Journal of Gambling Behavior* 3:98-114.
1996   Role of Dissociative Experiences in Problem Gambling. Paper presented at the Second European Conference on Gambling and Policy Issues, Amsterdam, September 4-7.

Bruce, A.C., and J.E.V. Johnson
1996   Decision-making under risk: Effect of complexity on performance. *Psychological Reports* 79(1):67-76.

Busch, C.M.
1983   The theory and measurement of three independent personality dimensions: Impulsivity, self-control, and caution. *Dissertation Abstracts* 44:1219.

Carlton, P.L., and P. Manowitz
1994   Factors determining the severity of pathological gambling in males. *Journal of Gambling Studies* 10:147-158.

Carlton, P.L., P. Manowitz, H. McBride, R. Nora, M. Swartzburg, and L. Goldstein
1987   Attention deficit disorder and pathological gambling. *Journal of Clinical Psychiatry* 48:487-488.

Castellani, B., and L. Rugle
1995   A comparison of pathological gamblers to alcoholics and cocaine abusers on impulsivity, sensation seeking, and craving. *International Journal of the Addictions* 30(3):275-289.

Ciarrocchi, J.W., N. Kirschner, and F. Fallik
1991 Personality dimensions of male pathological gamblers, alcoholics, and dually addicted gamblers. *Journal of Gambling Studies* 7:133-142.

Cloninger, C.R.
1987 Neurogenetic adaptive mechanisms in alcoholism. *Science* 236:410-416.

Clotfelter, C.T., and P.J. Cook
1989 *Selling Hope: State Lotteries in America.* Cambridge, MA: Harvard University Press.

Comings, D.E.
1998 The molecular genetics of pathological gambling. *CNS Spectrums* 3(6): 20-37.

Comings, D.E., R.J. Rosenthal, H.R. Lesieur, L.J. Rugle, D. Muhleman, C. Chiu, G. Dietzand, and R. Gade
1996 A study of the dopamine D_2 receptor gene in pathological gambling. *Pharmacogenetics* 6:223-234.

Condas, G.P., Jr.
1990 Assessment of the difference in personality characteristics between pathological and nonpathological gamblers. *Dissertation Abstracts* 51:2044.

Coulombe, A., R. Ladouceur, R. Desharnais, and J. Jobin
1992 Erroneous perceptions and arousal among regular and occasional video poker players. *Journal of Gambling Studies* 8(3):235-244.

Coventry, K.R., and A.C. Norman
1997 Arousal, sensation-seeking and frequency of gambling in off-course horse racing bettors. *British Journal of Psychology* 88:671-681.

Crockford, D.N., and N. el-Guebaly
1998 Psychiatric comorbidity in pathological gambling: A critical review. *Canadian Journal of Psychiatry* 43:43-50.

Cronbach, L.J., and P.E. Meehl
1955 Construct validity in psychological tests. *Psychological Bulletin* 52(4):281-302.

Culleton, R.P.
1989 The prevalence rates of pathological gambling: A look at methods. *Journal of Gambling Behavior* 5(1):22-41.

Cunningham-Williams, R.M., L.B. Cottler, W.M. Compton, and E.L. Spitznagel
1998 Taking chances: Problem gamblers and mental health disorders— Results from the St. Louis Epidemiological Catchment Area (ECA) Study. *American Journal of Public Health* 88(7):1093-1096.

Custer, R.L.
1980 *The Profile of Pathological Gamblers.* Washington, DC: National Foundation for Study and Treatment of Pathological Gambling.
1982 An overview of compulsive gambling. Pp.107-124 in *Addictive Disorders Update: Alcoholism, Drug Abuse, Gambling,* P.A. Carone, S.F. Yolles, S.N. Kieffer, and L.W. Krinsky, eds. New York: Human Sciences Press, Inc.

Custer, R.L., and L.F. Custer
  1978 Characteristics of the Recovering Compulsive Gambler: A Survey of 150 Members of Gamblers Anonymous. Paper presented at the Fourth Annual Conference on Gambling, Reno, Nevada, December.
Custer, R.L., and H. Milt
  1985 *When Luck Runs Out.* New York: Facts on File Publications.
Davies, J.B.
  1996 Reasons and causes: Understanding substance users' explanations for their behavior. *Human Psychopharmacology* 11:S39-S48.
Davis, G., and D. Brisset
  1995 Comparing the Pathological and Recreational Gambler: An Exploratory Study. Unpublished report. Minnesota Department of Human Services, December.
Devereux, E.C.
  1979 Gambling. In *The International Encyclopedia of the Social Sciences, Vol. 17.* New York: Macmillan.
Dickerson, M.G., M. Walker, S.L. England, and J. Hinchy
  1990 Demographic, personality, cognitive and behavioral correlates of off-course betting involvement. *Journal of Gambling Studies* 6:165-182.
Dohrenwend, B.P.
  1995 "The problem of validity in field studies of psychological disorders" revisited. Pp. 3-20 in *Textbook in Psychiatric Epidemiology*, M. T. Tsuang, M. Tohen, and G.E. Zahner, eds. New York: Wiley-Liss.
Ebstein, R.P., O. Novick, R. Umansky, B. Priel, Y. Osher, D. Blaine, E.R. Bennett, L. Nemanov, M. Katz, and R.H. Belmaker
  1996 Dopamine D4 receptor (D4DR) exon III polymorphism associated with the human personality trait of novelty seeking. *Nature Genetics* 12(January):78-80.
Faigman, D.L., D.H. Kaye, M.S. Saks, and J. Sanders
  1997 *Modern Scientific Evidence: The Law and Science of Expert Testimony, Volume 1.* St. Paul, MN: West Publishing Co.
Gaboury, A., and R. Ladouceur
  1989 Erroneous perceptions and gambling. *Journal of Social Behavior and Personality* 4:411-420.
Gaboury, A., R. Ladouceur, G. Beauvais, L. Marchand, et al.
  1988 Cognitive dimensions and behaviors among regular and occasional blackjack players. *International Journal of Psychology* 23(3):283-291.
Gamblers Anonymous
  1997 Gamblers Anonymous: Sharing Recovery Through Gamblers Anonymous. Los Angeles: Gamblers Anonymous.
Goldstein, J.M., and J.C. Simpson
  1995 Validity: Definitions and applications to psychiatric research. Pp. 229-242 in *Textbook in Psychiatric Epidemiology*, M.T. Tsuang, M. Tohen, and G. E. Zahner, eds. New York: Wiley-Liss.

Graham, J.R., and B.H. Lowenfeld
1986   Personality dimensions of the pathological gambler. *Journal of Gambling Behavior* 2:58-66.
Griffiths, M.D.
1994   The role of cognitive bias and skill in fruit machine gambling. *British Journal of Psychology* 85:351-369.
Hickey, John E., C.A. Haertzen, and J.E. Henningfield
1986   Simulation of gambling responses on the Addiction Research Center Inventory. *Addictive Behaviors* 11:345-349.
Jacobs, D.F.
1987   Evidence for a common dissociative-like reaction among addicts. *Journal of Gambling Behavior* 4:27-37.
1988   A general theory of addictions: Rationale for and evidence supporting a new approach for understanding and treating addictive behaviors. Pp. 35-64 in *Compulsive Gambling: Theory, Research and Practice*, H.J. Shaffer, S. Stein, B. Gambino, and T.N. Cummings, eds. Lexington, MA: Lexington Books.
1989a   Illegal and undocumented: A review of teenage gambling and the plight of children of problem gamblers in America. In *Compulsive Gambling: Theory, Research and Practice*, H.J. Shaffer, S.A. Stein, B. Gambino, and T.N. Cummings, eds. Lexington, MA: Lexington Books.
1989b   Special issue: Gambling and the family. *Journal of Gambling Behavior* 5(4).
Kallick, M., D. Suits, T. Dielman, and J. Hybels
1979   *A Survey of American Gambling Attitudes and Behavior*. Research report series, Survey Research Center, Institute for Social Research. Ann Arbor: University of Michigan Press.
Khantzian, E.J.
1975   Self-selection and progression in drug dependence. *Psychiatry Digest* 36:19-22.
1977   The ego, the self, and opiate addiction: Theoretical and treatment considerations. *NIDA Research Monograph* 12.
1985   The self-medication hypothesis of addictive disorders: Focus on heroin and cocaine dependence. *American Journal of Psychiatry* 142(11):1259-1264.
Knapp, T.J.
1976   A functional analysis of gambling behavior. In *Gambling and Society: Interdisciplinary Studies on the Subject of Gambling*, W.R. Eadington, ed. Springfield, IL: Charles C. Thomas.
Koepp, M.J., R.N. Gunn, A.D. Lawrence, V.J. Cunningham, A. Dagher, T. Jones, D.J. Brooks, C.J. Bench, and P.M. Grasby
1998   Evidence for striatal dopamine release during a video game. *Nature* 393:266-268.

Kuley, N., and D. Jacobs
  1988   The relationship between dissociative-like experiences and sensation seeking among social and problem gamblers. *Journal of Gambling Behavior* 4:197-207.
Ladouceur, R., D. Dube, I. Giroux, N. Legendre, et al.
  1995   Cognitive biases in gambling: American roulette and 6/49 lottery. *Journal of Social Behavior and Personality* 10(2):473-479.
Ladouceur, R., A. Gaboury, M. Dumont, and P. Rochette
  1988   Gambling: Relationship between the frequency of wins and irrational thinking. *Journal of Psychology* 122:409-412.
Ladouceur, R., and M. Mayrand
  1984   Evaluation of the "illusion of control": Type of feedback, outcome sequence, and number of trials among regular and occasional gamblers. *Journal of Psychology* 117(1):37-46.
Langer, E.J.
  1975   The illusion of control. *Journal of Personality and Social Psychology* 32:311-328.
Langer, E.J., and J. Roth
  1975   Heads I win, tails it's chance: The illusion of control as a function of the sequence of outcomes in a purely chance task. *Journal of Personality and Social Psychology* 32:951-955.
Leary, K., and M.G. Dickerson
  1985   Levels of arousal in high and low frequency gamblers. *Behavioral Research and Therapy* 23:197-207.
Lesieur, H.R.
  1984   *The Chase: Career of the Compulsive Gambler.* Rochester, VT: Schenkman Books.
  1988   Altering the DSM-III criteria for pathological gambling. *Journal of Gambling Behavior* 4(1):38-47.
  1989   Gambling, pathological gambling and crime. Pp. 89-110 in *The Handbook of Pathological Gambling*, T. Galski, ed. Springfield, IL: Charles C. Thomas.
  1994   Epidemiological surveys of pathological gambling: Critique and suggestions for modification. *Journal of Gambling Studies* 10(4):385-398.
Lesieur, H.R., and S.B. Blume
  1987   The South Oaks Gambling Screen (SOGS): A new instrument for the identification of pathological gamblers. *American Journal of Psychiatry* 144(9):1184-1188.
  1991   When Lady Luck loses: Women and compulsive gambling. Pp. 181-197 in *Feminist Perspectives on Addictions*, N. van den Bergh, ed. New York: Springer.
Lesieur, H.R., S.B. Blume, and R. Zoppa
  1986   Alcoholism, drug abuse and gambling. *Alcoholism: Clinical and Experimental Research* 10:33-38.

Lesieur, H.R., and R. Klein
1987   Pathological gambling among high school students. *Addictive Behaviors* 12:129-135.
Lesieur, H.R., and R.J. Rosenthal
1991   Pathological gambling: A review of the literature (prepared for the American Psychiatric Association Task Force on DSM-IV Committee on Disorders of Impulse Control Not Elsewhere Classified). *Journal of Gambling Studies* 7:5-39.
1994   Self-Reported Physiological and Dissociative Experiences Among Pathological Gamblers. Paper presented at the Conference on Gambling Behavior of the National Council on Problem Gambling, Seattle, July. (Also presented at the First European Conference on Gambling and Policy Issues, Cambridge, UK, August, 1995.) Institute for Problem Gambling, Middletown, CT.
1998   Analysis of pathological gambling Pp. 393-401 in *DSM-IV Sourcebook: Volume 4*, T.A. Widiger, A.J. Frances, H.A. Pincus, R. Ross, M.B. First, W. Davis, and   M. Kline, eds. Washington, DC: American Psychiatric Association.
Livingston, J.
1974   *Compulsive Gamblers: Observations on Action and Abstinence.* New York: Harper Torchbooks.
Lopes, L.L.
1987   Between hope and fear: The psychology of risk. *Advances in Experimental Social Psychology* 20:255-295.
Lorenz, V.C., and R.A. Yaffee
1986   Pathological gambling: Psychosomatic, emotional, and marital difficulties as reported by the gambler. *Journal of Gambling Behavior* 2:40-49.
Lukas, S.E.
1998   Brain Imaging of Altered Mood States: Implications for Understanding the Neurobiological Bases of Gambling. Paper prepared for the National Research Council, Committee on the Social and Economic Impact of Pathological Gambling. McLean Hospital, Cambridge, MA.
Malagady, R.G., L.H. Rogler, and W.W. Tryon
1992   Issues of validity in the diagnostic interview schedule. *Journal of Psychiatric Research* 26(1):59-67.
Marlatt, G.A., J.S. Baer, D. Donovan, and D.R. Kivlahan
1988   Addictive behaviors: Etiology and treatment. In *Annual Review of Psychology* (39:223-252), M.R. Rosenzweig and L.W. Porter, eds. Palo Alto: Annual Reviews, Inc.
Marston, A.R., D.F. Jacobs, R.D. Singer, and K.F. Widaman
1988   Characteristics of adolescents at risk for compulsive overeating on a brief screening test. *Adolescence* 23(89):59-65.
McCormick, R.A., A.M. Russo, L.F. Ramirez, and J.I. Taber
1984   Affective disorders among pathological gamblers seeking treatment. *American Journal of Psychiatry* 141:215-218.

McCormick, R.A., J. Taber, N. Kruedelbach, and A. Russo
  1987 Personality profiles of hospitalized pathological gamblers: The California Personality Inventory. *Journal of Clinical Psychology* 43:521-527.
McGue, M., W. Slutske, J. Taylor, and W.G. Iacono
  1997 Personality and substance use disorders: I. Effects of gender and alcoholism subtype. *Alcoholism: Clinical and Experimental Research* 21:513-520.
Meyer, G.
  1989 *Glucksspieler in Selbsthilfegruppen: Erste Ergebnisse Einer Empirischen Untersuchung.* Hamburg: Neuland.
Monroe, R.R.
  1970 *Episodic Behavioral Disorders: A Psychodynamic and Neurophysiologic Analysis.* Cambridge, MA: Harvard University Press.
Moran, E.
  1969 Taking the final risk. *Mental Health* 3:21-22 (London).
Moravec, J.D., and P.H. Munley
  1983 *The Moral Order: An Introduction to the Human Situation.* Beverley Hills, CA: Sage Press.
Morse, S.
  1994 Culpability and control. *University of Pennsylvania Law Review* 142:1587
  1998 Excusing and the new excuse defenses: A legal and conceptual review. In *Crime and Justice: A Review of Research,* Vol. 23, M. Tonry, ed. Chicago: University of Chicago Press.
Neese, R.M., and K.C. Berridge
  1997 Psychoactive drug use in evolutionary perspective. *Science* 278:63-66.
O'Donnell, R., and L.R. Rugle
  1996 Gambling Severity and Dissociation in a Group of Inpatient Gamblers. Paper presented at the Tenth National Conference on Gambling Behavior, Chicago, September.
Prochaska, J.O., C.C. DiClemente, and J.C. Norcross
  1992 In search of how people change: Applications to addictive behaviors. *American Psychologist* 47:1102-1114.
Quinn, J.P.
  1892 *Fools of Fortune or Gambling and Gamblers, Comprehending a History of the Vice in Ancient and Modern Times, and in Both Hemispheres: An Exposition of Its Alarming Prevalence and Destructive Effects, with an Unreserved and Exhaustive Disclosure of Such Frauds, Tricks and Devices as Are Practiced by "Professional" Gamblers, "Confidence Men" and "Bunko Steerers."* Chicago: Anti-Gambling Association.
Rachlin, S., A.L. Halpern, and S.L. Porthow
  1984 The volitional rule, personality disorders and the insanity defense. *Psychiatric Annals* 14(2):139-141, 145-147.
Reid, R.L.
  1986 The psychology of the near miss. *Journal of Gambling Behavior* 2:32-39.

Rosecrance, J.D.
1985   Compulsive gambling and the medicalization of deviance. *Social Problems* 32:275-284.
1988   Active gamblers as peer counselors. *International Journal of the Addictions* 23(7):751-766.
Rosenthal, R.J.
1986   The pathological gambler's system of self-deception. *Journal of Gambling Behavior* 2:108-120.
1989   Pathological gambling and problem gambling: Problems of definition and diagnosis. Pp 101-125 in *Compulsive Gambling: Theory, Research, and Practice*, H.J. Shaffer, S.A. Stein, et al., eds. Lexington, MA: Lexington Books.
1992   Pathological gambling. *Psychiatric Annals* 22(2)(February):72-78.
Rosenthal, R.J., and H.R. Lesieur
1992   Self-reported withdrawal symptoms and pathological gambling. *American Journal on Addictions* 1:150-154.
Rosenthal, R.J., and V.C. Lorenz
1992   The pathological gambler as criminal offender: Comments on evaluation and treatment. *Psychiatric Clinics of North America* 15(3)(September):647-660.
Rostand, J.
1939   Pensées d'un Biolgiste. (Reprinted in *The Substance of Man, A Biologist's Thoughts*, Doubleday, Garden City, NY, 1962).
Roy, A., R. Custer, V. Lorenz, and M. Linnoila
1989   Personality factors and pathological gambling. *Acta Psychiatrica Scandinavica* 80:37-39.
Rugle, L.
1998   The Biopsychosocial Model of Pathological Gambling. Draft manuscript in *Gambling: Trivial Intensity*. Trimeridian Inc., Carmel, IN.
Rugle, L., and R. Rosenthal
1993   Impulsivity and pathological gambling. Paper presented at the Symposium on Pathological Gambling, 146th Annual Meeting of the American Psychiatric Association. San Francisco, California, May.
Rule, B.G., and D.G. Fischer
1970   Impulsivity, subjective probability, cardiac response and risk-taking. *Personality* 1:251-260.
Rule, B.G., R.W. Nutler, and D.G. Fischer
1971   The effect of arousal on risk-taking. *Personality* 2:239-247.
Shaffer, H.J.
1986   Assessment of addictive disorders: The use of clinical reflection and hypotheses testing. *Psychiatric Clinics of North America* 9(3):385-398.
1996   Understanding the means and objects of addiction: Technology, the Internet, and gambling. *Journal of Gambling Studies* 12(4):461-469.
1997a The most important unresolved issue in the addictions: Conceptual chaos. *Substance Use and Misuse* 32(11):1573-1580.

1997b	The psychology of stage change. Pp. 100-106 in *Substance Abuse: A Comprehensive Textbook*, 3rd ed., J.H. Lowinson, P. Ruiz, R.B. Millman, and J.G. Langrod, eds. Baltimore, MD: Williams and Wilkins.

Shaffer, H.J., and M.N. Hall
1996	Estimating prevalence of adolescent gambling disorders: A quantitative synthesis and guide toward standard gambling nomenclature. *Journal of Gambling Studies* 12:193-214.

Shaffer, H.J., and S.B. Jones
1989	*Quitting Cocaine: The Struggle Against Impulse.* Lexington, MA: Lexington Books.

Shaffer, H.J., R. LaBrie, K.M. Scanlan, and T.N. Cummings
1994	Pathological gambling among adolescents: Massachusetts gambling screen (MAGS). *Journal of Gambling Studies* 10(4):339-362.

Shaffer, H.J., S.A. Stein, et al., eds.
1989	*Compulsive Gambling: Theory, Research, and Practice.* Lexington, MA: Lexington Books.

Shaffer, H.J., M.N. Hall, and J.V. Bilt
1997	*Estimating the Prevalence of Disordered Gambling Behavior in the United States and Caanda: A Meta-Analysis.* Cambridge, MA: Harvard Medical School Division on Addictions.

Sher, K.J.
1990	*Children of Alcoholics: A Critical Appraisal of Theory and Research.* Chicago: University of Chicago Press.

Sher, K.J., K.S. Walitzer, and P. Wood
1991	Characteristics of children of alcoholics: Putative risk factors, substance abuse and abuse, and psychopathology. *Journal of Abnormal Psychology* 100(November):427-448.

Skinner, B.F.
1953	*Science and Human Behavior.* New York: Macmillan.
1969	*Contingencies of Reinforcement: A Theoretical Analysis.* Engelwood Cliffs, NJ: Prentice-Hall, Inc.

Specker, S.M., G.A. Carlson, K.M. Edmonson, P.E. Johnson, and M. Marcotte
1996	Psychopathology in pathological gamblers seeking treatment. *Journal of Gambling Studies* 12:67-81.

Steinberg, M.A., T.A. Kosten, and B.J. Rounsaville
1992	Cocaine abuse and pathological gambling. *American Journal on Addictions* 1(2):121-132.

Steiner, J.
1970	An experimental study of risk-taking. *Proceedings of the Royal Society of Medicine* 63(12):1271.

Stinchfield, R.D.
1998	Reliability, Validity, and Classification Accuracy of the South Oaks Gambling Screen (SOGS). University of Minnesota Medical School.

Stinchfield, R.D., and K.C. Winters
1996	*Treatment Effectiveness of Six State-Supported Compulsive Gambling*

Treatment Programs in Minnesota, April 1996. Minneapolis, MN: Department of Psychiatry, University of Minnesota.

Stoltz, T.
1989 Cognitive factors in pathological gambling. *Dissertation Abstracts* 51:1537.

Szasz, T.S.
1970 *The Manufacture of Madness: A Comparative Study of the Inquisition and the Mental Health Movement.* New York: Dell Publishing Company.
1987 *Insanity: The Idea and Its Consequence.* New York: John Wiley and Sons, Inc.
1991 Diagnoses are not diseases. *Lancet* 338:1574-1576.

Templer, D.I., G. Kaiser, and K. Siscoe
1993 Correlates of pathological gambling in prison inmates. *Comprehensive Psychiatry* 34:347-351.

Thompson, W.N., R. Gazel, and D. Rickman
1996 The social costs of gambling in Wisconsin. *Wisconsin Policy Research Institute Report*, Vol. 9, No. 6.

Vaillant, G.E.
1983 Natural history of male alcoholism: Is alcoholism the cart or the horse to sociopathy? *British Journal of the Addictions* 78(3):317-326.

Volberg, R.A.
1993 *Gambling and Problem Gambling Among Adolescents in Washington State.* Albany, NY: Gemini Research.
1994 The prevalence and demographics of pathological gamblers: Implications for public health. *American Journal of Public Health* 84:237-241.
1997 Gambling and Problem Gambling in Mississippi: A Report to the Mississippi Council on Compulsive Gambling. Social Research Report Series 97-1, Social Science Research Center, Mississippi State University.
1998 Methodological Issues on Research on Problem Gambling. Paper prepared for the Committee on the Social and Economic Impact of Pathological Gambling. Gemini Research, Northampton, MA.

Volberg, R.A., and J. Boles
1995 *Gambling and Problem Gambling in Georgia.* Report to the Georgia Department of Human Resources. Roaring Spring, PA: Gemini Research.

Von Hattingberg, H.
1914 Analerotik, angstlust und eigensinn. *Internationale Zeitsschrift fur Psychoanalyse* 2:244-258.

Wakefield, J.C.
1992 The concept of mental disorder: On the boundary between biological facts and social values. *American Psychologist* (47):373-388.

Walker, M.B.
1992 Irrational thinking among slot machine players. *Journal of Gambling Studies* 8:245-261.

Walker, M.B., and M.G. Dickerson
  1996   The prevalence of problem and pathological gambling: A critical analysis. *Journal of Gambling Studies* 12(2):233-249.
Weider, H., and E. Kaplan
  1969   Drug use in adolescents. *Psychoanalytic Study of the Child* 24:399-431.
Wildman, R.W. II
  1998   *Gambling: An Attempt at an Integration.*   Edmonton, Alberta, Canada: Wynne Resources.
Winters, K.C., S. Specker, and R.D. Stinchfield
  1997   *Diagnostic Interview for Gambling Severity (DIGS).*   Minneapolis: University of Minnesota Medical School.
Winters, K.C., R.D. Stinchfield, and J. Fulkerson
  1993   Toward the development of an adolescent gambling severity scale. *Journal of Gambling Studies* 9(1):63-84.
Wray, I., and M. Dickerson
  1981   Cessation of high frequency gambling and "withdrawal" symptoms. *British Journal of Addiction* 76:401-405.
Zinberg, N.E.
  1975   Addiction and ego function. *Psychoanalytic Study of the Child* 30:567-588.
  1984   *Drug, Set, and Setting: The Basis for Controlled Intoxicant Use.* New Haven: Yale University Press.
Zuckerman, M.
  1979   *Sensation Seeking: Beyond the Optimal Level of Arousal.* Hillsdale, NJ: L. Erlbaum Associates.
  1983   A biological theory of sensation seeking. In *Biological Basis of Sensation Seeking, Impulsivity, and Anxiety,* M. Zuckerman, ed. Hillsdale, NJ: Lawrence Erlbaum Associates.
Zuckerman, M., R.N. Bone, R. Neary, D. Mangelsdorff, and B. Brustman
  1972   What is the sensation seeker? Personality trait and experience correlates of the Sensation-Seeking Scales. *Journal of Consulting and Clinical Psychology* 39(2):308-321.

3

Pathological and Problem Gamblers in the United States

The perception of increased pathological and problem gambling is currently driving interest and concern among policymakers, treatment professionals, industry officials, gambling researchers, and the public. Data describing the extent of pathological and problem gambling are useful for many purposes, including planning public health services and medical services. This chapter discusses the prevalence of pathological and problem gamblers among the general U.S. population and specific subpopulations. As limited by the available data, the discussion is often framed in terms of the proportion of pathological and problem gamblers reported in studies of U.S. residents. Of particular concern is determining prevalence among reportedly vulnerable demographic groups, such as men, adolescents, the poor, the elderly, and minorities (including American Indians). We also attempt to examine trends in relation to the increased availability of legal gambling opportunities in the last decade. This chapter also makes comparisons with the prevalence rates of alcohol and drug abusers, to help put the magnitude of excessive gambling and related problems into perspective.

The committee thanks Matthew N. Hall and Joni Vander Bilt for their assistance in providing literature and data for this chapter.

LIMITATIONS OF PREVALENCE RESEARCH

In Chapter 2 we described the difficulties involved in defining and measuring pathological gambling using various assessment instruments. Here it is important to note that comparing and interpreting prevalence findings is problematic when different studies use different screening and/or diagnostic instruments or criterion levels to measure differing levels of intemperate gambling and associated problems. Unfortunately, such differences are common in the research literature on pathological and problem gambling (Volberg, 1998b), which creates problems in estimating prevalence rates in the United States.

Another important limitation of the available prevalence research pertains to the different facets of the concept of prevalence. A prevalence estimate requires specification of the population or geographical area represented and the time frame over which prevalence is defined (Walker and Dickerson, 1996). Most of the prevalence research on pathological and problem gambling is specific about the population or area represented, but the time frames within which gambling behavior is assessed vary widely. This variation is troublesome because the information of greatest policy relevance is generally the prevalence of current pathological or problem gambling, that is, estimates over a relatively recent but behaviorally representative time frame (e.g., the past year). The time frame most common in available research, however, is lifetime. Thus, many of those who are counted in prevalence research as being pathological or problem gamblers may have met screening or diagnostic criteria at some point during their lives, but did not manifest gambling problems at the time of the study.

Measuring pathological and problem gambling also requires distinguishing incidence from prevalence: incidence is the number of new cases arising in a given time period, and prevalence is the average total number of cases during a given time period, factoring in new cases and deleting cases representing cures and deaths. Incidence is especially pertinent to policy questions involving the effects of increased gambling opportunities and changes in technology, industry practices, and regulation. There is almost no research that examines the incidence of pathological or problem gambling cases over a representative, recent time period.[1] Nor are there longitudinal studies that provide trend data for population cohorts or that track the progression of individuals into or out of the states of pathological or problem gambling. Finally, literature on pathological and problem gambling rarely distinguishes, in an epidemiological sense, the difference between rates of pathological and problem gambling and proportions of pathological and problem gamblers. This distinction is made throughout the chapter to the extent allowed by the data available to the committee.

DETERMINING NATIONAL PREVALENCE

Perhaps the most serious limitation of existing prevalence research is that the volume and scope of studies are not sufficient to provide solid estimates for the national and regional prevalence of pathological and problem gamblers, or to provide estimates of changes in prevalence associated with expanded gambling opportunities and other recent secular trends. Only three studies have attempted to measure the prevalence of pathological or problem gambling in the United States for more than one or a few states. A national study was undertaken by the University of Michigan Survey Research Center in 1975 (Commission on the Review of the National Policy Toward Gambling, 1976; Kallick et al., 1979). At that time, illegal gambling was believed to be widespread, and the nation was facing the prospect of increased legalization of gambling. Accordingly, the survey concentrated on assessing American gambling practices and attitudes toward gambling. The scale that attempted to measure "compulsive gambling" was only one small component of the larger gambling survey (Commission on the Review of the National Policy Toward Gambling, 1976).

From the responses of 1,736 adults about behaviors over their lifetimes, "it was estimated that 0.77 percent of the national sample could be classified as 'probable' compulsive gamblers,

---

[1]The one notable exception is the Epidemiologic Catchment Area (ECA) Study (see Cunningham et al., 1996; Cunningham-Williams et al., 1998).

with another 2.33 percent identified as 'potential' compulsive gamblers" (Commission on the Review of the National Policy Toward Gambling, 1976). A combined total of 3.10 percent of the population was therefore estimated to be probable or potential compulsive gamblers sometime during their lives. Although the findings of the survey were considered important, the researchers advised caution in interpreting the results because it was not clear that their measures could distinguish compulsive (i.e., pathological) gambling from other possible disorders (Commission on the Review of the National Policy Toward Gambling, 1976).

A second attempt to estimate the prevalence of pathological or problem gambling in the United States and Canada was the recent meta-analysis by Shaffer and colleagues (Shaffer et al., 1997) under a grant received from the National Center for Responsible Gaming. As opposed to original research, which involves collection of new data, meta-analytic research empirically integrates the findings of previously conducted independent studies. On the basis of predetermined criteria, Shaffer et al. selected 120 studies of gambling prevalence in various states and provinces of the United States and Canada for inclusion in the meta-analysis. These studies represented adults and youth in the general population, college students, adults and youth in treatment or prison settings, and a variety of other special populations.

To standardize the different terms used in the studies analyzed, Shaffer et al. (1997) defined four levels of gambling: Level 0 referred to nongamblers; Level 1 described social or recreational gamblers who did not experience gambling problems; Level 2 represented gamblers with less serious levels of gambling problems (problem gambling); and Level 3 represented pathological gambling.

This meta-analysis concluded that combined pathological and problem gambling—what they termed disordered gambling—was a robust phenomenon, although the majority of Americans and Canadians gamble with little or no adverse consequences. The study found that lifetime prevalence rates among adults in the general population for both nations together were estimated at 1.60 percent for Level 3 gamblers and 5.45 percent for Levels 2 and 3 combined. Past-year prevalence rates were estimated at 1.14 percent for Level 3 gamblers and 3.94 percent for Levels 2 and 3 combined. Prevalence rates among youth and other special populations were found to be substantially higher (Shaffer et al., 1997).

As part of its review of the pathological gambling literature, the committee undertook an analysis of the Shaffer et al. meta-analysis data for 49 of the original 120 studies that were based on samples of the general population (not clinical or institutional) drawn from U.S. residents.[2] Of these 49, 20 were conducted during the past 10 years, all at the state level. Although these 20 surveys do not represent all states and territories within the United States, or any reasonable purposive sampling of them, they nonetheless provide the best recent information about the prevalence of pathological and problem gambling in the United States that is currently available. As described in more detail in the following sections, the median prevalence rates found in those studies were as follows:

- Lifetime prevalence rates: 1.5 percent for Level 3 gamblers and 5.4 percent for Levels 2 and 3 combined.
- Past-year prevalence rates: 0.9 percent for Level 3 gamblers and 2.9 percent for Levels 2 and 3 combined.

Most recently, a third national prevalence study was commissioned by the National Gambling Impact Study Commission. The study was conducted by the National Opinion Research Center (NORC) of the University of Chicago. Preliminary results, released while this report was in its final stages, estimated the lifetime prevalence rate of Type E (i.e., pathological) adult gamblers to be 0.9 percent. The past-year prevalence rate for Type E adult gamblers was estimated to be 0.6 percent (National Opinion Research Center, 1999). The NORC study estimates are discussed in more detail later in this chapter.

---

[2]A few state and regional surveys have been conducted since publication of the Shaffer et al. meta-analysis in December 1997, but they vary sufficiently in methods and coverage that meaningful comparison is difficult. No attempt, therefore, was made to include them in this analysis.

PATHOLOGICAL AND PROBLEM GAMBLERS
IN THE U.S. ADULT POPULATION

Table 3-1 identifies the general population studies included in the Shaffer et al. (1997) meta-analysis that furnished gambling prevalence data for U.S. adult samples from 1975 to 1997 (exclusive of persons in treatment, prisoners, and other specialized groups).[3] The majority of these surveys were conducted at the state level in the past 10 years, but a few regional studies are also included. Table 3-1 also shows that a variety of survey instruments for identifying pathological and problem gamblers was used in these studies. However, the South Oaks Gambling Screen (SOGS) and its variants have dominated practice so completely that it has been the de facto standard operationalization of pathological and problem gambling for adult populations. As discussed in Chapter 2, the SOGS instrument has been criticized as a measure of pathological or problem gambling in the general population, chiefly because it was originally developed for use in clinical settings (Lesieur and Blume, 1987) and may produce a high rate of false positives (Culleton, 1989). In particular, there is some evidence that the threshold values for pathological and problem gambling generally applied to SOGS scores yield overestimates of prevalence relative to the results of classification using the criteria from the DSM (Shaffer et al., 1997; Volberg, 1998b).

Not shown in Table 3-1, but relevant to interpretation of the limited available prevalence research, are the uneven methodological characteristics of the prevalence studies. Response rate, for instance, varied from 36 to 98 percent, with a median of 68 percent. These prevalence studies were also inconsistent in their coverage of the gambling items. Some surveys asked all questions of all respondents, and others asked certain questions only of those who responded affirmatively to a prior question. (For example, if people had never had financial problems from gambling, they might not be asked how much money they lost from gambling.) Finally, the data analysis in these studies consisted chiefly of frequency distributions and simple cross-tabulations,

---

[3]The meta-analysis reference number for each study listed in Table 3-1 is the same used by Shaffer et al. (1997).

with little examination of missing data or other potentially biasing characteristics.

One useful approach for integrating information across studies of varying methodological quality is to use meta-analytic techniques to adjust for methodological differences, in an attempt to minimize any distortion in the cross-study mean that stems from those differences. For instance, Shaffer et al. coded nine items related to the quality of study methods and combined them into a composite methodological quality score. They found, however, that there was neither a statistically significant relationship between that score and reported prevalence rates nor meaningful differences between unweighted prevalence means and those weighted by methodological quality. In light of these findings and the relatively small number of recent U.S. studies pertinent to the committee's analysis, no attempt was made to develop adjustments for method differences among studies.

With the limitations of coverage and methodological quality in mind, the prevalence findings from the studies listed in Table 3-1 are discussed in the remaining portions of this section.

Gambling Activities

Rather high proportions of the adult populations in the states surveyed have participated in at least some gambling during their lives. Among the 20 surveys identified in Table 3-1 that were conducted in the past 10 years (i.e., 1988-1997), the percentage of respondents reporting lifetime participation in some form of gambling ranged from 64 to 96 percent, with a median of 87 percent. However, there was great variation across the years in which studies were conducted, across different types of gambling activities, and between states.

More indicative of the prevalence of currently active gamblers are the survey data for participation in gambling activities in the past year. Unfortunately, this information was less often collected than lifetime data. Eleven of the studies in Table 3-1 that were conducted in the past 10 years reported gambling during the prior year. The proportion of respondents in those studies who reported any type of gambling in the past year ranged from 49 to 88 percent, with a median of 72 percent. If this is representative,

TABLE 3-1 General Adult Population Surveys of Gambling Conducted in the United States, 1975-1997

Year of Survey	State	Type of Survey	Instrument	Sample Size	Author	Meta-Analysis Ref Number[a]
1989	California	Telephone	SOGS	1,250	Volberg	94
1977	Connecticut	Face-to-face	3-item scale	568	Abrahamson	125
1986	Connecticut	Telephone	DIS	1,224	Laventhol and Horwath	56
1991	Connecticut	Telephone	SOGS	1,000	Christiansen/Cummings	10
1996	Connecticut	Telephone	SOGS	992	WEFA Group	154
1994	Georgia	Telephone	SOGS	1,550	Volberg and Boles	99
1990	Indiana	Telephone	DSM-IV mod	1,015	Laventhol and Horwath	55
1988	Iowa	Telephone	SOGS	750	Volberg and Steadman b	94, 105
1995	Iowa	Telephone	SOGS-R	1,500	Volberg a	95
1995	Louisiana	Telephone	SOGS-R	1,818	Volberg b	96, 113
1988	Maryland	Telephone	SOGS	750	Volberg and Steadman a	94, 104
1989	Massachusetts	Telephone	SOGS	750	Volberg	94
1990	Minnesota	Telephone	SOGS-M	1,251	Laundergan et al.	54
1994	Minnesota	Telephone	SOGS-M	1,028	Emerson and Laundergan	23, 24
1996	Mississippi	Telephone	SOGS	1,014	Volberg b	98
1981	Missouri	Face-to-face	DIS	2,954	Cunningham et al.	16
1992	Montana	Telephone	SOGS-R	1,020	Volberg	89

1975	Nevada	Face-to-face	ISR	296	Kallick et al.	43
1988	New Jersey	Telephone	SOGS	1,000	Volberg and Steadman a	94, 104
1996	New Mexico	Telephone	DSM-IV mod	1,279	University of New Mexico	140
1986	New York	Telephone	SOGS	1,000	Volberg and Steadman	103
1996	New York	Telephone	SOGS/DSM-IV	1,829	Volberg a	97
1992	North Dakota	Telephone	SOGS-R	1,517	Volberg and Silver	102
1985	Ohio	Telephone	CC/CS	801	Culleton	86
1991	South Dakota	Telephone	SOGS mod	1,560	Volberg et al.	107
1993	South Dakota	Telephone	SOGS-R	1,767	Volberg and Stuefen	106
1992	Texas	Telephone	SOGS	6,308	Wallisch	109
1995	Texas	Telephone	SOGS	7,015	Wallisch	110
1992	Washington	Telephone	SOGS	1,502	Volberg	92
1995	Wisconsin	Telephone	DSM-IV mod	1,000	Thompson	85
1984	Mid-Atlantic	Telephone	ISR/IGB	534	Culleton	15, 78
1975	National	Face-to-face	ISR	1,736	Kallick et al.	43
1990	Not reported	Not reported	2-item scale	900	Ubell	148

SOGS: South Oaks Gambling Screen
SOGS-M: SOGS multifactor method
SOGS-R: SOGS modified for adolescents
DSM: Diagnostic and Statistical Manual criteria
DSM mod: modified DSM criteria

DIS: Diagnostic Interview Schedule
ISR: Institute of Survey Research "compulsive gambler" items
IGB: Inventory of Gambling Behavior
CC: Custer criteria
CS: Clinical signs

[a] Reference number from source document.

SOURCE: Shaffer et al. (1997) database.

then approximately three-quarters of the adult population in the United States has participated in some form of gambling in any recent year.

Table 3-2 summarizes the information available from studies conducted in the past 10 years regarding the lifetime and past-year participation in various specific forms of gambling. These findings must be interpreted with some caution, since relatively few studies contributed to each category and the coverage and content of the surveys varied considerably. For example, illegal gambling showed the highest percentages of lifetime participation reported for any gambling activity (ranging from 56 percent in Mississippi to 65 percent in New York)—a curious finding given legalized forms of gambling in those states—but was reported in only two studies, both conducted in 1996. As Table 3-2 indicates, lottery gambling and illicit gambling were generally reported as having the highest proportions of respondents who have participated sometime during their lifetime. Following these are charitable games, casino gambling, pari-mutuel betting, sports betting, video lottery, and card games, all with rather similar participation rates. Games of skill and gambling in financial markets (i.e., speculating) had the lowest lifetime participation rates.

The more limited information from these surveys on past-year participation in specific types of gambling is similar to that for lifetime participation, but with lower proportions in all categories. Lottery participation was highest, with the lowest proportions found among games of skill, pari-mutuel betting, gambling in financial markets, and charitable games.

Pathological and Problem Gamblers

Table 3-3 summarizes the prevalence rates of Level 2 (problem) and Level 3 (pathological) gamblers identified in the general population surveys conducted during the past 10 years, virtually all of which were conducted at the state level. The lifetime prevalence of pathological gamblers (Level 3) across the 18 studies reporting that information ranged from 0.1 percent to 3.1 percent, with a median value of 1.5 percent. Estimates of combined lifetime problem and pathological gambler prevalence (Levels 2 and

TABLE 3-2 Percentage of the Adult Population Reporting Lifetime and Past-Year Gambling for Different Types of Gambling (Surveys Conducted 1988-1997)

Type of Gambling	Lifetime			Past Year		
	No. of Studies	Range, %	Median, %	No. of Studies	Range, %	Median, %
Any gambling	17	64-96	87	11	49-88	72
Lottery	11	28-81	64	10	5-40	24
Video lottery terminal	9	09-54	26	6	6-44	26
Casino	8	19-66	36	7	6-44	27
Charitable	7	13-67	38	3	4-40	04
Pari-mutuel	11	15-37	30	9	4-12	08
Sports	11	20-45	29	9	9-26	17
Cards	9	20-49	26	5	10-20	18
Skill	6	13-25	18	2	11-11	11
Financial markets	9	07-20	12	5	5-7	5
Illicit	2	56-65	60	4	4-39	18

SOURCE: Summarized from the studies identified in Table 3-1 that reported pertinent data and were conducted during the last 10 years (1988-1997).

TABLE 3-3 Percentage Classified as Pathological or Problem Gamblers in Adult Population Samples (Surveys Conducted 1988-1997)

Ref Number[a]	Year	State	Lifetime (All Respondents)			Past Year (All Respondents)			Past Year (Gamblers Only)	
			Levels 2 & 3	Level 2	Level 3	Levels 2 & 3	Level 2	Level 3	Levels 2 & 3	Level 3
94	1989	California			1.2					
154	1996	Connecticut	5.4	4.2	1.2	2.8	2.2	0.6	3.2	0.7
99	1994	Georgia	4.4	2.8	1.6	2.3	1.5	0.8	3.5	1.2
55	1990	Indiana	5.6	5.5	0.1					
95	1995	Iowa	5.4	3.5	1.9	3.3	2.3	1.0	4.6	1.4

[a]	Year	State								
96	1995	Louisiana	7.0	4.5	2.5	4.8	3.4	1.4	6.6	1.9
104	1988	Maryland	3.9	2.4	1.5					
94	1989	Massachusetts			2.3					
24	1994	Minnesota								
98	1996	Mississippi	6.8	3.7	3.1	4.4	3.2	1.2	6.8	1.8
89	1992	Montana	3.6	2.3	1.3	4.9	2.8	2.1	10.0	4.3
104	1988	New Jersey	4.2	2.8	1.4	2.2	1.5	0.7		
140	1996	New Mexico				14.7	11.2	3.4		
97	1996	New York	7.3	4.7	2.6	3.6	2.2	1.4	4.5	1.8
102	1992	North Dakota	3.5	2.5	1.0	2.0	1.3	0.7	2.7	1.0
106	1993	South Dakota	2.3	1.4	0.9	1.2	0.7	0.5		
110	1995	Texas	5.4	3.6	1.8	3.0	2.2	0.8	4.4	1.2
92	1992	Washington	5.0	3.5	1.5	2.8	1.9	0.9	3.5	1.1
85	1995	Wisconsin			0.9					
148	1990	Not reported	12.9	12.0	2.0					

[a] Reference number from source document.

SOURCE: Shaffer et al. (1997) database.

3) ranged from 2.3 percent to 12.9 percent across 15 studies, with a median of 5.4 percent.

From a policy standpoint, the most relevant data are those reflecting pathological or problem gambling prevalence in the past year, that is, relatively recent activity. Percentages of past-year pathological and problem gamblers were reported in only 13 studies, all conducted between 1992 and 1996. All but one of these (New Mexico Department of Health, 1996) used the SOGS or a variant. The New Mexico data were based on a modified DSM-IV instrument and showed substantially higher rates for both problem and pathological gambling. If the New Mexico study is set aside as an outlier in the distribution, the remaining prevalence estimates cluster fairly closely. Problem gambling (Level 2) ranged from 0.7 to 3.4 percent (median = 2.2 percent); pathological gambling (Level 3) ranged from 0.5 to 2.1 percent (median = 0.9 percent); and combined pathological and problem gambling ranged from 1.2 to 4.9 percent (median = 2.9 percent).

It is possible to calculate the prevalence of pathological and problem gamblers *among those who gamble* by examining the rates for only those survey respondents who reported any gambling in the past year. The last two columns in Table 3-3 show these estimates.[4] Over the 10 samples for which such computations could be made, the proportion of pathological and problem gamblers combined ranged from 2.7 percent in North Dakota to 10 percent in Mississippi. The 10 percent prevalence rate reported in Mississippi was notably higher than in other states. If it is set aside as a possible statistical outlier, a more conservative prevalence estimate results, ranging from 2.7 percent in North Dakota to 6.8 percent in Minnesota. This indicates that, since 1990, approximately 3 to 7 percent of those who gambled in the year before being surveyed reported Level 2 (problem) or Level 3 (pathological) gambling symptoms.

---

[4]These numbers represent the proportion of (a) past-year problem and pathological or (b) pathological gamblers, respectively, among only those who have gambled in the last year. The other numbers in Table 3-3 represent the proportions of problem and/or pathological gamblers among all respondents in the sample, whether or not they have gambled within the indicated time frame.

Looking only at pathological gamblers (Level 3) among those who reported having gambled in the year prior to being surveyed, the Mississippi estimate of 4.3 percent is again notably higher than in other states. Setting aside that value, the prevalence estimates in the other states surveyed ranged from 0.7 percent in California to 1.9 percent in Louisiana. Thus, approximately 1 to 2 percent of those who gambled in the year prior to being surveyed reported symptoms consistent with pathological gambling.

While this report was in its final stages, preliminary results were released from the national survey conducted by NORC for the National Gambling Impact Study Commission. As only the third national survey of gambling problems ever carried out, this is an important contribution to research on problem gambling. The NORC survey used a newly developed screening instrument, called "NORC DSM SCREEN for Gambling Problems" (NODS), for gambling problems based on DSM-IV criteria that has little direct overlap with the items in the SOGS, the instrument on which most of the prevalence research over the last decade has been based. This screen was not administered to all respondents, but rather only to those who acknowledged losing $100 or more in a single day or who have been $100 or more behind across an entire year of gambling. Based on this screen, the NORC results sorted some gamblers into a Type D, said to correspond to the Shaffer et al. (1997) category of problem gamblers, and a Type E, said to correspond to the Shaffer et al. category of probable pathological gamblers.

These differences in procedure, instrumentation, and categorization make comparison with the largely SOGS-based surveys in Table 3-3 questionable. Nor is the NODS or the procedures by which it was administered and scored sufficiently well validated to accept its estimates of the prevalence of pathological and problem gambling as definitive. Nonetheless, for the category of pathological gambling, the NORC estimates are similar to those reported here. NORC estimated the lifetime prevalence of pathological gamblers at 0.9 percent (compared with 1.5 percent estimated from the studies in Table 3-3) and the past-year prevalence at 0.6 percent (compared with 0.9 percent from Table 3-3). Since the NORC sample yielded only about 22 respondents classified as lifetime pathological gamblers and about 14 as past-year pathological gamblers, its estimates may not depart from those derived from Table 3-3 by more than would be expected from sampling error (no confidence intervals were reported in the NORC preliminary results).

In the category of problem gambling, however, the NORC estimates are much more discrepant from those derived from the surveys in Table 3-3. The NORC lifetime prevalence estimate is 1.2 percent (compared with 3.5 (median) percent calculated from Table 3-3) and their past-year estimate is 0.4 percent (compared with 2.2 (median) percent calculated from Table 3-3). Again, the numbers of respondents represented in the NORC figures are quite small, so these differing estimates may be within the range of sampling error. If not, however, then additional inquiry will be required to determine why these discrepancies are observed.

Primary Types of Gambling

Pathological and problem gambling may be associated with certain types of gambling more than others. If so, the proportion of respondents classified as pathological and problem gamblers who participate in some games should be higher than the comparable proportion of gamblers without problems participating in the same games. Eleven of the studies summarized in Table 3-3 reported the proportions of gamblers who had participated in various types of gambling activities at some time, usually during the past year or in their lifetime.[5] Table 3-4 reports the range and median of the differentials between the percentage of gamblers without problems (Level 1) and the percentage of problem and pathological gamblers (Levels 2 and 3 combined) who participated in each type of gambling across the 11 studies.

In general, the percentage of pathological and problem gamblers participating in each gambling activity was larger than the percentage of gamblers without problems for all forms of gambling. However, pathological and problem gamblers were most disproportionately active in bingo and charitable games, lotteries

---

[5]Laundergran et al. (1990); Reilly and Guida (1990); Volberg (1992, 1993, 1995a, 1995b, 1996a, 1997); Volberg and Boles (1995); Volberg and Silver (1993); Volberg and Stuefen (1994).

TABLE 3-4   Participation Rates in Different Types of Gambling for Nonproblem and Problem and Pathological Gamblers Combined

Gambling Activity	Number of Studies	Range of % Differences Between Level 1 and Level 2/3 Combined	Median % Difference Between Level 1 and Level 2/3 Combined
Bingo, charitable games	3	12-24	21
Lottery, general	9	8-29	20
Instant/daily lottery, pulltabs	11	7-33	16
Racetrack, horse races	3	10-27	18
Sports betting	11	6-35	16
Casino, casino games	8	7-24	15
Card games	6	8-34	12
Games of skill	2	12-13	12
Video poker	2	7-18	12

SOURCE: Summarized from the studies identified in Table 3-3 that reported pertinent data and were conducted during the last 10 years (1988-1997).

(both general and the instant variety), racetrack betting, sports betting, and casino games.

Gambling Expenditures

Eight of the studies listed in Table 3-3 reported the responses of gamblers to questions about their net monthly gambling expenditures. Although expense reporting has dubious accuracy, the data nonetheless provide some indication of the order of magnitude of the gambling expenditures of pathological and problem gamblers relative to other persons who gamble but are not classified as problem gamblers. For the gamblers without problems in these studies, the mean reported monthly expenditures ranged from $24 to $131 across the studies, with a median of $43. For the pathological and problem gamblers, the range across studies was from $121 to $660, with a median of $188. Thus, by self-report, pathological and problem gamblers spend approximately 4.5 times as much per month as gamblers without problems on their gambling activities.

Comparisons with Other Addictions Among Adults

To put the pathological and problem gambling prevalence rates in perspective, it is instructive to compare them with the rates for other addictive behaviors. The prevalence of alcohol dependence provides one relevant comparison. Like gambling, many people have access to alcohol and engage in drinking, but most of them do not abuse alcohol or become dependent. Drug dependence provides a different sort of comparison. Illicit drugs, being illegal, are not as widely available as alcohol and gambling, but many are highly addictive.

The National Comorbidity Survey (Kessler et al., 1994) provides data collected in 1990-1992 from a national probability sample of noninstitutionalized persons ages 15 to 54 for DSM-III-R psychiatric disorders. Table 3-5 shows the prevalence rates for alcohol and drug dependence compared with those for pathological gambling. In addition, the prevalence rates for alcohol dependence and abuse combined and for drug dependence and abuse combined are compared with the rates for pathological and problem gambling (Levels 2 and 3) combined. As Table 3-5 shows, the estimated prevalence rates for gambling problems are lower in all categories than those for alcohol and drug problems.

Increased Gambling Availability and Trends in Prevalence Rates

Over the past 20 years, there has been a steady expansion in the availability of legal gambling. Currently, legal forms of gambling are available in all the U.S. states except Hawaii, Tennessee, and Utah; 37 states have lotteries; the great majority permit gambling on charitable games, including bingo and pari-mutuel betting; and in 1998 casinos or casino-style gambling was permitted in 21 states (National Opinion Research Center, 1999). Such rapid expansion in the availability of gambling provides an opportunity to examine the extent to which increased availability is associated with increased prevalence rates for pathological and problem gambling. When comparing the 1975 survey lifetime prevalence estimate of 0.77 percent for probable compulsive gambling (Commission on the Review of the National Policy on Gambling, 1976) with the preliminary lifetime prevalence estimate of

TABLE 3-5 Comparison of U.S Adult Pathological and Problem Gambling with Alcohol and Drug Dependence and Abuse

	Pathological Gambling	Alcohol Dependence	Drug Dependence
12-Month	0.9%	7.2%	2.8%
Lifetime	1.5%	14.1%	7.5%
Source	Committee analysis of Shaffer et al. 1997 data	National Comorbidity Survey (NCS): Kessler et al., 1994	National Comorbidity Survey (NCS): Kessler et al., 1994
	Pathological and Problem Gambling	Alcohol Dependence and Abuse	Drug Dependence and Abuse
12-Month	2.9%	9.7%	3.6%
Lifetime	5.4%	23.5%	11.9%
Source	Committee analysis of Shaffer et al. 1997 data	National Comorbidity Survey (NCS): Kessler et al., 1994	National Comorbidity Survey (NCS): Kessler et al., 1994

0.9 percent for Type E pathological gamblers by the NORC survey (National Opinion Research Center, 1999), we see an increase of 0.13 percent. When the 1975 national estimate is compared with the committee's lifetime prevalence estimate of 1.5 percent we see an increase of .73 percent. However, each of these studies employed different operationalizations or measures of pathological gambling in their estimates. In addition, relatively few prevalence surveys have been conducted in the same state at two points in time so that trends during this period of expansion might be examined. Table 3-1 shows that the adult population in six states has been surveyed in different years using similar instruments (all SOGS variants): Connecticut (1991, 1996), Iowa (1988, 1995), Minnesota (1990, 1994), New York (1986, 1996), South Dakota (1991, 1993), and Texas (1992, 1995). Although the time periods represented and the changes in gambling opportunities in each of these states are different, this set of surveys nonetheless provides the best available evidence about trends in the prevalence of pathological gamblers over a period in which gambling opportunities were generally increasing. The prevalence rate estimates from these surveys are presented in Table 3-6.

Of these repeated surveys, the cases of Iowa, Minnesota, Texas, and Connecticut are especially interesting. In each of these states, the survey dates straddled the introduction of significant new legal gambling opportunities. In Iowa, riverboat casinos were opened and slot machines were permitted at the state's racetracks (Cox et al., 1997); in Minnesota, American Indian casino gambling was established (Emerson and Laundergan, 1996); in Texas, a state lottery was instituted, and in Connecticut, American Indian gambling was established with the opening of the immense Foxwoods Casino. In all of these states, the prevalence rates for pathological, problem, and pathological and problem gambling combined showed increases for past-year and/or lifetime gambling activities. All the increases were statistically significant in Iowa; all the increases except for pathological gambling were statistically significant in Minnesota; but only the increases for lifetime pathological gambling and past-year problem gambling were statistically significant in Texas. In Connecticut, pathological gambling decreased and problem gambling increased, but only the decrease in pathological gambling was statistically significant.

In the remaining two cases of repeated surveys (New York and South Dakota), no major new forms of gambling were introduced between surveys, but there was probably a general increase in the availability of legal gambling because of the national trends in this direction. In these states, the prevalence of pathological or problem gamblers showed statistically significant increases only in New York. The rates in South Dakota showed some decreases, although these were not statistically significant.

Because the differences in the prevalence rates found in surveys done at different times might be due to differences in response rates, sampling procedures, or a host of other such factors, these findings should not be overinterpreted. There are very few studies that permit an assessment of whether the prevalence of problem and pathological gambling is associated with changes

TABLE 3-6 Percentage of (Level 3) Pathological and/or (Level 2) Problem Gamblers in Adult Population Samples in States with Repeated Surveys

Ref Number[a]	Year	State	Lifetime (All Respondents)			Past Year (All Respondents)			Past Year (Gamblers Only)	
			Levels 2 & 3	Level 2	Level 3	Levels 2 & 3	Level 2	Level 3	Levels 2 & 3	Level 3
10	1991	Connecticut	6.3	3.6	2.7					
154	1996	Connecticut	5.4	4.2	1.2	2.8	2.2	0.6	3.2	0.7
105	1988	Iowa	1.7	1.6	0.1					
95	1995	Iowa	5.4	3.5	1.9	3.3	2.3	1.0	4.6	1.4
54	1990	Minnesota	2.5	1.6	0.9	4.0	1.4			
24	1994	Minnesota	4.4	3.2	1.2	6.8	1.8			
103	1986	New York	4.2	2.8	1.4					
97	1996	New York	7.3	4.7	2.6	3.6	2.2	1.4	4.5	1.8
107	1991	South Dakota[b]	2.8	1.8	1.0	1.4	0.8	0.6		
106	1993	South Dakota[b]	2.3	1.4	0.9	1.2	0.7	0.5		
109	1992	Texas	4.8	3.5	1.3	2.5	1.7	0.8	5.1	1.6
110	1995	Texas	5.4	3.6	1.8	3.0	2.2	0.8	4.4	1.2

[a] Reference number from source document.
[b] The South Dakota surveys asked about gambling problems within the past six months rather than past year.

SOURCE: Shaffer et al. (1997) database.

in the availability of legal gambling. The nature of the changes observed in those studies, however, was consistent with the view that increased opportunity to gamble results in more pathological and problem gambling.

In addition, a large majority of the statistically significant differences found in these studies were in the direction of increases in pathological and problem gambling. This pattern suggests that, during the recent decade, the prevalence of pathological and problem gambling has generally either stayed constant or increased. Further support comes from comparisons made by Volberg (1996a) and in the Shaffer et al. (1997) meta-analysis. Both observed that the results of state-level prevalence studies conducted in more recent years have shown higher prevalence rates than those conducted in the 1980s.

VULNERABLE POPULATIONS

Several populations are of particular interest because of the possibility that they may be especially likely to develop gambling problems or, if such problems develop, because they may be especially vulnerable to their harmful effects. Other populations are of interest because the relative prevalence of pathological and problem gamblers among them may shed light on the risk factors and causes of pathological gambling. Among the populations of particular interest for one or the other of these reasons are adolescents, the elderly, men, minorities, and the poor. There are substantial numbers of studies of adolescent prevalence, but the research on other possible vulnerable populations is more limited. The discussion below first reviews the studies of adolescent problem gambling and then examines what little has been identified that bears on the other populations of interest.

Adolescents

Table 3-7 provides descriptive information on the studies compiled by Shaffer et al. (1997) that report on pathological or problem gambling among U.S. adolescents. Table 3-8 summarizes the available data on the percentage of gambling behavior among adolescents assessed over the full history of their experience (lifetime) and for the year prior to the survey (past year). The percentage of adolescents who report having ever gambled during their lifetimes ranges from 39 to 92 percent in those surveys, with the 39 percent value being an outlier (next highest is 62 percent). The median is 85, indicating that a high percentage of adolescents have gambled at some time in their lives. The curious fact that estimates in Table 3-8 for a few lifetime proportions and medians are more uniform across studies than those reported for past-year proportions stems from different subsets of studies and, in some cases, different instruments within studies.

Not all of the studies contributing to Table 3-8 reported the percentage of adolescents participating in specific types of gambling but, among those that did, card games, lotteries, and games of skill were the most common. Although less frequently collected and reported, data on gambling in the past year give a more meaningful estimate of the prevalence of active adolescent gamblers. As Table 3-8 shows, the estimates for any gambling during the past year ranged from 52 to 89 percent over the six studies providing this information. The median value of 73 percent suggests that most adolescents not only gamble, but also have gambled fairly recently. The estimates for specific types of gambling show that the most frequent activities are card games and sports betting. (Appendix C provides information by state on the minimum legal age required to place a bet.)

Pathological and Problem Gamblers

Table 3-9 summarizes the information about the percentage of pathological and problem gamblers among adolescents defined over their lifetimes and for the past year that is available from the studies identified in Table 3-7 (conducted between 1988 and 1997) and for which reported lifetime proportions (necessarily) exceed past-year proportions. The committee urges caution when considering these data, because they stem from different subsets of studies and, in some cases, different instruments within studies. Recognizing these difficulties, nine of the studies conducted in the past 10 years estimated the prevalence of past-year adolescent pathological and problem gambling combined (Levels 2 and 3) and reported these as proportions of those sampled. As shown in

TABLE 3-7 Surveys of Adolescents and College Students Conducted in the United States, 1975-1998

Year of Survey	State	Sample	Survey	Instrument[a]	Study Author	Sample Size	Meta-Analysis Ref Number
1989	Connecticut	High school	Not reported	DSM-III-R	Steinberg	1,592	149
1996	Connecticut	High school	Paper/pencil	SOGS-RAb/MAGS	Steinberg	3,886	149
1995	Connecticut	College	Paper /pencil	SOGS-P	Devlin and Peppard	238	19
1995	Florida	High school	Paper/pencil	SOGS-RA	Lieberman and Cuadrado	1,882	64
1996	Georgia	Adolescent	Telephone	SOGS/SOGS-M	Volberg b	1,007	151
1997	Louisiana	Middle/high	Paper/pencil	SOGS-RAn	Westphal et al.	12,066	157
1995	Massachusetts	Middle/high	Paper/pencil	DSM-IV/MAGS	Vagge	466	87
1993	Massachusetts	High school	Paper/pencil	DSM-IV/MAGS	Shaffer et al.	856	75
1994	Massachusetts	High school	Paper/pencil	DSM-IV/MAGS	Shaffer and Hall	854	74
1994	Massachusetts	High school	Paper/pencil	GAPS	Allen	1,500	126
1994	Michigan	College	Paper/pencil	SOGS	Lumley and Roby	1,147	138
1995	Minnesota	High school	Paper/pencil	SOGS mod	Zitzow	277	123
1990	Minnesota	High school	Telephone	SOGS-RAb,n	Winters et al.	532	117, 119
1992	Minnesota	High sch/coll	Telephone	SOGS-RAb,n	Winters et al.	532	117, 119
1995	Minnesota	College	Paper/pencil	SOGS	Winters et al.	868	114
1990	Minnesota	Adolescent	Combination	SOGS-RAb	Winters et al.	1,094	115, 116

1988	Nevada	College	Not reported	SOGS	219	Lesieur et al.	60
1992	Nevada	College	Not reported	SOGS/DSM-III-R,IV	544	Oster and Knapp	70
1994	Nevada	College	Not reported	SOGS/DSM-III-R	350	Oster and Knapp	70
1987	New Jersey	College	Paper/pencil	SOGS	636	Frank	28, 29
1988	New Jersey	College	Not reported	SOGS	227	Lesieur et al.	60
1986	New Jersey	Combination	Paper/pencil	DSM-III mod	892	Lesieur and Klein	62
1990	New Jersey	Adolescent	Telephone	DSM-IV	858	Reilly and Guida	71
1988	New York	College	Not reported	SOGS	446	Lesieur et al.	60
1997	New York	Adolescent	Telephone	SOGS-M/MAGS/DSM	1,103	Volberg	156
1988	Oklahoma	College	Not reported	SOGS	583	Lesieur et al.	60
1988	Texas	College	Not reported	SOGS	299	Lesieur et al.	60
1992	Texas	Adolescent	Telephone	SOGS-M/SOGS mod	924	Wallisch	108
1995	Texas	Adolescent	Telephone	SOGS-M	3,079	Wallisch	110
1993	Washington	Adolescent	Telephone	SOGS-M/SOGS-RAb	1,054	Volberg	88
1986	Wisconsin	College	Paper/pencil	Self assess	604	Cook	12
1988	Combination	College	Not reported	SOGS	1,771	Lesieur et al.	60
1985	Not reported	College	Other	SOGS/DSM-III-R	384	Lesieur and Blume	57, 58

[a] SOGS: South Oaks Gambling Screen; SOGS-P: SOGS Plus; SOGS-RA: SOGS modified for adolescents, n = narrow criteria, b = broad criteria; SOGS-M: SOGS multifactor method; MAGS: Massachusetts Gambling Screen; GAPS: Modified MAGS; DSM: Diagnostic and Statistical Manual criteria; DSM mod: modified DSM criteria.

SOURCE: Shaffer et al. (1997) database.

TABLE 3-8 Percentages of Adolescents Reporting That They Have Participated in Various Types of Gambling

Form of Gambling	Lifetime			Past Year		
	Range	Median	Number of Studies	Range	Median	Number of Studies
Any gambling	39-92	85	21	52-89	73	6
Cards	21-59	53	17	32-71	42	9
Casino	3-84	27	13	1-71	10	6
Financial markets	15-23	18	7	—	—	—
Illicit	2-10	9	3	—	—	—
Lottery	15-69	42	19	10-65	28	11
Pari-mutuel	7-41	20	15	4-29	9	8
Skill	12-51	41	17	22-60	31	10
Sports betting	11-49	31	17	16-53	40	10
Video lottery terminal	24-28	26	3	—	—	—

NOTE: The estimates are independent and not necessarily from the same studies (i.e., some studies reported only lifetime proportions, and some studies reported both lifetime and past-year proportions of various forms of gambling participation).

SOURCE: Summarized from studies identified in Table 3-7 that reported pertinent data.

column eight of Table 3-9, estimates ranged from 11.3 to 27.7 percent, with a median of 20 percent. For pathological gamblers only, these studies presented past-year estimates ranging from 0.3 to 9.5 percent, with a median of 6.1 percent. Sixteen studies provided estimates of the proportion of lifetime adolescent pathological and problem gamblers. The range of estimates across these studies was from 7.7 to 34.9 percent, with a median of 15.5 percent. For pathological gamblers only, the estimates ranged from 1.2 percent to 11.2 percent, with a median of 5.0 percent. Acknowledging again the difficulty in interpreting these data, we observe that, in comparison to the proportions of adult pathological and problem gamblers presented earlier, by the prevailing operationalizations, the proportion of pathological gamblers among adolescents in the United States could be more than three times that of adults (5.0 versus 1.5 percent).

It is important to emphasize, however, that the proportions reported in the adolescent studies and those found in the adult studies using the prevailing measures and criteria are not always directly comparable. In particular, many of the studies of adolescents use adaptations of the pathological and problem gambling instruments especially tailored for adolescents. Moreover, even the same survey items may have different meaning for adolescents, for example, regarding debt incurred. These circumstances introduce the possibility that adolescent and adult scales measure different underlying constructs. In addition, there may be different thresholds for youthful and adult gambling problems— the same gambling behavior that might not be problematic for an adult could be considered excessive for an adolescent. In many studies, therefore, the criteria for classifying adolescents as pathological or problem gamblers are not the same as those used for adult samples. Thus, although studies of adolescents provide credible indications that the proportion of pathological and problem gamblers is higher among adolescents than among adults, the matter of how much higher depends on the definitions and interpretations applied to the respective groups.[6]

---

[6]This problem of applying similar definitions to both adolescents and adults has been similarly raised in the substance abuse literature. For example, there are several lines of validity evidence for alcohol dependence criteria for adults, but the evidence is less defensible when applied to adolescent drinkers (Martin and Winters, in press).

TABLE 3-9 Percentage Classified as Pathological and/or Problem Gamblers in Adolescent Samples (Surveys Conducted in 1988-1997)

Ref #	Year	State	Sample	Lifetime			Past Year		
				Levels 2 & 3	Level 2	Level 3	Levels 2 & 3	Level 2	Level 3
149	1989	Connecticut	High school	9.9	8.2	1.7	—	—	—
149	1996	Connecticut	High school	—	—	—	18.1	9.4	8.7
19	1995	Connecticut	College	—	2.5	—	—	—	—
64	1995	Florida	High school	—	—	—	27.7	23.0	4.7
151	1996	Georgia	Adolescent	10.1	6.7	3.4	—	—	—
157	1997	Louisiana	Middle/high	—	—	—	16.0	10.0	6.0
87	1995	Massachusetts	Middle/high	—	—	—	19.1	14.8	4.3
75	1993	Massachusetts	High school	—	—	—	—	—	4.4
74	1994	Massachusetts	High school	—	—	—	20.0	13.0	7.0
126	1994	Massachusetts	High school	—	—	—	11.3	10.9	0.3
138	1994	Michigan	College	30.8	27.7	3.1	—	—	—

123	1995	Minnesota	High school	19.5	12.3	7.2	—	—	—
119	1990	Minnesota	High school	—	—	—	24.8	16.6	8.2
119	1992	Minnesota	High sch/coll	—	—	—	24.2	14.7	9.5
114	1995	Minnesota	College	7.7	4.8	2.9	—	—	—
115	1990	Minnesota	Adolescent	—	—	—	26.1	19.9	6.2
60	1988	Nevada	College	16.0	12.4	3.6	—	—	—
70	1992	Nevada	College	34.9	23.7	11.2	—	—	—
70	1994	Nevada	College	25.4	17.4	8.0	—	—	—
60	1988	New Jersey	College	16.0	10.0	6.0	—	—	—
71	1990	New Jersey	Adolescent	18.9	7.7	1.2	—	—	—
60	1988	New York	College	18.0	10.4	7.6	—	—	—
60	1988	Oklahoma	College	11.0	6.0	5.0	—	—	—
60	1988	Texas	College	12.0	7.0	5.0	—	—	—
108	1992	Texas	Adolescent	16.7	11.7	5.0	—	—	—
110	1995	Texas	Adolescent	12.2	9.9	2.3	—	—	—
60	1988	Combination	College	15.0	9.5	5.5	—	—	—

SOURCE: Shaffer et al. (1997) database.

Given these problems of comparison, the most direct indication that the prevalence rates among adolescents are indeed greater than those among adults comes from research in which the same instruments and criteria are used to assess adolescents and adults in the same survey. For instance, the lower age strata in the adult studies should resemble adolescent samples, even though they rarely include people younger than 18 years old. Pathological and problem gambling rates are not generally reported for distinct age groups. What is reported is the proportion of respondents in each age group among problem gamblers and, separately, among gamblers without problems. These can be compared for a number of the studies listed in Table 3-1.

One study (Reilly and Guida, 1990) presented a comparison for the age group 15-18 that showed a disproportionate number of problem gamblers relative to older age groups. Three other studies (Volberg, 1996a, 1997; New Mexico Department of Health, 1996) broke out the 18-20 age group; in all cases, the proportions were higher for problem gamblers than for those without problems. Another group of studies reported comparisons for the age group 18-24 (Emerson and Laundergan, 1996; Kallick et al., 1979; Laundergan et al., 1990; Wallisch 1993, 1996), all but one of which showed an overrepresentation of younger persons among problem gamblers. These age breakouts from the adult studies therefore support the studies of adolescent populations in revealing more gambling problems among younger respondents.

As noted earlier, while this report was in its final stages, preliminary results were released from the national survey conducted by NORC for the National Gambling Impact Study Commission. One component of that study was a survey of 500 youths ages 16 and 17. Using the instrument and procedures developed for the study, NORC estimated the prevalence among youth of pathological and problem gamblers combined at 1.5 percent. However, this estimate was based on responses by youth who reported they had lost $100 or more in a single day or as a net yearly loss. When this financial limitation was removed, the percentage of pathological and problem gamblers under their categorization increased to about 3 percent. In both cases, these figures are quite discrepant from the estimates derived from the studies in Table 3-9, i.e., 6.1 percent for past-year pathological gambling among youth and 15.5 percent for lifetime pathological and problem gambling. As we have discussed, however, the great variation among studies in procedures, instrumentation, and definitions makes it quite difficult to either compare or integrate findings regarding the prevalence of problem gambling among adolescents. The NORC study adds further variation to this situation. There remains considerable question about how pathological and problem gambling should be defined and measured among youth, and no general consensus on these matters seems to be emerging in the research.

Comparisons with Drug and Alcohol Problems

Some perspective on the magnitude of the prevalence rates for pathological and problem gambling among adolescents is provided by comparing them with the rates for other problem behaviors in the same population. Six of the studies identified in Table 3-7 not only examined the prevalence of gambling problems but also asked respondents about other problem behaviors (Volberg, 1993, 1998a; Volberg and Boles, 1995; Allen, 1995; Steinberg, 1997; Westphal et al., 1997). These studies provide especially comparable information on other problem behaviors because of the common samples, methods, instruments, and so forth used to collect the data on both issues.

Among these six studies, three reported the percentages of adolescents who said they had used marijuana in the past month (Volberg, 1993, 1998a; Volberg and Boles, 1995). These values ranged from 3 to 9 percent. The percentages using other drugs in the past month ranged from 1 to 2.5 percent. By comparison, in those same studies the proportions found to have the most serious (Level 3) gambling problems in the past year ranged from 1 to 4 percent. Combined with those classified as at-risk or problem gamblers (Level 2), the totals ranged from 10 to 23 percent, although it is important to note that the time periods differ.

Five of these studies reported the percentages of their adolescent samples that used alcohol once a month or more or ever had an alcohol problem (Steinberg, 1997; Volberg, 1993, 1998a; Volberg and Boles, 1995; Westphal et al., 1997). These proportions ranged from 8 to 23 percent. In these same studies, the

TABLE 3-10 Comparison of U.S. Adolescent Pathological Gambling, Alcohol Use, and Drug Use Rates

Gambling	Alcohol Use	Drug Use
1-6% pathological gambling, past year	8-23% use alcohol once a month or more, or have ever had an alcohol problem	3-9% marijuana use, past month
9-23% pathological or problem gambling, past year		1-2.5% use of other drugs, past month

proportion of pathological gamblers ranged from 1 to 6 percent, and the proportion of problem and pathological gamblers combined ranged from 9 to 23 percent.

Although the number of studies on this issue is limited, it appears that the rates of past-year pathological and problem gambling combined among adolescents in the United States are comparable to the rates of monthly alcohol use among adolescents, and with rates of adolescents ever having had a problem with alcohol. In addition, the rates of past-year pathological gambling among adolescents are nearly comparable to past-month marijuana use, and they equal or exceed past-month use of other illicit drugs by that population. These results are summarized in Table 3-10.

The Elderly and Other Age Groups

Seventeen of the studies identified in Table 3-1 provided breakdowns for gamblers without problems and for problem and pathological gamblers in a form that permitted comparison across age groups.[7] As discussed above, virtually all of those break-

---

[7]Emerson et al. (1994); Kallick et al. (1979); Laundergan et al. (1990); Reilly and Guida (1990); Volberg (1992, 1993, 1995a, 1996a, 1997); Volberg and Boles (1995); Volberg and Silver (1993); Volberg and Stuefen (1994); Volberg et al. (1991); Wallisch (1993, 1996); New Mexico Department of Health (1996).

downs showed that the younger cohorts were overrepresented among pathological and problem gamblers in comparison to their proportions among gamblers without problems. In only 3 of the 17 studies did any age group over age 30 appear in greater proportions among pathological and problem gamblers than among gamblers without problems (Kallick et al., 1979; Emerson et al., 1994; Reilly and Guida, 1990). These instances occur roughly in the 40-60 age group, not in the most elderly categories, and the differences are relatively modest. In the remaining 14 studies, all groups over age 30 are proportionately larger among the gamblers without problems than among the problem or pathological gamblers. This evidence does not indicate that either middle-aged or elderly age cohorts are generally especially susceptible to gambling problems. The age relations appear to be confined almost exclusively to younger age groups. For a discussion of age and cohort effects and the difficulty of disentangling these from genuine longitudinal effects during research on age-related trends in problem and pathological gambling, see Chapter 4.

Gender

Eighteen of the studies identified in Table 3-1 provided gender breakouts for gamblers without problems in comparison to pathological or problem gamblers.[8] In all but one (New Mexico Department of Health, 1996), the proportion of men was greater among pathological and problem gamblers than among gamblers without problems. Among the gamblers without problems, the percentages of men across the available studies ranged from 40 to 64 percent, with a median of 47 percent. Among the pathological and problem gamblers, the proportions ranged from 45 to 80 percent, with a median of 62 percent. Correspondingly, the proportions of women among the gamblers without problems ranged from 38 to 60 percent, with a median of 53 percent; among patho-

---

[8]Cunningham et al. (1996); Emerson et al. (1994); Kallick et al. (1979); Emerson et al. (1994); Reilly and Guida (1990); Volberg (1992, 1993, 1995a, 1996a, 1997); Volberg and Boles (1995); Volberg and Silver (1993); Volberg and Stuefen (1994); Volberg et al. (1991); Wallisch (1993, 1996); New Mexico Department of Health (1996).

logical and problem gamblers, the percentages ranged from 20 to 55 percent, with a median of 38 percent. Overall, therefore, men are much more likely to be pathological or problem gamblers than are women. It may be, however, that within this overall trend there are some types of gambling for which women are more likely than men to show problems. Unfortunately, the available research provides too few breakouts of gender by type of gambling to examine this issue.

Minorities

Eighteen of the studies identified in Table 3-1 provided breakouts of the comparative proportions of at least one ethnic group for gamblers without problems and problem and pathological gamblers.[9] Of those, 17 studies included either white or nonwhite as one category. These studies suggest that, in general, minorities who gamble are at risk for developing gambling problems. In every case, the proportion of minorities among the pathological and problem gamblers was greater than the proportion among gamblers without problems. Those percentages ranged from 5 to 63 percent, with a median of 31 percent, of the pathological and problem gamblers being minorities. By comparison, among the gamblers without problems the proportion of minorities ranged from 2 to 36 percent, with a median of 15 percent. These studies clearly indicate that minority groups are overrepresented among pathological and problem gamblers and would appear therefore to be at higher risk. The reasons for this overrepresentation are unknown, because the studies did not generally provide the numbers of minority respondents who gambled so that the rates of pathological or problem gambling within or across groups could be calculated. Less information was available about specific minority groups. Eight studies broke

---

[9]Cunningham et al. (1996); Emerson et al. (1994); Kallick et al. (1979); Laundergan et al. (1990); Reilly and Guida (1990); Volberg (1992, 1993, 1995a, 1996a, 1997); Volberg and Boles (1995); Volberg and Silver (1993); Volberg and Stuefen (1994); Volberg et al. (1991); Wallisch (1993, 1996); New Mexico Department of Health (1996).

out the proportion of African Americans in the nonproblem, problem, and pathological gambling groups. The median values were 18 percent among pathological and problem gamblers and 11 percent among gamblers without problems. The five studies that reported the proportions of Hispanics had a median of 28 percent among pathological and problem gamblers and 22 percent among gamblers without problems. Only three studies reported on the percentage of American Indians among the gambling groups. Across those studies, American Indians were represented among pathological and problem gamblers ranging from 3 to 7 percent, compared with only 1 to 4 percent of the gamblers without problems. These studies are too few in number to allow meaningful comparisons across groups.

Income, Employment, and Education

Seventeen of the studies in Table 3-1 provided income distributions with two or more brackets for gamblers without problems compared with pathological and problem gamblers.[10] The most common breakout was to distinguish household income above and below $25,000 per year. Dividing all the income categories reported by any of the studies into these two broad categories showed some tendency for lower-income persons to be overrepresented among pathological and problem gamblers. In particular, the median percentage of the pathological and problem gamblers with income under $25,000 per year was 33 percent compared with 27 percent of the gamblers without problems.

Only seven of the studies in Table 3-1 compared problem and pathological gamblers and gamblers without problems with regard to employment status.[11] Employed persons were represented in about equal proportions among the pathological and

---

[10]Emerson et al. (1994); Laundergan et al. (1990); Reilly and Guida (1990); Volberg (1992, 1993, 1995a, 1996a, 1997); Volberg and Boles (1995); Volberg and Silver (1993); Volberg and Stuefen (1994); Volberg et al. (1991); Wallisch, (1993, 1996); New Mexico Department of Health (1996).

[11]Emerson et al. (1994); Laundergan et al. (1990); Volberg (1997); Volberg and Boles (1995); Wallisch (1993, 1996); New Mexico Department of Health (1996).

problem gamblers (median = 64 percent) as among the gamblers without problems (median = 61 percent). By contrast, there were larger differentials for persons who were disabled (three studies: median = 6 versus 2 percent), those in school including college (four studies: median = 13 versus 5 percent), and those who were retired (four studies: median = 3 versus 11 percent). Thus disabled persons and those in school were overrepresented among pathological and problem gamblers and retired persons were underrepresented.

Eighteen studies provided breakouts of educational background for the groups of gamblers without problems and problem and pathological gamblers.[12] These data show that education has a moderately strong relationship to the risk for problem and pathological gambling. Persons who had completed only high school or less were overrepresented among pathological and problem gamblers in these studies. Across 22 comparisons, a median value of 23 percent of the pathological or problem gamblers had a high school education or less compared with a median of 13 percent among gamblers without problems.

CONCLUSIONS

Although a substantial majority of the U.S. population gambles, not everyone does, and of those who do, relatively few experience adverse effects sufficient to qualify them as problem gamblers; fewer still can be considered pathological gamblers. The best current estimates of pathological and problem gambling among the general adult U.S. population and selected subpopulations can be found in the studies included in the meta-analysis conducted by the research team at Harvard Medical School, Division on Addictions (Shaffer et al., 1997). Based on its analysis of the U.S. prevalence studies that had been conducted in the past 10 years, the committee estimates that approximately 0.9 percent

---

[12]Cunningham et al. (1996); Emerson et al. (1994); Laundergan et al. (1990); Reilly and Guida (1990); Volberg (1992, 1993, 1995a, 1996a, 1997); Volberg and Boles (1995); Volberg and Silver (1993); Volberg and Stuefen (1994); Volberg et al. (1991); Wallisch (1993, 1996); New Mexico Department of Health (1996).

of the adults in the United States meet the SOGS criteria as pathological gamblers on the basis of their gambling activities in the past year. For pathological and problem gambling combined, the committee estimates that the prevalence rate for past-year activity was approximately 2.9 percent.

Applying these rates to the U.S. census estimates of the number of residents age 18 or older in 1997 (196 million) indicates that currently about 1.8 million adults are pathological gamblers and 5.7 million are either pathological or problem gamblers. In relation to drug and alcohol dependence, the current prevalence of pathological gamblers is equivalent to about one-third the estimated rate of drug-dependent persons under DSM-III-R criteria and one-eighth the estimated rate of alcohol-dependent persons.

The few instances of repeated surveys in the same state show either significant increases in the prevalence of pathological and problem gamblers or no significant change, indicating that the national trend over the last decade may be upward. In addition, some of the greatest increases shown in these repeated surveys came over periods of expanded gambling opportunities in the states studied. Although sparse, such evidence is consistent with the view that expansions in the availability of gambling have resulted in increased numbers of pathological and problem gamblers.

The most recent gambling surveys also show that the prevalence rates for pathological and problem gamblers vary substantially for different population subgroups in the states studied. The rates are higher for adolescents than for any of the older age groups and higher for men than for women. Prevalence rates were also higher for minorities than for whites and were somewhat higher for lower-income and less-educated people than for their higher-income and more-educated counterparts. Across subpopulations, therefore, we would expect the prevalence rates for pathological and problem gambling to be highest for minority men, especially adolescents, with relatively low levels of income and education.

The gambling behavior of adolescents has been more frequently studied than that of other vulnerable populations. On the basis of the available studies, the committee estimates that the current prevalence rate for pathological gambling among adolescents is approximately 6.1 percent and for pathological and problem gamblers combined, about 20 percent. Taken at face value, these figures indicate considerably higher levels of pathological and problem gambling among adolescents than adults. And although the evidence consistently shows higher rates among adolescents, it is difficult to determine how much higher those rates are. Differences between survey instruments, in criteria for classification as a pathological or problem gambler, and in the significance of certain symptoms (e.g., incurring debt) complicate any attempt to directly compare adolescent and adult prevalence rates.

Nonetheless, the best available evidence indicates that pathological and problem gambling among adolescents is a significant problem. The proportions of adolescents classified as pathological and problem gamblers in recent studies examining this issue are roughly comparable to the proportions who use alcohol once a month or more or who use illicit drugs.

Although we have characterized the findings of the research currently available, it is important to emphasize how inadequate that research base is for drawing confident conclusions about the prevalence of pathological and problem gambling in the U.S. population or in important subpopulations. Only three national prevalence surveys have been conducted since 1977, and each estimated in a way quite different from ways used to operationalize and measure the prevalence of pathological (and problem) gambling in the past 10 years. All consideration of more recent periods must therefore rely on a modest number of state-level surveys. Moreover, the states covered in those surveys do not constitute a representative sample of U.S. states or even a reasonable purposive sample. Further limitations apply to the assessment of trends in pathological and problem gambling during the recent decades of great expansion in the availability of legal gambling opportunities. Prevalence surveys have been conducted at more than one time in only a handful of states, and in some of those cases the same instrument and sampling procedures were not used on both occasions.

Further complications are associated with the relatively unstandardized constructs, operational definitions, screening instruments, and criteria that have been used in research on pathological and problem gambling. This variation makes most attempts to compare prevalence rates across states, regions, periods of time, and subpopulations problematic. For purposes of constructing national prevalence estimates for pathological and problem gambling and breaking out important subpopulations, the existing research provides only limited and uncertain information. As a basis for informed policy discussion, therefore, the available prevalence data are incomplete. The findings presented in this chapter are best viewed as rough estimates of the likely orders of magnitude for the prevalence of pathological and problem gamblers, not as definitive estimates.

Nevertheless, these finding indicate that pathological and problem gambling is an important enough social issue to warrant a sizeable investment in epidemiological and other studies. It would be useful to undertake a variety of studies that use a common set of instruments, definitions, and design criteria. Studies of high caliber would also distinguish between prevalence and incidence while accounting for conditional risk factors; they would also distinguish between the proportion of pathological and problem gamblers and rates of pathological and problem gambling in both general and subpopulations; and they would be consistent in their use of screening instruments validated for use in general populations to measure pathological and problem gambling longitudinally.

REFERENCES

Allen, T.F.
    1995   *The Incidence of Adolescent Gambling and Drug Involvement.* Providence: Rhode Island College School of Social Work.
Christiansen/Cummings Associates Inc.
    1992   *Legal Gambling in Connecticut: Assessment of Current Status and Options for the Future, Volume One.* Report to the State of Connecticut Division of Special Revenue. New York: Christiansen/Cummings Associates Inc.
Commission on the Review of the National Policy Toward Gambling
    1976   *Gambling in America: Final Report of the Commission on the Review of the National Policy Toward Gambling.* Washington, DC: Commission on the Review of the National Policy Toward Gambling.

Cook, D.R.
1987   Self-identified addictions and emotional disturbances in a sample of
       college students. *Psychology of Addictive Behaviors* 1(1):55-61.
Cox, S., H.R. Lesieur, R.J. Rosenthal, and R.A. Volberg
1997   *Problem and Pathological Gambling in America: The National Picture.*
       Columbia, MD: National Council on Problem Gambling.
Culleton, R.P.
1989   The prevalence rates of pathological gambling: A look at methods.
       Journal of Gambling Behavior 5(1):22-41.
Culleton, R.P., and M.H. Lang
1985   The prevalence rate of pathological gambling in the Delaware Valley in
       1984. Report to People Acting to Help, Philadelphia PA. Camden, NJ:
       Forum for Policy Research and Public Service, Rutgers University.
Cunningham, R.M., L.B. Cottler, and W.M. Compton
1996   *Taking Chances: Problem Gamblers and Mental Health Disorders—Results
       from the St. Louis Epidemiologic Catchment Area (ECA) Study.* St. Louis,
       MO: Washington University School of Medicine, Department of
       Psychiatry.
Cunningham-Williams, R.M., L.B. Cottler, W.M. Compton, and E.L. Spitznagel
1998   Taking chances: Problem gamblers and mental health disorders–Results
       from the St. Louis Epidemiological Catchment Area (ECA) Study.
       American Journal of Public Health 88(7):1093-1096.
Devlin, A.S., and D.M. Peppard
1996   Casino use by college students. *Psychological Reports* (78):899-906.
Emerson, M.O., and J.C. Laundergan
1996   Gambling and problem gambling among adult Minnesotans: Changes
       1990 to 1994. *Journal of Gambling Studies* 12(3):291-304.
Emerson, M.O., J.C. Laundergan, and J.M. Schaefer
1994   *Adult Survey of Minnesota Problem Gambling Behavior; a Needs Assessment:
       Changes 1990 to 1994.* Report to the Minnesota Department of Human
       Services, Mental Health Division. Duluth: University of Minnesota
       Center for Addiction Studies.
Frank, M.L.
1990   Underage gambling in Atlantic City casinos. *Psychological Reports*
       67:907-912.
1993   Underage gambling in New Jersey. Pp. 387-394 in *Gambling Behavior
       and Problem Gambling,* W.R. Eadington and J.A. Cornelius, eds. Reno,
       NV: Institute for the Study of Gambling and Commercial Gaming.
Kallick, M., D. Suits, T. Dielman, and J. Hybels
1979   *A Survey of American Gambling Attitudes and Behavior.* Research report
       series, Survey Research Center, Institute for Social Research. Ann
       Arbor: University of Michigan Press.
Kessler, R.C., K.A. McGonagle, S. Zhao, C.B. Nelson, M. Hughes, S. Eshleman, H-
U. Wittchen, and K.S. Kendler
1994   Lifetime and 12-month prevalence of DSM-III-R psychiatric disorders
       in the United States. *Archives of General Psychiatry* 51(1):8-19.

Laundergan, J.C., J.M. Schaefer, K.F. Eckhoff, and P.L. Pirie
  1990   *Adult Survey of Minnesota Gambling Behavior: A Benchmark, 1990.* St. Paul: State of Minnesota Department of Human Services, Mental Health Division.
Laventhol and Horwath, David Cwi and Associates, and Public Opinion Laboratory
  1990   *A Study of Pathological and Problem Gambling Among Citizens of Indiana Associated with Participation in the Indiana State Lottery.* Indianapolis: Laventhol and Horwath.
Laventhol and Horwath, David Cwi and Associates, and Survey Research Associates, Inc.
  1986   *The Effects of Legalized Gambling on the Citizens of the State of Connecticut.* Newington: State of Connecticut Division of Special Revenue.
Lesieur, H.R.
  1988   Altering the DSM-III criteria for pathological gambling. *Journal of Gambling Behavior* 4(1):38-47.
Lesieur, H.R., and S.B. Blume
  1987   The South Oaks gambling screen (SOGS): A new instrument for the identification of pathological gamblers. *American Journal of Psychiatry* 144(9):1184-1188.
Lesieur, H.R., J. Cross, M. Frank, M. Welch, C.M. White, G. Rubenstein, K. Mosely, and M. Mark
  1991   Gambling and pathological gambling among university students. *Addictive Behaviors* 16:517-527.
Lesieur, H.R., and R. Klein
  1987   Pathological gambling among high school students. *Addictive Behaviors* 12:129-135.
Lieberman, L., and M. Cuadrado
  1996   *Summary Data on Florida High School Student Gambling in Five Counties.* Altamonte Springs: Florida Council on Compulsive Gambling, Inc.
Martin, C., and K.C. Winters
  in   Diagnosis and assessment of alcohol use disorders among adolescents.
  press *Alcohol Health and Research World.*
National Opinion Research Center
  1999   *Overview of the National Survey and Community Database Research on Gambling Behavior: Report to the National Gambling Impact Study Commission.* Chicago, IL: National Opinion Research Center.
New Mexico Department of Health and University of New Mexico Center on Alcoholism, Substance Abuse and Addictions
  1996   *New Mexico Survey of Gambling Behavior.* Santa Fe: New Mexico Department of Health and University of New Mexico Center on Alcoholism, Substance Abuse and Addictions.
Oster, S., and T.J. Knapp
  1994   Casino Gambling by Underage Patrons: Two Studies of a University Student Population. Paper presented at the Ninth International Conference on Gambling and Risk-Taking, Las Vegas, NV, June 2.

Reilly, P., and F. Guida
  1990   *Pathological Gambling Prevalence in New Jersey 1990 Final Report.* Report to the New Jersey Department of Higher Education. Piscataway: University of Medicine and Dentistry of New Jersey.
Shaffer, H.J., and M.N. Hall
  1994   *The Emergence of Youthful Addiction: The Prevalence of Pathological Gambling Among Adolescents at Agawan High School.* Massachusetts Council on Compulsive Gambling: Technical Report Series 031594-HS100. Boston: Massachusetts Council on Compulsive Gambling.
Shaffer, H.J., M.N. Hall, and J.V. Bilt
  1997   *Estimating the Prevalence of Disordered Gambling Behavior in the United States and Canada: A Meta-Analysis.* Cambridge: Harvard Medical School Division of Addictions.
Shaffer, H.J., R. LaBrie, K.M. Scanlan, and T.N. Cummings
  1994   Pathological gambling among adolescents: Massachusetts gambling screen (MAGS). *Journal of Gambling Studies* 10(4):339-362.
Sommers, I.
  1988   Pathological gambling: Estimating prevalence and group characteristics. *International Journal of the Addictions* 23(5):477-490.
Steinberg, M.A.
  1997   *Connecticut High School Problem Gambling Surveys 1989 & 1996.* Guilford: Connecticut Council on Problem Gambling.
Thompson, W.N., R. Gazel, and D. Rickman
  1996   The social costs of gambling in Wisconsin. *Wisconsin Policy Research Institute Report* 9(6):1-44.
Transition Planning Associates
  1985   *A Survey of Pathological Gamblers in the State of Ohio.* Philadelphia, PA: Transition Planning Associates.
Vagge, L.M.
  1996   The Development of Youth Gambling. Unpublished honors thesis, Harvard-Radcliffe Colleges.
Volberg, R.A.
  1992   *Gambling Involvement and Problem Gambling in Montana.* Albany, NY: Gemini Research.
  1993   *Gambling and Problem Gambling Among Adolescents in Washington State.* Albany, NY: Gemini Research.
  1994   The prevalence and demographics of pathological gamblers: Implications for public health. *American Journal of Public Health* 84:237-241.
  1995a *Gambling and Problem Gambling in Iowa: A Replication Study.* Report to the Iowa Department of Human Services. Roaring Spring, PA: Gemini Research.
  1995b *Wagering and Problem Wagering in Louisiana.* Report to the Louisiana Economic Development and Gaming Corporation. Roaring Spring, PA: Gemini Research.
  1996a *Gambling and Problem Gambling in New York: A 10-year Replication Survey,*

1986 to 1996. Report to the New York Council on Problem Gambling. Roaring Spring, PA: Gemini Research.

1996b Prevalence studies of problem gambling in the United States. *Journal of Gambling Studies* 12(2):111-128.

1997 *Gambling and Problem Gambling in Mississippi: A Report to the Mississippi Council on Compulsive Gambling.* Social Science Research Center, Mississippi State University.

1998a *Gambling and Problem Gambling Among Adolescents in New York.* Albany: New York Council on Problem Gambling, Inc.

1998b Methodological Issues in Research on Problem Gambling. Paper commissioned by National Research Council, Committee on the Social and Economic Impact of Pathological Gambling, Washington, DC. Gemini Research, Northampton, MA.

Volberg, R.A., and J. Boles

1995 *Gambling and Problem Gambling in Georgia.* Report to the Georgia Department of Human Resources. Roaring Spring, PA: Gemini Research.

Volberg, R.A., and E. Silver

1993 *Gambling and Problem Gambling in North Dakota.* Report to the North Dakota Department of Human Services, Division of Mental Health. Albany, NY: Gemini Research.

Volberg, R.A., and H.J. Steadman

1988a Prevalence estimates of pathological gambling in New Jersey and Maryland. *American Journal of Psychiatry* 146(12):1618-1619.

1988b Refining prevalence estimates of pathological gambling. *American Journal of Psychiatry* 145(4):502-505.

1989 *Problem Gambling in Iowa.* Delmar, NY: Policy Research Associates, Inc.

Volberg, R.A., and R.M. Stuefen

1994 *Gambling and Problem Gambling in South Dakota: A Follow-up Survey.* Vermillion: Business Research Bureau, University of South Dakota.

Volberg, R.A., R.M. Stuefen, and M.K. Madden

1991 *Gaming in South Dakota: A Study of Gambling Participation and Problem Gambling and a Statistical Description and Analysis of Its Socioeconomic Impacts.* Vermillion: Business Research Bureau, University of South Dakota.

Walker, M.B., and M.G. Dickerson

1996 The prevalence of problem and pathological gambling: A critical analysis. *Journal of Gambling Studies* 12(2):233-249.

Wallisch, L.S.

1993 *Gambling in Texas: 1992 Texas Survey of Adult Gambling Behavior.* Austin: Texas Commission on Alcohol and Drug Abuse.

1996 *Gambling in Texas: 1995 Surveys of Adult and Adolescent Gambling Behavior.* Austin: Texas Commission on Alcohol and Drug Abuse.

Westphal, J.R., and J. Rush

1996 Pathological gambling in Louisiana: An epidemiological perspective. *Journal of the Louisiana State Medical Society* 148:353-358.

Westphal, J.R., J.A. Rush, and L. Stevens
  1997   Statewide baseline survey for pathological gambling and substance abuse Louisiana adolescents. Baton Rouge: Louisiana Department of Health and Hospitals, Office of Alcohol and Drug Abuse.
Winters, K.C., P.L. Bengtson, D. Dorr, and R.D. Stinchfield
  1998   Prevalence and risk factors of problem gambling among college students. *Psychology of Addictive Behaviors* 12(2):127-135.
Winters, K.C., and R.D. Stinchfield
  1993   *Gambling Behavior Among Minnesota Youth: Monitoring Change from 1990 to 1991/1992.* Minneapolis: Center for Adolescent Substance Abuse, University of Minnesota.
Winters, K.C., R.D. Stinchfield, and J. Fulkerson
  1990   *Adolescent Survey of Gambling Behavior in Minnesota: A Benchmark.* Minneapolis: Center for Adolescent Substance Abuse, University of Minnesota.
  1993a Patterns and characteristics of adolescent gambling. *Journal of Gambling Studies* 9(4):371-386.
  1993b Toward the development of an adolescent gambling severity scale. *Journal of Gambling Studies* 9(1):63-84.
Winters, K.C., R.D. Stinchfield, and L.G. Kim
  1995   Monitoring adolescent gambling in Minnesota. *Journal of Gambling Studies* 11(2):165-183.
Zitzow, D.
  1996   Comparative study of problematic gambling behaviors between American Indian and non-Indian adolescents within and near a northern plains reservation. *American Indian and Alaskan Native Mental Health Research* 7(2):14-26.

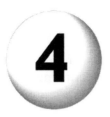

Research on the Origins of
Pathological and Problem Gambling

tiology is the study of causal pathways. Because of the
complex analyses and study designs that must be used,
this type of research represents the crown jewel of health
research. The outcomes of such research often lead to successful
treatments and preventive interventions. The process of discov-
ering causal associations and pathways to understand how different factors, exposures, or disease-causing situations relate to
each other usually involves multidisciplinary teams of psychiatrists, psychologists, statisticians, sociologists, economists, and
epidemiologists.

This chapter begins by describing considerations for undertaking or evaluating etiological research on pathological gambling, as well as the current state of knowledge regarding the
causal pathways of pathological gambling. Risk factors for and
correlates of pathological gambling, including psychosocial, environmental, genetic, and biological ones, are discussed and
evaluated in terms of commonly accepted criteria for determining the strength of an association. Cooccurring disorders and
their similar risk factors are also discussed. Throughout the chapter, substantial deficiencies in current research on pathological
gambling are noted.

ETIOLOGICAL CONSIDERATIONS IN UNDERTAKING RESEARCH ON PATHOLOGICAL GAMBLING

Etiological research is complex, and a number of aspects are essential to consider in undertaking it. They include the accuracy of diagnostic labels, the associations and causal relationships among potential risk factors, the uniqueness of risk factors, and age and cohort effects. In order to review the available evidence, the committee developed criteria to determine a causal association between a given risk factor and pathological gambling.

Diagnostic Labels

Considerable discussion has already been devoted to the definition, measurement, and prevalence of pathological gambling. When discussing the etiology of an illness, it is useful to revisit its label, because a label, as suggested by Nathan (1967), reflects the state of knowledge about the illness at the time it is labeled. In addition, etiological explanations keen on identifying causal pathways necessarily take labels into consideration, because they often describe the clinical site and clinical picture of an illness. For example, lung cancer, myocardial infarction, and lymphatic leukemia are medical labels that describe both the clinical site and the clinical picture of those illnesses. Medical labels such as tuberculosis and human immunodeficiency virus (HIV) can also specify the diagnosis, cause, or etiology of a physical illness.

Precise diagnostic labels are less common in psychiatry. However, with the American Psychiatric Association's introduction of the *Diagnostic and Statistical Manual of Mental Disorders* (DSM), research on the more common mental disorders has flourished and has led to a concomitant explosion in research on risk factors (Goodwin and Guze, 1974). Research on the diagnostic classification of pathological gambling has lagged behind, and it has been identified as an area in serious need of etiological research.

Associations and Causal Relationships

As with other areas of research, when designing, undertaking, or evaluating etiological research on pathological gambling, one must understand and distinguish between associations and causal relationships among many potential risk factors. A risk factor is something that has a possible role in the initiation of a disease, the progression of a disease to a further state, or in the waning of a disease (which is then a protective factor). Demographic, biological, personality, family, peer, and genetic factors, among other possible risk factors, may interact over time to influence the course of outcomes, symptoms, and behaviors. Risk factors are most useful for research when they refer to a specific phenomenon that provides a feasible point of intervention. Some factors may be related exclusively to initiation; others may be related only to subsequent progression into problem or pathological gambling. Although important, such etiological distinctions have been rarely made in the relatively recent and limited literature on pathological and problem gambling.

The literature on posttraumatic stress disorder (PTSD) offers an analytic model for distinguishing risk factors. Breslau and Davis (1987) demonstrated that it was the original exposure to a precipitating event, and not reexposure, that led to symptoms of PTSD among Vietnam veterans. In another study, Breslau and colleagues (1991), in an examination of young urban adults, identified risk factors for exposure to traumatic events (i.e., low education levels, being male, early conduct problems, and extraversion) that were distinct from risk factors for the actual disorder once exposed (i.e., early separation from parents, neuroticism, preexisting anxiety or depression). Distinguishing risk factors is crucial in etiology research, as is identifying common risk factors for the progression of an illness. In the study just described, a family history of a psychiatric disorder or a substance abuse problem was identified as a common risk factor for exposure to traumatic events and acquiring PTSD.

Unique Risk Factors

Equally important to consider in etiological research on pathological and problem gambling is which factors for chronic, long-term gambling are unique to this disorder and not just predictors of excessive deviant behavior of all kinds. Again, the PTSD literature provides a template for research on pathological and problem gambling. For example, Breslau and Davis (1992) identified several unique risk factors for chronic compared with nonchronic PTSD.

Age and Cohort Effects

Etiological research must also consider how the effects of age and being in a cohort (a group of people born in the same year or decade) increase or decrease one's risk for initiating gambling or developing a gambling problem. Although these effects are infrequently considered in existing pathological and problem gambling research, Erikson's stages of development (Erickson, 1963, 1968, 1982) are one explanatory model that accounts for aging effects and could potentially be applied when investigating gambling behaviors. Specifically, the model hypothesizes that, as people age, they move through several developmental stages that correspond to certain stage-related tasks. When applied to gambling behavior, the implication is that, at certain developmental stages, the motivation for and expectations about gambling might change. A recent review demonstrated that gambling among young people occurs on a developmental continuum of gambling involvement ranging from no gambling experimentation to gambling with serious consequences (Stinchfield and Winters, 1998). These effects pertain to how risk factors and outcomes change with age and differ among groups of people (Mok and Hraba, 1991).

Cohort effects pertain to specific events that affect groups of people born during the same time period (Mok and Hraba, 1991). When applied to gambling behavior, this means that increases in gambling opportunities during a certain period in history may affect a certain age group of people. For example, a cohort of same-age people who are passing through the age of risk for gambling problems when gambling opportunities are expanding may experience greater and increasing exposure to, involvement in, and social acceptance of gambling during their lifetimes than a cohort of same-age people at risk during periods of fewer gambling opportunities. In addition, circumstances can affect more than one cohort in the same way or in different ways. A classic example of an event that changed the trajectory of same-age people is the drug revolution of the late 1960s and early 1970s. During this period, expanded drug use affected both teens and young adults, marking this time period as a historical risk factor for drug abuse.

As opportunities to gamble continue to increase throughout most of the United States, it is likely that certain birth cohorts will be affected differently, perhaps in unanticipated ways. For example, in a random telephone survey of 1,011 Iowa residents stratified into eight age cohorts (ranging from 18-24 through 85 and older), it was found, even after controlling for other variables, that older cohorts are less likely to gamble than younger cohorts (Mok and Hraba, 1991).

Criteria to Determine the Strength of an Association

Mindful of the considerations discussed above, and in order to evaluate the research evidence that various risk factors are associated with pathological gambling, the committee adopted a number of general criteria, which are commonly accepted by epidemiologists throughout the world (Hill et al., 1963), for determining the strength of an association:

1. The event or exposure precedes the outcome of pathological gambling;
2. Findings are consistent—that is, they have been replicated in other studies, with other samples, or in other cultures;
3. There is a strong association between the risk factor and pathological gambling;
4. The association between the risk factor and pathological gambling is biologically plausible based on scientific research findings in such areas as behavioral genetics or neurobiology;
5. Findings remain consistent when different study methods and designs are used (e.g., case control and cohort epidemiological studies, experimental studies, biological studies); and
6. Associations examined are specific to pathological gambling and are not generally found in other disorders as well.

To suggest that a causal association might exist between risk factors, events, or situations and pathological gambling, it would be necessary for at least one of these criteria to be met. However, satisfying one or more of the criteria would not be sufficient to positively determine if there is a causal relationship between an exposure and pathological or problem gambling. In many gambling studies, the first criterion (that a risk factor necessarily precedes the outcome of pathological or problem gambling) is unknown. Without this principal evidence, an exposure, a situation, or an event is not proven to be causal.

Furthermore, many studies reviewed by the committee collected data without exploring when and to what extent subjects were exposed to potential risk factors, or the age of onset of their pathological or problem gambling. Again from an etiological standpoint, these methodological limitations make it impossible to determine whether suspected risk factors might "cause" pathological or problem gambling, or whether they are only correlated or associated with these behaviors. Thus, much of the evidence presented or implied in the literature as causal to pathological and problem gambling is, by commonly accepted etiological standards, better defined merely as evidence for an association. Still, despite the generally deficient state of etiological research on pathological and problem gambling, there does exist some tangible evidence to suggest certain risk factors and associations.[1]

PSYCHOSOCIAL AND ENVIRONMENTAL RISK FACTORS

Determining psychosocial and environmental risk factors for pathological and problem gambling is guided by the following question: Is the risk for pathological or problem gambling associated with sociodemographic factors, such as age, gender, ethnicity, and family effects, or is it associated with the availability of gambling to the gambler? In this section, we pay special attention to studies having sufficient sample sizes to generalize findings to larger groups within the population and studies that examine: (1) sociodemographic, family, and peer influences that

---

[1]Some demographic risk factors pertaining to pathological and problem gamblers in vulnerable populations were previously discussed in Chapter 3.

are associated with initiation into gambling, (2) the risk of progression from gambling without problems to problem or pathological gambling, (3) individual factors among multiple factors associated with pathological or problem gambling, and (4) factors that predict chronicity of symptoms of pathological gambling.

Age

In the United States and throughout much of the world, many people begin gambling as children. For example, in a small study of British adolescents ages 13 and 14, the mean age of initiation into gambling for social recreation or entertainment was found to be 8.3 years for boys and 8.9 years for girls (Ide-Smith and Lea, 1988). The literature has also weakly supported a young age of onset of pathological and problem gambling following initiation to gambling (Kallick et al., 1979; Lesieur and Klein, 1987). In a retrospective study, for example, it was found that adult pathological gamblers remembered their gambling addiction to have started when they were between ages 10 and 19 (Dell et al., 1981). In 1990, Griffiths found that adolescents addicted to slot machines began gambling significantly earlier (at 9.2 years of age) than nonaddicted adolescents (who began at 11.3 years of age) (Griffiths, 1990a). In 1997, Gupta and Derevensky (1998a) found that pathological gamblers started gambling, on average, at age 10.9 and nonpathological gamblers at age 11.5.

Studies of teens indicate that young age of onset of gambling is more than an artifact of reporting bias. According to a summary of independent studies of high school students conducted between 1984 and 1988 (Jacobs, 1989b; Lesieur and Klein, 1985; Jacobs et al., 1989), 36 percent of teenage respondents reported gambling before age 11; 46 percent began gambling between ages 11 and 15; and 18 percent began after age 15. Between 6 and 25 percent of the teenagers in these studies reportedly wanted to stop gambling but could not.

These findings are consistent with a study of 892 eleventh and twelfth graders at four high schools in New Jersey, in which 91 percent reported having gambled during their lifetime and 5.7 percent met criteria for pathological gambling as measured by the DSM-III (Lesieur and Klein, 1987). In a school newspaper survey of over 1,100 students at an inner-city, largely minority Atlantic City high school, 62 percent reported having gambled at area casinos, and 9 percent reported gambling at least once a week (Arcuri et al., 1985). In another study among students from six colleges and universities in New York, New Jersey, Oklahoma, Texas, and Nevada (Lesieur et al., 1991), using the South Oaks Gambling Screen (SOGS), the lifetime gambling rate was found to be 85 percent, the rate of problem gambling was 15 percent, and the rate of probable pathological gambling was 5.5 percent (Lesieur and Blume, 1987).[2] Comparable lifetime gambling rates were found in a Minnesota study of 1,094 youths ages 15-18 (including 684 from a random telephone sample and 410 from a school sample) in which the rate of problem gambling was found to be 6.3 percent and the age of onset for over half the subjects was reported to be before or during the sixth grade (Winters et al., 1993a). Finally, in a recent review of 12 U.S. and 5 Canadian adolescent gambling studies, Jacobs found that in the past 10 years the number of teenagers ages 12 to 17 reporting serious gambling problems has increased from 50 to 66 percent. The age of onset for gambling has dropped so that now, throughout America, the majority of 12-year-olds have already gambled (Jacobs, in press).

Studies of those who seek help for themselves or others indicate that gambling severity and frequency varies by age. A recent analysis of problem gambling help-line calls in Texas revealed that the frequency of calls increased with age, peaked at ages 35 to 44, and declined for callers age 45 and older (Cox, 1998). In fact, adults age 55 and older who called about their own gambling problems (14 percent of all callers) were comparable in frequency to those age 18 and younger who called about their own gambling problems (13 percent of all callers). The percentage of calls about a problem gambler from a friend, family member, or other concerned person followed a similar age pattern. Although interesting and clinically meaningful, these help-line data alone do

---

[2]The SOGS covers betting for money on a wide variety of gambling activities, including cards, sports, dogs, dice games, bingo, and slot and other machines.

not contradict the notion that younger and older people have gambling problems.

Gender

Etiological studies of pathological and problem gambling have generally focused on men from Gamblers Anonymous (GA) and men from the Veterans Administration hospital system (Mark and Lesieur, 1992). Consequently, men in the general population have been underrepresented in studies, and women are critically underrepresented as well. Many early studies that did include women were based on small numbers of women or relied on anecdotal reports of women in Gamblers Anonymous (Lesieur and Blume, 1991). Yet many studies inappropriately generalize findings about men to women (Mark and Lesieur, 1992). Although men typically begin gambling earlier than women, women appear to experience the onset of problem gambling earlier in the course of their gambling disorder than men (Mark and Lesieur, 1992), but controlled studies are rare (Custer, 1982; Livingston, 1974; Custer and Milt, 1985).

The American Psychiatric Association reports in three editions of the *Diagnostic and Statistical Manual of Mental Disorders* (DSM) that the rate of pathological gambling is twice as high among men than among women (American Psychiatric Association, 1987, 1994, 1980). Although no epidemiological evidence substantiated this finding at the time the manuals were first published, some studies have found rates that high (e.g., Cunningham-Williams et al., 1998; Volberg and Abbott, 1997; Volberg, 1994), and other studies consistently show that men gamble more and have higher rates of pathological gambling than do women, even if not at twice the rate (e.g., Lesieur et al., 1991).

Ethnicity and Socioeconomic Status

Most studies of pathological and problem gambling have focused on white male gamblers. Consequently, there exists little population-based literature or data pertaining to women or non-white ethnic and cultural groups (Mark and Lesieur, 1992; Volberg, 1994). Specifically, studies among black, Hispanic, Asian, and American Indian gamblers have been lacking. The few studies that include diverse populations have in general failed to distinguish the specific racial or ethnic background of the minority group being included, thus limiting conclusions regarding specific subgroups. A few studies have specifically compared gambling among minority and majority populations (Volberg and Abbott, 1997; Zitzow, 1996; Cunningham-Williams et al., 1998). Since the passage of the Indian Gaming Regulatory Act of 1988, gambling among and sponsored by American Indians on reservations has increased substantially (Rose, 1992). In the Zitzow study, American Indian adolescents exhibited more serious problems from gambling, earlier onset of gambling problems, and greater frequency of gambling problems than their non-Indian peers. The Volberg study found that indigenous populations reported more gambling involvement, gambling expenditures, and gambling-related problems than white populations from the same areas. However, the sampling strategies and questionnaires of these two studies were not identical (Volberg and Abbott, 1997). Thus, the Cunningham-Williams et al. study, using a sample of the St. Louis general population, remains one of the few studies of race that controlled for race and other factors. The finding that problem gambling (but not pathological gambling) is more likely to affect whites than African Americans remains unchallenged. Among African Americans in this study, problem gambling was more common than gambling without problems or social and recreational gambling (Cunningham-Williams et al., 1998).

Studies have also generally failed to disentangle race and ethnicity from issues of poverty and sociodemographic status. A series of analyses of Georgia residents identified 10 sociodemographic variables that correctly discriminated nearly 80 percent of nongamblers from (nonproblematic) social and recreational gamblers; 84 percent of the cases of nongamblers from problem gamblers; and 94 percent of gamblers without problems from pathological gamblers. When compared with nongamblers, problem gamblers tended to be nonwhite (race/ethnicity was not specified), male, and single, and to have low self-esteem (Volberg and Abbott, 1997). An earlier multistate analysis found that the only significant difference between probable pathological gamblers from different states is that those from the East Coast states and California are significantly more likely to be nonwhite than those from Iowa (Volberg, 1994).

Family and Peer Influences on Children and Adolescents

Family and peer influences on children and adolescents to gamble may also constitute a risk factor for pathological and problem gambling. Studies reveal that gamblers, especially pathological and problem gamblers who begin gambling as children or adolescents, are frequently introduced to gambling by family members or their peers (Jacobs, 1989b, 1989a; Jacobs et al., 1989). Often the first exposure to gambling for American youths is gambling in a relaxed family setting with cards, dice, and board games. Other forms of gambling exposure reported by adolescents include playing lotteries, playing games of skill such as bowling or billiards for money, sports betting, racetrack betting, and gambling in casinos (Lesieur and Klein, 1987; Kuley and Jacobs, 1988; Steinberg, 1989), which themselves may be potentially influenced by family members and friends.

An association between personal gambling and peer gambling has been observed in several studies of adolescent gamblers (Derevensky and Gupta, 1996; Gupta and Derevensky, 1998a, 1998b; Jacobs, 1989a; Wynne et al., 1996; Stinchfield and Winters, 1998). These findings are consistent with theoretical and empirical literature substantiating that peers have a strong influence on other adolescent risky behaviors, such as substance use, driving without safety belts, and early sexual behavior (Jessor and Jessor, 1977; Billy and Udry, 1985; Newcomb and Bentler, 1989). Moreover, peer gambling may influence an individual's involvement in gambling in a direct way, through social factors that include peer pressure, or through indirect processes, in which an individual is attracted to a peer group for several reasons, including gambling behavior. But there is still some question as to whether peers have a strong influence on early gambling or other risky adolescent behaviors. At this point, all we can say for sure is that family and peer influences as psychosocial variables are correlates or predictors of gambling behavior.

Family Studies

Family studies indicate that pathological gambling may be familial. Adult problem gamblers are three to eight times more likely to report having at least one parent with a history of problem gambling compared with gamblers without problems (Gambino et al., 1993). Also, a similar familial pattern has been observed with college students (Winters et al., 1998) and adolescents (Winters et al., 1993a).

Previous research provides mounting evidence that children of alcoholics and of drug abusers are at increased risk for the development of alcohol and drug problems as they progress into adulthood (Goodwin, 1976; Gross and McCaul, 1991). Similar hypotheses about the familial and intergenerational influence of problem gambling on the gambling behavior of offspring have begun to be examined. A sample of predominately white male patients at a Veterans Administration hospital in Boston was asked about their perceptions of addictive behaviors among their parents and grandparents (Gambino et al., 1993). Nearly 25 percent indicated that their parents had problems with gambling, and 10 percent indicated this about their grandparents. Gambling was the second most prevalent behavior reported after drinking. Those who perceived that their parents had gambling problems were three times more likely to score as probable pathological gamblers on the South Oaks Gambling Screen. Those who also perceived that their grandparents had gambling problems had a 12-fold increased risk.

With a randomized sample of 844 adolescents from four southern California high schools, Jacobs and colleagues found that children who described their parents as pathological gamblers were more likely to report substance use than children who did not identify parents as pathological gamblers (Jacobs et al., 1989). They were also more likely to be overeaters, to be moderate-to-heavy gamblers, and to report resultant gambling problems. However, results such as these may suffer from differential recall bias—that is, people who have had gambling problems are more likely to attribute their gambling behavior to family involvement in gambling and related problems.

Biology-Based Studies

Pathological gambling, classified by the American Psychiatric Association as a disorder of impulse control, has been found to have many similarities to such addictive disorders as alcoholism and drug dependence (Moran, 1970; Lesieur, 1984; Miller, 1980; Wray and Dickerson, 1981; Levison et al., 1983; Rosenthal and Lesieur, 1992). Similarities include an aroused euphoric state comparable to the high derived from cocaine or other drugs, the presence of craving, the development of tolerance (increasingly larger bets or greater risks are needed to satisfy the gambler, or the same bet or win has less effect than before), and the experience of withdrawal-like symptoms when not betting or gambling (Comings et al., 1996). These similarities have caused researchers in search of the origins of pathological gambling to apply relatively new and sophisticated technologies used in other health research, including twin studies, genetics, brain imaging, and other biology-based strategies. Although only a few studies of pathological gambling involve these technologies, several promising avenues of investigation are emerging.

Twin Studies

Eisen and colleagues (1997) investigated gambling involvement among 3,359 twin pairs using DSM-III-R criteria, assessed via phone interview. Their original evaluation found that inherited factors explained between 35 and 54 percent of the liability for five individual symptoms of pathological gambling behavior. In addition, familial or genetic factors explained 56 percent of the report of three or more symptoms of pathological gambling, and 62 percent of the diagnosis of pathological gambling (four or more symptoms). This study presented novel evidence that genetic factors have an influence on symptoms of pathological gambling and the development of the disorder.

Winters and Rich (in press) found in a much smaller-scale twin study that, among males, a significant and moderate heritability effect was observed for high-action gambling such as casinos, but not for other types of games. These recent study findings are consistent with that of the earlier classic study of identical twins reared apart by Tellegen (1988); it revealed substantial heritability for impulsiveness as measured by his multidimensional personality questionnaire.

Neurobiological Mechanisms

Data are accumulating at this time on the association between receptor genes and pathological gambling, for example low-platelet monoamine oxidase activity and high urinary and spinal fluid levels of norepinephrine or its metabolite among pathological gamblers. There is recent evidence that pathological gamblers are more likely than others to carry the D_2A1 allele (Comings et al., 1996; Comings, 1998), which has also been linked to a spectrum of other addictive and impulsive disorders (Blum et al., 1996). The implications of these findings and their relevance are explored further.

Theoretically, specific human genes can be linked to biochemical reward and reinforcement mechanisms in the brain, which in turn can be associated with impulsive or addictive behaviors. For example, alcoholism, substance abuse, smoking, compulsive overeating, attention-deficit disorder, Tourette's syndrome, and pathological gambling may be linked in the brain by cells and signal molecules that are "hard wired" together to provide pleasure and rewards from certain behaviors. If an imbalance occurs in the chemicals that participate in this reward system, the brain may substitute craving and compulsive behavior for satiation (Blum et al., 1996). Recently, research has identified an association between the Taq A1 variant of the human dopamine D_2 receptor gene (DRD_2) and drug addiction, some forms of severe alcoholism, and other impulsive or addictive behaviors (Comings et al., 1996).

Because the impulsive and addictive disorders that are associated with this variant are also related to pathological gambling, research was conducted to determine if a similar relationship might be present with pathological gambling. Based on this premise, genetic research on pathological gambling theorizes that variants in the DRD_2 gene, and perhaps other genes, might be associated with biochemical reward and dysfunctioning reinforcement mechanisms that effectively lead pathological gamblers to behave self-destructively.

Dopaminergic dysfunction, one type of biochemical dysfunction affecting reward and reinforcement systems in the brain, has been at the center of recent genetic studies on pathological gambling. These studies provide preliminary molecular evidence suggesting a genetic pathway to pathological gambling that is similar to that for impulse control and addictive disorders. For example, research findings suggest that the D_2 A1 allele gene type is associated with behaviors that cooccur with pathological gambling, including cocaine abuse, suggesting a possible link between dopamine receptor genes and pathological gambling. Candidate genes for association include the dopamine D_2, dopamine D_1, and dopamine D_4 receptor genes (Comings et al., 1996; Comings, 1998; Perez de Castro et al., 1997).

The Comings laboratory independently collected blood DNA samples from 171 white pathological gamblers recruited from inpatient and outpatient treatment programs, Gamblers Anonymous, and attendees from conferences on problem gambling. Researchers also collected self-reports of gambling behaviors and blood specimens from 102 people in the sample (about 60 percent). A correlation was found between the number of symptoms of pathological gambling and the presence of the D_2 A1 allele gene type. The allele gene was present in a larger proportion of the sample that also met the criteria for a substance use disorder.

The scholarly community has criticized this work on several specific grounds: Does the dopamine dysfunction predict initiation into problem gambling, or only into pathological gambling among gamblers? Because the researchers did not assess substance abuse separately from gambling or for any specific substance, it would be difficult to state with any certainty how substance abuse, in general, is related specifically to the same receptor as pathological gambling. In addition, the investigators may have misclassified respondents by using a self-administered questionnaire, modified from a structured, diagnostic face-to-face interview assessment tool, to determine psychiatric symptoms and disorders.

In other studies, the D_4 receptor gene has also been targeted as a potential marker for pathological gambling, since there is some indication that it might be associated with novelty-seeking in general, which itself is associated with pathological gambling

(Benjamin et al., 1995; Novick et al., 1995) and dependence on opiates (Kotler et al., 1997). Although controversial (Malhotra et al., 1996), this finding, like the one on the D_2 A1 allele gene type, suggests a genetic predisposition that affects the dopamine pathway, resulting in a possible association with pathological gambling. However, these genetic findings are similarly associated with a range of other disorders, such as attention-deficit hyperactivity disorder, oppositional defiant disorder, antisocial personality disorder, Tourette's syndrome, and conduct disorder.

It is important to note that serious controversy surrounds the entire knowledge base on the relationship between dopamine receptor genes and addictive behaviors, with some psychiatric researchers doubtful that such an association has been demonstrated (e.g., Gelernter et al., 1991, 1993a, 1993b; Cook et al., 1992; Freimer et al., 1996). Thus, firm conclusions about the significance of the work on the relationship between receptor genes and pathological gambling cannot be drawn at this time.

For example, the lack of specificity of association between the dopamine genes and pathological gambling is a concern that must be addressed, so that researchers can better understand the nature of this finding. In view of the general difficulties of establishing genetic relationships to rare behaviors, however, it would be premature to rule out the possibility that some complex interactions involving multiple genes and life experiences play a role in pathological gambling.

The serotonergic (5-HT) neurotransmitter system, part of the system that allows impulses to travel within the central nervous system, has been found to be associated with impulsive, compulsive, mood, and other disorders (Branchey et al., 1984; Brown et al., 1982; Comings et al., 1995, 1996). This system has also been implicated in the development and maintenance of alcohol abuse (Krystal et al., 1994) and cocaine abuse (Lee and Meltzer, 1994). These findings have led investigators to evaluate its association with pathological gambling, since these disorders often cooccur with pathological gambling. Moreno and colleagues have reported a blunted prolactin response among a small sample of gamblers, suggestive of serotonin receptor hyposensitivity (Moreno et al., 1991). DeCaria and colleagues found an enhanced prolactin response in pathological gamblers suggestive of serotonin receptor hypersensitivity (DeCaria et al., 1998). Although these findings are contradictory, they both implicate the serotonin system in pathological gambling. More research is warranted to determine the specific mechanisms through which this dysfunction occurs and how it may affect gambling behavior and other conditions that cooccur with pathological gambling.

Other studies that implicate serotonin have measured platelet monoamine oxidase (MAO) levels. Platelet MAO activity, a peripheral marker of 5-HT function, was found to be lower in gamblers compared with nongamblers (Carrasco et al., 1994). In 1996, with a slightly larger sample (27 gamblers and 27 matched controls), Blanco and colleagues found evidence to support the Carrasco finding (Blanco et al., 1996). A similar finding has been reported for sensation-seekers, risk-takers, and depressed persons (Murphy et al., 1997; von Knorring et al., 1984; Ward et al., 1987; Buchsbaum et al., 1977). However, these studies must be viewed with caution because low-platelet MAO can also be found in smokers, and smoking is highly prevalent among persons with each of these conditions.

It should also be noted that there are studies that have failed to support a central role for serotonin. In several studies, the metabolites 5-HT and 5-HIAA in the cerebral spinal fluid of pathological gamblers were unchanged (Roy et al., 1988, 1989; Bergh et al., 1997). Studies did find, however, evidence of increased noradrenergic activity. The metabolite of noradrenaline, MHPG, was increased in pathological gamblers (Roy et al., 1988, 1989). Bergh et al. (1997) confirmed that finding and reported an increase in the concentration of noradrenaline.

The clinical severity of pathological gambling has been associated with a growth hormone response to a noradrenergic agonist (clonidine) challenge (DeCaria et al., 1998). Specifically, the level of gambling behavior and cravings to gamble were associated with a growth hormone response, implicating a dose-response relationship between gambling problem severity and levels of this biological marker. This finding is of interest because the noradrenergic system has been associated with increased arousal and pathological gambling (Anderson and Brown, 1984; Dickerson et al., 1987).

Early in pathological gambling research, attention focused on plasma endorphin levels among treatment-seeking gamblers (stratified by type of game played) and nongamblers. For example, Blaszczynski and colleagues (1986), in a study of plasma endorphin levels, found that, with one exception, gamblers did not differ from nongamblers on baseline B-endorphin levels. Racetrack bettors, compared with poker machine players, had lower baseline levels. Although this finding has not yet spurred additional studies in this area, it highlights a critical need to consider the type of game played in pathological gambling research.

In summary, a great deal has been learned about the neurobiology factors contributing to drug abuse. Particular attention has been paid to the role of the mesolimbic dopamine pathway in mediating the acute reinforcing effects of most and possibly all drugs of abuse. In fact, drug effects may lead to adaptation in the brain's systems after prolonged drug exposure, and this may lead to addiction. Other brain neurotransmitters may be implicated in drug reinforcement mechanisms. The question is whether these same mechanisms are involved in pathological gambling.

Currently evidence is accumulating for the role of biological factors in the etiology of pathological gambling. In order to present convincing evidence of an association between gambling and biological factors, controlled studies are needed that evaluate gambling history (duration and onset) and environmental factors. Diverse populations also need to be studied. Studies with strong research designs will enable investigators to determine the independent contribution of molecular biological, genetic, and social factors in the development of pathological and problem gambling.

Brain-Imaging Studies [3]

In conjunction with epidemiological, biological, and molecular studies of pathological gambling, the field is now beginning to utilize sophisticated imaging techniques to uncover the brain mechanisms underlying pathological gambling. With evidence

---

[3]The committee thanks Scott Lukas for his written contributions to this section.

that gambling and drug abuse represent similar subsets of addictive behaviors (Jacobs, 1989a; Gupta and Derevensky, 1998a, 1998b), methods for detecting brain changes among substance abusers can be applied to pathological gamblers. In the mid-1980s, Hickey and colleagues (1986) measured changes in mood state in gamblers as they simulated winning at gambling. The resultant euphoria was indistinguishable from that produced by psychoactive stimulants. More recently, Koepp and colleagues demonstrated that brain dopamine levels were elevated while subjects played a video game for money (Koepp et al., 1998). Since nearly all abused drugs have an effect on the dopamine system, these findings may suggest that gambling (or at least winning while gambling) somehow influences the same basic reward circuits of the brain (Goyer and Semple, personal communication to the committee, 1998). Studies that control for lifetime drug abuse are important, however, since drugs may have a permanent effect on brain circuitry.

Because various stimuli may reinforce and maintain stimulus-seeking behavior, researchers hypothesize that a shared brain mechanism is at work in a variety of activities, including gambling. However, a problem emerges when scientists attempt to identify and measure this mechanism. Measuring brain functions in stimulus-seeking situations requires a valid method of communicating behaviors and feelings. It is important that the research methods used to collect these data minimize verbal communication so as to increase the likelihood that the behavioral responses of study subjects adequately reflect the activity of the underlying brain mechanism. To this end, drug studies have used joysticks and switch closure devices to collect relevant data (Lukas et al., 1995; Lukas and Mendelson, 1988; Koukkou and Lehmann, 1976; Lukas et al., 1986; McEachern et al., 1988; Volavka et al., 1973). Implementing such laboratory-type settings for pathological gambling research could be both challenging and restrictive. Investigations into the role of the brain in pathological gambling are further complicated by how little is known about the specific mechanisms that underlie brain dysfunction.

In evaluating any brain function measure, it is important to make the distinction between trait and state categories. Most trait theorists conceptualize traits as dimensional and as relatively stable dispositions, but not as fixed characteristics that cannot change over long time periods.   State categories refer to conditions at a given point in time. With respect to trait changes, many investigators have documented specific brain wave changes in individuals with chronic schizophrenia (Goldstein et al., 1963, 1965; Sugerman et al., 1964), depression (D'Elia and Perris, 1973; Von Knorring and Goldstein, 1984), neuroticism (Hoffman and Goldstein, 1981), hyperemotionality (Wiet, 1981), and anxiety (Koella, 1981). To some extent, these changes have been used diagnostically, but their utility in this regard (especially for an individual) is questionable. Changes in state have been studied electrophysiologically for quite some time. Recently other brain imaging techniques such as positron emission tomography (PET) and magnetic resonance imaging (MRI) have also been used to quantify brain states.

This technology allows scientists to examine features of the brain heretofore unavailable to them, but it does not solve all of the problems inherent in this type of research. For example, the mercurial nature of human behavior—its rapidly changing, unpredictable quality—and the difficulty inherent in quantifying various mood states make drawing conclusions difficult. Despite this problem, brain states, such as mental fatigue, menstrual tension, pain, sexual arousal, meditation, and drug-induced intoxication, have been quantified in this way quite successfully.

Of particular relevance to scientists studying the brain mechanisms that underlie stimulus-seeking behavior are changes occurring immediately *after* a reinforcing stimulus is administered. In drug use, for example, it is useful to think of such pleasurable, drug-induced behaviors as feeling extremely good, high, or even euphoric as existing on a continuum with other drug or nondrug-related behaviors. The fact that individuals can have cravings for various foods (chocolate, candy, sweets) and for a variety of activities (jogging, gambling, sex) suggests that a neurobiological basis for craving may be similar regardless of the item craved.

Regardless of the source of the change in state, measures of brain electrical activity are well suited for the task. For example, the electroencephalogram (EEG) is available for measurement on a continual basis (i.e., the subject is not required to do anything). Thus, the measurements obtained are free of confounding elements that are often associated with techniques that require a response. With the advent of computer and interfacing technology, methods for recording, quantifying, and displaying brain electrical activity have improved dramatically in the last decade. Lukas (1998) suggests the following research strategies to increase knowledge of the biological basis and etiology of pathological gambling:

- Using EEG, PET, or MRI technology to characterize the changes in brain function that are associated with: (a) *winning* during a simulated gambling session, (b) *losing* during a simulated gambling session, (c) different types of gambling (e.g., racetrack, casino, lottery), and (d) the presentation of gambling-related cues.
- Comparing and contrasting the above profiles with the direct effects of psychoactive stimulants, such as amphetamines and cocaine.
- Investigating the generalizability of different gambling-related cues to determine if individual differences exist and dictate the degree of craving.
- Examining the effects of changing reinforcers or simulated gambling behavior.
- Exploring the utility of offering alternative reinforcers in exchange for not engaging in gambling behavior.
- Exploring the utility of using cue desensitization techniques to interrupt the classic conditioned responses to an individual's preferred method of gambling.
- Evaluating the extent to which pretreatment with alcohol (a) increases or decreases gambling behavior or (b) modifies the euphoric effects of winning and the dysphoric effects of losing during a gambling session.

PATHOLOGICAL GAMBLING
AND OTHER DISORDERS

Comorbidity is the medical term used to describe the cooccurrence of two or more disorders in a single individual. To qualify as comorbid, each suspected disorder is required to demonstrate the characteristic pattern and etiological basis typically present when each disorder is found by itself (el-Guebaly, 1995). Comorbid illnesses may be described as lifetime comorbid or currently comorbid. Lifetime comorbidity may describe a situation in which the diagnostic criteria for two or more illnesses were met at some time, although not necessarily at the same time during one's lifetime. Simultaneous comorbidity occurs when criteria for two or more illnesses are met at the same time.

The cooccurrence of other disorders with pathological gambling may be one of the most important and influential indicators of the pathways into and out of pathological gambling. This is because common factors found for different disorders may signal shared familial, environmental, or biological vulnerabilities. Elucidating these factors may improve understanding about prevention and treatment of the comorbid conditions studied. The internal medicine profession is further along in its search for clues about comorbid conditions than are researchers in the field of pathological gambling. For example, it is widely known that hypertension and diabetes cooccur. Interest in the comorbidity of psychiatric disorders has been increasing as the public health consequences of certain disorders begin to be more heavily scrutinized. In addition, information about the cooccurrence of psychiatric disorders improves the field's understanding of the neurophysiology, genetics, and risk factors associated with these disorders. The occurrence of one disorder with another in an epidemiological study can indicate that one disorder causes another, that there is a common underlying risk factor associated with both disorders, or that comorbid disorders are not independent but simply two phenotypes of the same underlying illness. This ultimately increases understanding of the etiology of the disorders and benefits the development and implementation of treatment strategies (Regier et al., 1990).

As Berkson (1946) showed in his classic mathematical application of hospital data, when information on comorbid disorders comes from studies of treated cases, the data may lead to false associations stemming from the increased likelihood that people with multiple disorders seek treatment and have a better chance of being included in studies. Thus, studies of clinical or treated populations must be viewed cautiously, as any findings of the cooccurrence of illness may be a result of this selection inclusion or Berkson's bias (Berkson, 1946). DSM-IV warns against diagnosing certain disorders if some other specific disorders are already present. In Chapter 2 we mentioned a partial exclusion for pathological gambling in cases for which the clinician believes the symptoms were better accounted for by a manic episode.

Historically, exclusion criteria were designed to ensure that, when studying a given disorder, the group to be studied would be homogeneous to allow for specific and significant findings regarding the risk factors under study. Exclusion criteria originated from the European literature of diagnostic hierarchy, which determined that disorders were hierarchically rated, and that the presence of a disorder from the hierarchy would preclude a diagnosis lower on the hierarchy (Boyd et al., 1984). Jaspers (1946) assumed that this hierarchy corresponded to the idea that no more than one illness could be diagnosed in any one person.

Following a change in DSM diagnostic criteria that only one disorder could be diagnosed per patient, the National Institute of Mental Health funded the Epidemiologic Catchment Area (ECA) study, a landmark study of psychiatric disorders (Cunningham-Williams et al., 1998). In this study, nonclinical interviewers interviewed nearly 20,000 randomly selected people in five sites (data on pathological gambling were collected at only one site, St. Louis, MO). The study showed for the first time, in an unbiased sample, that psychiatric illnesses do occur together, confirming what clinicians—some of whom had treated pathological gamblers—had known for years. Hence, in order to understand what therapies might best reduce or ameliorate suffering from a psychiatric disorder, it is vital to understand who is at risk for a psychiatric disorder and what the cooccurring illnesses are.

Evaluating studies of conditions that cooccur with pathological gambling requires careful formulation of research questions, such as: Does gambling precede the onset of other disorders? Do gambling symptoms cluster simultaneously with the other disorder or develop progressively? Do certain disorders exacerbate pathological gambling? Is there a pattern of symptom clustering? Is the severity of one disorder related to the other? And is a standard assessment instrument used to collect data for both gambling and the comorbid condition? Very few pathological gambling studies have addressed even one of these questions. Thus, the field is ripe for etiological research, especially on the topics described in the following sections.

Substance Use Disorders

A review of the literature on comorbidity shows that substance use disorders are most commonly associated with progression to problem gambling and pathological gambling. The evaluation of the literature is especially interesting given the conditional probability related to both disorders. Specifically, substance abuse or dependence cannot develop in an individual who has never used drugs. Similarly, people cannot get into trouble with gambling if they have never gambled. Thus, investigators must clearly define the exposure conditions for people at risk for both drug abuse or dependence and problem or pathological gambling when reporting comorbidity findings. Specifically, investigators should state the rate of drug abuse only among drug users and should report a conditional rate among nongamblers, gamblers without problems, and pathological gamblers. Rarely has this been done.

A review by Crockford and el-Guebaly (1998) found that rates of lifetime substance use disorders among pathological gamblers in both community and clinical samples ranged from 25 to 63 percent. Other studies reported rates of pathological gambling ranging from 9 to 30 percent among substance abusers (Lesieur et al., 1986; McCormick, 1993). Rather than assess substance use disorders (a task that requires an assessment of the consequent problems from drug use), investigators instead have relied only on the use of substances and gambling. Crockford and others have found that heavy alcohol use is highly associated with increased gambling spending and multiple gambling problems (Crockford and el-Guebaly, 1998; Smart and Ferris, 1996; Spunt et al., 1995). Lesieur et al. (1986) demonstrated that the rate of pathological gambling increased with the number of substances used. The study was important because it attempted to find a typology of gambling by assessing gambling problems among alcohol users only, among drug users without alcohol use, and among multiple substance users.

In a study of 298 individuals seeking cocaine treatment, those who also had gambling problems were twice as likely as those without gambling problems to have more drug overdoses, greater past treatment for alcohol and for drugs, and more drug use in the past month (Steinberg et al., 1992). They were 1.5 times as likely as those without gambling problems to use opiates and solvents. Studies have found that persons admitted to chemical dependence treatment programs are three to six times more likely to be problem gamblers than people from the general population (Lesieur and Heineman, 1988; Lesieur et al., 1986; Steinberg et al., 1992; Lesieur and Rosenthal, 1998). Natural history studies of gambling and substance abuse are rare. Ramirez and colleagues found that substance use predated the onset of gambling problems in their study addressing the age of onset of these behaviors (Ramirez et al., 1983). The results might have been different if the onset of drug or alcohol problems, rather than use only, had been evaluated.

Given the reported high prevalence rates of alcoholism among American Indians, one concern since passage of the Indian Gaming Regulatory Act of 1988 is the suspected increase in the comorbidity of alcoholism and gambling for this population. In the first study exploring this relationship (Elia and Jacobs, 1993), researchers, using the South Oaks Gambling Screen among a small sample of 85 patients on an alcohol treatment ward of the Ft. Meade Veterans Administration hospital, found that American Indians compared with whites had a higher rate of probable pathological gambling (22 compared with 7.3 percent) and had more problems from gambling (41 compared with 21.3 percent).

Studies of pathological and problem gambling among general population samples are needed to minimize the bias inherently attributable to treatment samples. The St. Louis component of the ECA study showed that, after adjusting for the effects of a number of variables, gambling without problems and problem gambling were associated with substance use, abuse, and dependence (Cunningham-Williams et al., 1998). In another study, a random sample of Texans was interviewed by telephone about both their gambling and their substance use behaviors (Feigelman et al., 1998). The study found that persons with both conditions were more likely than individuals with a single disorder to be psychosocially dysfunctional. These results demonstrate a new direction in gambling research: to discover risk-related typologies for a better understanding of who seeks treatment and of how to prevent gambling problems in the first place. Telephone interviews may not be the best way to obtain information about illegal behaviors, such as drug abuse, however, because people are generally reluctant to acknowledge or provide details of crimes they have committed. As telephone technology improves, it may soon offer a confidential medium for collecting sensitive information that is vitally needed to learn more about the disorders that cooccur with pathological and problem gambling.

Mood Disorders

Early clinical case observations found an association between depression and gambling. In general, these case reports were limited by methodological flaws inherent in small case studies of help-seekers (Moran, 1970; Bishay, 1979). However, a review of these studies documents their importance for informing subsequent comorbidity research (Crockford and el-Guebaly, 1998). Pathological gamblers in some studies did report more depression than nongamblers. Depression scales that measure current depressed mood were commonly used. Given that gambling may stem from attempts to relieve or change subjective states (Jacobs, 1988), it is not surprising that negative affect, or the tendency to experience psychological distress and negative mood states, is frequently associated with gambling severity. However, weaknesses in the studies finding an association between depression scores and gambling need to be addressed. These weaknesses include small samples, minority group exclusion (they are mostly whites), gender exclusion (they are mostly male), and Berkson's bias (gamblers entering treatment for pathological gambling) (Moravec and Munley, 1983; Blaszczynski et al., 1989; Blaszczynski and McConaghy, 1989; Lyons, 1985; Ferrioli and Ciminero, 1981; Roy et al. 1988).

Published studies using diagnostic criteria for depression among gamblers are rare compared with studies that use depression scales. However, the data collected in studies using diagnostic criteria, even if not substantial, are important because they correspond to the diagnostic nomenclature used by clinicians around the world and address criteria that meet a certain threshold of severity. In fact, because there is a perceived similarity between some of the symptoms of pathological gambling and affective disorders, the DSM-III-R states that, during a manic or hypomanic episode, loss of judgment and excessive gambling may follow the onset of the mood disturbance. When manic-like mood changes occur in pathological gamblers, they are generally related to winning streaks, and they are usually followed by depressive episodes because of subsequent losses. Periods of depression tend to increase as the disorder progresses. Although somewhat reasonable, the current understanding of this progression is informed only by anecdotal information and case histories of patients who have entered treatment.

In one of the first studies to distinguish whether a depression or a gambling disorder came first (i.e., whether pathological gambling was a primary or secondary disorder), McCormick et al. (1984) found that 76 percent of gamblers in treatment met the criteria for a major affective disorder. They also found that gambling preceded depression 86 percent of the time, and even the onset of pathological gambling preceded depression. In another study of gamblers both in and out of treatment, the investigators found, using a structured diagnostic interview, that gamblers in treatment, compared with untreated controls, were about three times more likely to meet criteria for major depression (Specker et al., 1996).

Perhaps the only general population study that has examined the relationship between problem gambling and depression was the ECA study described above. Unfortunately, of the five sites that were involved in the ECA study, only in St. Louis did investigators ask questions to assess pathological gambling. The study found that problem gamblers were at least three times as likely to meet criteria for depression, schizophrenia, alcoholism, and antisocial personality disorder than nongamblers (Cunningham-Williams et al., 1998; Cunningham-Williams, 1998). Because the diagnostic instrument used ascertains the age of onset of psychiatric symptoms, the investigators were able to determine that the depression preceded the gambling problems, unlike the Specker et al. study.

Studies have shown no association between problem gambling and depression, perhaps as a result of methodological weaknesses. For example, Thorson et al. (1994) were unable to find an association between scores on a depression scale (Radloff, 1977) and reported gambling behaviors among nonaddicted adults selected from residents living in Douglas County, Nebraska. The prevalence of gambling was low in this sample, even with the broad inclusion of such activities as entering magazine contests and purchasing stocks and bonds with other, more common forms of gambling like lottery and casino betting. The authors did not evaluate the association between gambling frequency and the amount of depression, which further weakened the association.

Studies have also explored the association between bipolar disorder and pathological gambling. For example, McCormick found that 38 percent of Veterans Administration patients hospitalized for gambling were diagnosed with hypomania (McCormick, 1993). Specker and colleagues found no difference between pathological gamblers and controls for bipolar and dysthymia disorders (Specker et al., 1996). One early study of psychiatric disorders, conducted by Winokur and colleagues (1969), found a high prevalence of problem gambling among families of individuals with bipolar disorder. However, with the exception of the last study mentioned, these findings are based on extremely small sample sizes involving men in clinical settings. As such, conclusions pertaining to associations between bipolar disorders and pathological gambling are not possible at this time.

Suicide

The literature reports a strong association between rates of suicidal thoughts or attempts and pathological gambling. One of the first studies to find this association was Moran's sample of 162 members of Gamblers Anonymous from the United Kingdom, in which 20 percent of subjects reported having attempted suicide and 77 percent had thought of committing suicide (Moran, 1969). Subsequently, other investigators have corroborated this finding (McCormick et al., 1984; Ladouceur et al., 1994). Frank and colleagues (1991) surveyed 162 members of Gamblers Anonymous by mail to gather information on their suicidal history: 34 reported never having had considered suicide, 77 reported suicidal thoughts, and 21 had attempted suicide (30 did not respond). The researchers found that respondents with a history of suicidal thoughts had an earlier age of onset of gambling compared with nonsuicidal gamblers and were more likely to have engaged in illicit behaviors to support their gambling. Kennedy and colleagues (1971) found that patients who attempted suicide reported gambling more money than nonsuicidal patients.

In another study, 58 male patients in an inpatient treatment program for pathological gamblers in Germany were compared with a control group of patients with other addictions. The gamblers were found to be younger, previously convicted of theft, highly indebted, susceptible to other addictive substances, especially alcohol, and in danger of committing suicide (Schwarz and Lindner, 1992). In yet another study, with a sample from the Compulsive Gambling Society of New Zealand, many gamblers who contacted a nationwide information and counseling hot line reported that they considered suicide as a solution to their gambling problems (Sullivan, 1994). In general, the high rate of suicide among these help-seeking gamblers could be attributed to the sample selection process, since a seriously depressed mood (i.e., suicidal thoughts) increases the likelihood of seeking treatment. The association may also be spurious, in that alcohol abuse and other substance abuse, which are highly comorbid disorders in gamblers, are also strongly associated with depression and suicidal thoughts (Vilhjalmsson et al., 1988).

Only two general population surveys have linked reported suicidal thoughts with pathological gambling. One, the St. Louis ECA study (Cunningham-Williams et al., 1998; Cunningham-Williams, 1998) surprisingly found that the association between the two was not statistically significant. A second study, conducted in 1993 in Canada, was modeled after the ECA study. In that study, investigators reported the rate of attempted suicide among the 30 pathological gamblers (out of 7,214 randomly selected residents of Edmonton) to be 13.3 percent. Although no rate for this behavior among gamblers without problems was reported, there is clearly an increased risk among the group of pathological gamblers in this study, especially when these rates are compared with suicide rates—below 4 percent—in general population studies. This is in contrast to the ECA, in which no significant difference in suicide rates was found, although the study designs were very similar. Studies using treatment populations tend to agree with the findings of the Edmonton study. No rate for this behavior among gamblers without problems, however, was provided, so there is no way to determine the increased risk among the group of pathological gamblers (Bland et al., 1993). These findings highlight a lack of association that is contrary to findings using help-seeking populations. They also stress the importance of carefully controlled studies to minimize the risk of making conclusions based on unrepresentative samples, such as a conclusion that pathological gambling leads to suicide. These findings do not suggest that pathological gamblers never think about or attempt suicide. Rather, these data demonstrate that findings from survey samples representative of the general population predictably differ from findings from surveys of treatment populations.

As with other evaluations of comorbid illnesses, there is the question of whether the gambling precedes or is consequent to depression and the suicidal thoughts or attempt. Although treatment samples have been used to address this issue, they constitute a convenience sample. In one study of 50 patients of an inpatient gambling treatment program, a correlation was found between significant depression and pathological gambling (McCormick et al., 1984). However, as expected from a treatment sample, the researchers were unable to reliably answer whether the depression was the result of, or the enabling factor for, the gambling activities. The research did indicate that relapse into gambling behavior for which help had been sought was common and was often accompanied by suicidal thoughts.[4]

In summary, although these above studies were generally analyzed without multivariate techniques, there appears to be a strong association between depression and gambling. It is not possible to tell, however, whether the depressed mood preceded gambling or was a consequence of gambling. And because the general population is underrepresented in nearly all studies of

---

[4]It is also possible that the depressed mood is a combination of major depression and dysthymia—what clinicians refer to as a double depression. Someone may begin gambling to alleviate a depressed mood, but later suffer a second, more acute depression as a consequence of the problems caused by gambling.

gambling-related suicide, such a connection from an etiological perspective must be viewed with caution.

Personality and Other Psychiatric Disorders

To date, very few studies have linked personality disorders with pathological gambling. Personality type and its dimensions such as neuroticism, aggressiveness, defensiveness, and socialization have been found to be related to pathological gambling, but the studies have generally been conducted with small samples (Malkin and Syme, 1986; McCormick et al., 1987; Specker et al., 1996). Recently however, Blaszczynski and Steel (1998) found that, of 82 gambling treatment seekers, 76 (93 percent) met diagnostic criteria for at least one personality disorder. In addition "multiple overlapping personality disorders per subject [were] more the rule than the exception" (p. 60). "On average, subjects met criteria for 4.6 DSM-III personality disorders" (p. 65). Consequently, the possibility that pathological gambling is a consequence and not independent of other psychiatric problems must be considered (Crockford and el-Guebaly, 1998).

Interest in the association of antisocial personality disorder (ASPD) with pathological gambling is strong, given that both disorders may be impairing to self, family, and society and each is characterized by persistent irresponsible, socially nonconforming, and risk-taking behaviors. Because these disorders are comprised of similar behaviors, there is an assumption that ASPD is comorbid with pathological gambling, although the evidence has come mainly from studies of gamblers in treatment for gambling or for substance abuse. It has also been reported that from 12 to 30 percent of U.S. and Great Britain and Australia prisoners who are assumed to have ASPD are probable pathological gamblers (Lesieur, 1987; Rosenthal and Lorenz, 1992; Templer et al., 1993; Kennedy and Grubin, 1990). In fact, as Lesieur and Klein (1985) reported in a sample of 230 male and 118 female prisoners, 30 percent were probable pathological gamblers, and 13 percent stated that gambling was either partially or wholly to blame for their detention. However, a spurious association between pathological gambling and ASPD may exist because substance use disorders, which are highly prevalent in these populations, are also associated with ASPD. In addition, research shows that, although gambling usually begins early in life, gambling problems generally occur later. Yet ASPD begins relatively early in life with childhood conduct disorder. It is also true that much pathological gambling may also be illegal gambling and as such might be associated with one or more DSM criteria for a diagnosis of ASPD.

Little is known about the association of anxiety disorders and problem gambling. Only two studies of pathological gamblers in treatment have reported an increased prevalence of anxiety among pathological gamblers, yet the numbers are so small that the meaning is questionable: namely, 12.5 percent in 24 cases of pathological gamblers in treatment (Roy et al., 1988) and 28 percent in 25 cases of Gamblers Anonymous members (Crockford and el-Guebaly, 1998).

Evidence is mounting to suggest an increase in attention-deficit hyperactivity disorder (ADHD) among pathological gamblers compared with nonpathological gamblers. In one study, Rugle and Melamed (1993) found that the groups differed on attention measures, with gamblers showing more attention deficits. Subjects had previously been screened to rule out head trauma, drug abuse, and other medical conditions that might contribute to attention problems. The gamblers also reported more childhood behaviors of ADHD than controls. However, as the authors pointed out, a specific diagnosis of ADHD was not assessed. Further evidence for an association between childhood ADHD and later pathological gambling comes from Specker et al. (1995), who found that pathological gamblers compared with controls were more likely to meet criteria for ADHD. These studies, though conducted with small samples and weak because of their potential retrospective bias, cannot be ignored. They indicate a potential association between early attention problems and later pathological gambling and should be replicated in larger, more representative samples. The data also speak to the need for longitudinal studies of young people, to determine the progression from attention problems to later problems, including pathological gambling.

General Population Studies

To the committee's knowledge, only two studies have assessed gambling and other psychiatric disorders among general population samples, and they are important for that reason. Both studies used the same diagnostic instrument. One study, the ECA, found that, of the associations found, that between gambling and ASPD was strongest (Cunningham-Williams et al., 1998). Problem gamblers were over six times more likely to meet criteria for ASPD than nongamblers. The association with alcohol use disorders was also strong and remained even after controlling for race, gender, age, and ASPD. Furthermore, among problem gamblers with alcohol use disorders, gambling problems occurred within two years of the onset of alcoholism in 65 percent of the cases. Although not one of the stronger associations, nicotine dependence was statistically significantly associated with gambling, with an odds ratio of 2 to 1 (meaning that those with nicotine dependence were twice as likely as those without nicotine dependence to be associated with gambling). Very few studies have reported on the noticeable cooccurrence of smoking and gambling (Smart and Ferris, 1996). Findings of the study pertaining to ASPD and suicidal thoughts have already been discussed. A second study, modeled after the ECA study, was conducted in Edmonton, Canada. Bland and colleagues found that gamblers were over three times more likely than nongamblers to meet criteria for alcohol and drug use disorders, affective disorder, agoraphobia, obsessive-compulsive disorder, and antisocial personality disorder (Bland et al., 1993). However, the associations presented did not control for either demographic or other psychiatric variables.

Thus, a review of the literature finds that only one study, the ECA report (Cunningham-Williams et al., 1998), was conducted with a general population sample in the United States, used diagnostic criteria, and controlled for the effects of other variables. Although this study has recently been published, it was conducted in the early 1980s and used an older version of the DSM criteria. Also, having been conducted only in a single Midwest city, the importance of replicating such a study nationwide cannot be overemphasized.

CONCLUSIONS

More and better research on the etiology of pathological gambling is needed. As the name of the illness suggests, pathological gambling merely describes a clinical picture. Because the available literature on pathological and problem gambling lacks sophisticated studies enabling this level of discrimination, the committee was not able to say whether the risk factors identified had their impact on initiating gambling or on progression to problem gambling or pathological gambling. Moreover, because risk factors for problem and pathological gambling have usually been dichotomized—that is, respondents either have or have not been exposed to a particular risk factor, and because the sample sizes are small—they are limited in their ability to inform public policy.

Although the past studies have limitations, they have provided the field with a foundation and guidepost for further development. It is now evident that the onset of gambling usually begins in the preteen or adolescent years (Custer, 1982; Griffiths, 1990b; Livingston, 1974) with such activities as baseball card flipping, pitching pennies, and shooting marbles. By adolescence there is poker and sports betting, as well as lottery, racetrack, and casino gambling. Although adolescents can gamble and not become problem or pathological gamblers, certain risk factors, including family member and peer influences, are important for this group. Preliminary evidence suggests that the earlier people begin gambling, the more likely they are to experience problems from gambling. This finding seems developmentally plausible and is consistent with the age of onset and severity for other public health problems, such as substance abuse. It is not clear whether an earlier start at gambling alone represents a risk factor for later pathological gambling, or whether other factors that might drive a person to gamble earlier are also related to developing gambling problems. Little detail is available about natural history of pathological gambling, how long it typically lasts, what causes recovery and relapse. Longitudinal studies would be valuable in answering these questions.

On the basis of the available evidence, we can conclude that men are more likely than women to become pathological and problem gamblers. We do not know yet if gender differences affect all stages of developing pathological gambling, gambling frequency, type of gambling involvement, and the chronicity of gambling problems. More research is also needed to identify risk factors for initiation into and progression of problem gambling behavior for minorities with high rates and to disentangle the complex association between race or ethnicity and socioeconomic status. More and better research is needed on communities in which gambling access and availability are limited, on the role of incentives for increased participation in gambling, and on identifying personal and environmental barriers to gambling. Such research will show the impact of these risk factors on initiation to gambling and the development of pathological gambling.

As yet, no longitudinal data exist on developmental trajectories of gambling behavior that adequately test aging and cohort effect theories of gambling progression or provide analytical models, such as Erikson's stages of development model, applied to gambling behaviors.

Research on cooccurring disorders in the field of psychiatry is evolving. As the studies noted above indicate, comorbidity research as it relates to gambling is in an early stage. Although studies conducted on treated cases point to important research avenues, results in treated populations may not be generalizable to the population at large. Very few studies of comorbidity evaluate disorders or syndromes, and very few control for the effects of other disorders or for sociodemographic variables. Evaluating comorbidity for descriptive purposes has been a useful first step. Now research is needed that addresses the history of the disorder, and that seeks biological etiologies for these changes. Antisocial personality disorder, substance use disorders, and depression seem to be the most prevalent disorders among pathological gamblers. To advance knowledge about comorbid disorders with pathological gambling, and to identify the disorders that are associated with initiation into gambling as well as progression into pathological and problem gambling, future research will need stronger designs and more rigorous methods. Such research can enhance knowledge and further understanding of how to prevent and treat pathological and problem gambling.

The study of pathological gambling, in its brief development, has no institutional base to sponsor research. The fact that the

American Psychiatric Association has adopted pathological gambling into its official nomenclature ensures that it will gain attention. In order to move the science forward, there need to be established funding sources that support the development of measurement tools to assess the consequences of each type of gambling activity and that test them in diverse populations, such as among men and women, young and old, rural and urban, and treated and untreated gamblers. Once the psychometric properties of these tools are firmly established, the field can move expeditiously to identify socioenvironmental, genetic, and family risk factors, as well as the neurobiological and molecular mechanisms that figure in the development of pathological gambling.

The committee concludes, from its review and critique of the literature, that the following specific areas are in critical need of immediate research attention:

• Longitudinal research that explores the transition from childhood to adolescence through later adulthood, to determine the natural history of pathological gambling, including initiation, progression, remission, and relapse.
• Research that controls for important sociodemographic variables in the study of risk for initiation into gambling and progression into problem gambling.
• Family and twin studies to determine familial risk factors for pathological gambling.
• Molecular genetic studies searching for genes that affect initiation into gambling and progression to pathological gambling.
• Brain imaging research to document the changes that occur during gambling situations.
• Studies that use adequate and diverse samples (racial or ethnic minorities, women, homeless, elderly, and teen populations, rural/urban).
• Research among individuals and communities that examines the effect of access and availability on gambling behaviors.
• Studies on comorbid gambling disorders (especially with mood disorders, substance use disorders, and ASPD), including onset, remission, symptom clustering, related severities of disor-

ders, standard assessments for gambling and other disorders, and multivariate analysis controlling for all comorbid conditions.

• Research on risk-taking and other dimensions of impulse control among gamblers—using adequate controls.

• Research that identifies whether certain games may be gateways to subsequent gambling problems, just as previous research indicates there are gateway drugs that precede the use of hard drugs.

• Studies to determine whether factors are risk factors or consequences of gambling. For example, studies of monozygotic twins with different histories of pathological gambling would be extremely useful.

• Research that encompasses multiple techniques obtaining data from the same participant, such as face-to-face interviews, computer-assisted methods, ethnography, and neurobiological and genetic strategies.

REFERENCES

American Psychiatric Association
  1980 *DSM-III: Diagnostic and Statistical Manual of Mental Disorders,* 3rd ed. Washington, DC: American Psychiatric Association.
  1987 *DSM-III-R: Diagnostic and Statistical Manual of Mental Disorders,* 3rd ed., revised. Washington, DC: American Psychiatric Association.
  1994 *DSM-IV: Diagnostic and Statistical Manual of Mental Disorders,* 4th ed. Washington, DC: American Psychiatric Association.
Anderson, G., and R. Brown
  1984 Real and laboratory gambling, sensation-seeking and arousal. *British Journal of Addiction* 75:401-410.
Arcuri A.F., D. Lester, and F.O. Smith
  1985 Shaping adolescent gambling behavior. *Adolescence* 20(80):935-938.
Benjamin, J., C. Paterson, B. Greenberg, D.L. Murphy, and D. Hamer
  1995 Dopamine D_4 receptor gene association with normal personality traits. *Psychiatric Genetics* 5:S36.
Bergh, C., T. Eklund, P. Soedersten, and C. Nordin
  1997 Altered dopamine function in pathological gambling. *Psychological Medicine* 27(2):473-475.
Berkson, J.
  1946 Limitations of the application of fourfold table analysis to hospital data. *Biometrics* 2:47-53.

Billy, J.O.G., and J.R. Udry
 1985   The influence of male and female best friends on adolescent sexual behavior. *Adolescence* 20:21-32.

Bishay, N.R.
 1979   Three different forms of depression in one family (letter). *British Journal of Psychiatry* 134:126.

Blanco, C., L. Orensanz-Munoz, C. Blanco-Kerez, and J. Saiz-Ruiz
 1996   Pathological gambling and platelet MAO activity: A psychobiological study. *American Journal of Psychiatry* 153:119-121.

Bland, R.C., S.C. Newman, H. Orn, and G. Stebelsky
 1993   Epidemiology of pathological gambling in Edmonton. *Canadian Journal of Psychiatry* 38:108-112.

Blaszczynski, A., and N. McConaghy
 1989   Anxiety and/or depression in the pathogenesis of addictive gambling. *International Journal of the Addictions* 24:337-350.

Blaszczynski, A., N. McConaghy, and A. Frankova
 1989   Crime, antisocial personality and pathological gambling. *Journal of Gambling Behavior* 5:137-152.

Blaszczynski, A., and Z.P. Steel
 1998   Personality disorders among pathological gamblers. *Journal of Gambling Studies* 14(1):51-71.

Blaszczynski, A., S. Winter, and N. McConaghy
 1986   Plasma endorphin levels in pathological gamblers. *Journal of Gambling Behavior* 2:3-15.

Blum, K., J.G. Cull, E.R. Braverman, and D.E. Comings
 1996   Reward deficiency syndrome: Addictive, impulsive and compulsive disorders including alcoholism, attention-deficit disorder, drug abuse and food bingeing may have a common genetic basis. *American Scientist* 84:132-145.

Boyd, J., J. Burke, E. Gruenberg, C. Holzer, D. Rae, L. George, M. Karno, R. Stoltzman, L. McEvoy, and G. Nesdadt
 1984   Exclusion criteria of DSM-III: A study of co-occurrence of hierarchy-free syndromes. *Archives of General Psychiatry* 41:983-989.

Branchey, L., M. Branchey, S. Shaw, and C.S. Lieber
 1984   Depression, suicide, and aggression in alcoholics and their relationship to plasma amino acids. *Psychiatry Research* 12:219-226.

Breslau, N., and G.C. Davis
 1987   Posttraumatic stress disorder: The etiologic specificity of wartime stressors. *American Journal Psychiatry* 144:578-583.
 1992   Posttraumatic stress disorder in an urban population of young adults: Risk factors for chronicity. *American Journal of Psychiatry* 149:671-675.

Breslau, N., G.C. Davis, P. Andreski, and E. Petersen
 1991   Traumatic events and posttraumatic stress disorder in an urban population of young adults. *Archives of General Psychiatry* 48:216-222.

Brown, G.L., M.F. Ebert, P.H. Goyer, et al.
1982   Aggression, suicide and serotonin relationships to CSF amine metabolism. *American Journal of Psychiatry* 139:741-746.
Buchsbaum, M.S., R.J. Haier, and D.L. Murphy
1977   Suicide attempts, platelet monoamine oxidase and the average evoked response. *Acta Psychiatrica Scandinavica* 56:69-79.
Carrasco, J.L., J. Saiz-Ruiz, E. Hollander, J. Cesar, et al.
1994   Low platelet monamine oxidase activity in pathological gambling. *Acta Psychiatrica Scandinavica* 90:427-431.
Comings, D.E.
1998   The molecular genetics of pathological gambling. *CNS Spectrums* 3(6):20-37.
Comings, D.E., D. Muhleman, G. Dietz, M. Sherman, and G. Forest
1995   Sequence of human tryptophan 2,3-deoxygenase: Presence of a glucocorticoid response-like element composed of a CTT repeat and an intronic CCCCT repeat. *Genomics* 29:390-396.
Comings, D.E., R.J. Rosenthal, H.R. Lesieur, et al.
1996   A study of the dopamine D_2 receptor gene in pathological gambling. *Pharmacogenetics* 6:223-234.
Cook, B.L., Z.W. Wang, R.R. Crowe, R. Hauser, and M. Freimer
1992   Alcoholism and the D_2 receptor gene. *Alcohol Clinical and Experimental Research* 16(4):806-809.
Cottler, L.B., W.M. Compton, D. Mager, E.L. Spitznagel, and A. Janca
1992   Posttraumatic stress disorder among substance abusers in the general population. *American Journal of Psychiatry* 149:664-670.
Cox, S.
1998   Problem Gamblers Helpline. Paper presented at the Problem Gambling Workshop of the Committee on the Social and Economic Impact of Pathological Gambling, Irvine, CA, June 1. Texas Council on Problem and Compulsive Gambling, Richardson.
Crockford, D.N., and N. el-Guebaly
1998   Psychiatric comorbidity in pathological gambling: A critical review. *Canadian Journal of Psychiatry* 43:43-50.
Cunningham-Williams, R.M.
1998   Comorbidity: Problem Gambling and Psychiatric and Substance Use Disorders. Paper presented at the Problem Gambling Workshop of the Committee on the Social and Economic Impact of Pathological Gambling, Irvine, CA, June 2. Washington University School of Medicine.
Cunningham-Williams, R.M., L.B. Cottler, W.M. Compton, and E.L. Spitznagel
1998   Taking chances: Problem gamblers and mental health disorders—Results from the St. Louis Epidemiological Catchment Area (ECA) Study. *American Journal of Public Health* 88(7):1093-1096.

Custer, R.L.
1982   An overview of compulsive gambling. Pp. 107-124 in *Addictive Disorders Update: Alcoholism, Drug Abuse, Gambling*, P.A. Carone, S.F. Yolles, S.N. Kieffer, and L.W. Krinsky, eds. New York: Human Sciences Press.

Custer, R.L., and H. Milt
1985   *When Luck Runs Out: Help for Compulsive Gamblers and Their Families.* New York: Facts on File Publications.

DeCaria, C.M., T. Begaz, and E. Hollander
1998   Serotonergic and noradrenergic function in pathological gambling. *CNS Spectrums* 3(6):38-47.

D'Elia, G., and C. Perris
1973   Cerebral functional dominance and depression. An analysis of EEG amplitude in depressed patients. *Acta Psychiatrica Scandinavica* 49(3):191-197.

Dell, L.J., M.F. Ruzika, and A.T. Palisi
1981   Personality and other factors associated with gambling addiction. *International Journal of Addictions* 16:149-156.

Derevensky, J.L., and R. Gupta
1996   Risk-taking and Gambling Behavior Among Adolescents: An Empirical Examination. Paper presented at the annual meeting of the National Counsel on Problem Gambling Conference, Chicago, IL. McGill University, Montreal, Canada.

Dickerson, M., J. Hinchy, and J. Falve
1987   Chasing, arousal and sensation seeking in off-course gamblers. *British Journal of Addiction* 82:673-680.

Eisen, J.L., D.A. Beer, M.T. Pato, T.A. Venditto, and S.A. Rasmussen
1997   Obsessive-compulsive disorder in patients with schizophrenia or schizoaffective disorder. *American Journal of Psychiatry* 154(2):271-273.

el-Guebaly, N.
1995   Substance use disorders and mental illness: The relevance of comorbidity (editorial). *Canadian Journal of Psychiatry* 40:2-3.

Elia, C., and D.F. Jacobs
1993   The incidence of pathological gambling among Native Americans treated for alcohol dependence. *International Journal of the Addictions* 28:659-666.

Erickson, E.
1963   *Childhood and Society.* New York: Norton.
1968   Generativity and ego integrity. Pp. 75-87 in *Middle Age and Aging*, B. Neugarten, ed. Chicago: University of Chicago Press.
1982   *The Life Cycle Completed.* New York: Norton.

Feigelman, W., L.S. Wallisch, and H.R. Lesieur
1998   Problem gamblers, problem substance users, and dual-problem individuals: An epidemiological study. *American Journal of Public Health* 88(3):467-470.

Ferrioli, M, and A. Ciminero
 1981 The treatment of pathological gambling as an addictive behavior. In *Proceedings of the Fifth National Conference on Gambling and Risk Taking*, W.R. Eadington, ed. Reno: University of Nevada, Bureau of Business and Economic Research.

Frank, M.L., D. Lester, and A. Wexler
 1991 Suicidal behavior among members of Gamblers Anonymous. *Journal of Gambling Studies* 7:249-254.

Freimer, N.B., V.I. Reus, M.A. Escamilla, L.A. McInnes, M. Spesny, P. Leon, S.K. Service, L.B. Smith, S. Silva, E. Rojas, A. Gallegos, L. Meza, E. Fournier, S. Baharloo, K. Blankenship, D.J. Tyler, S. Batki, S. Vinogradov, J. Weissenbach, S.H. Barondes, and L.A. Sankuijl
 1996 Genetic mapping using haplotype, association and linkage methods suggests a locus for severe bipolar disorder (BPI) at 18q22-q23. *Nature Genetics* 12(4):436-441.

Gambino, B., et al.
 1993 Perceived family history of problem gambling and scores on the SOGS. *Journal of Gambling Studies* 9:169-184.

Gelernter, J., S. O'Malley, N. Risch, H.R. Kranzler, J. Krystal, K. Merikangas, J.L. Kennedy, and K.K. Kidd
 1991 No association between an allele at the D_2 dopamine receptor gene and alcoholism. *Journal of the American Medical Association* 266(13):1801-1807.

Gelernter, J., D. Goldman, and N. Risch
 1993a The A1 allele at the D_2 dopamine receptor gene and alcoholism. A reappraisal. *Journal of the American Medical Association* 269(13):1673-1677.

Gelernter, J., J.L. Kennedy, D.K. Grandy, Q.Y. Zhou, O. Civelli, D.L. Pauls, A. Pakstis, R. Kurlan, R.K. Sunahara, and H.B. Niznik
 1993b Exclusion of close linkage of Tourette's Syndrome to D1 dopamine receptor. *American Journal of Psychiatry* 150(3):449-453.

Goldstein, L., H.B. Murphree, and C.C. Pfeiffer
 1963 Quantitative electroencephalography in man as a measure of CNS stimulation. *Annals of the New York Academy of Sciences* 107(3):1045-1056.

Goldstein, L., A.A. Sugerman, H. Stolberg, H.B. Murphree, and C.C. Pfeiffer
 1965 Electro-cerebral activity in schizophrenics and non-psychotic subjects: Quantitative EEG amplitude analysis. *Electroencephalography and Clinical Neurophysiology* 19(4):350-361.

Goodwin, D.W.
 1976 Adoption studies of alcoholism. *Journal of Operational Psychiatry* 7(1):54-63.

Goodwin, D.W., and S.B. Guze
 1974 *Psychiatric Diagnosis, First Edition.* New York: Oxford Press Inc.

Griffiths, M.D.
 1990a The acquisition, development, and maintenance of fruit machine gambling in adolescents. *Journal of Gambling Studies* 6(3):193-204.

1990b The cognitive psychology of gambling. *Journal of Gambling Behavior* 6:31-42.

Gross, J., and M.E. McCaul
1991 A comparison of drug use and adjustment in urban adolescent children of substance abusers. *International Journal of the Addictions* 25(4-A):495-511.

Gupta, R., and J.L. Derevensky
1998a An Examination of the Correlates Associated with Excessive Gambling Among Adolescents. Paper presented at the annual meeting of the National Council on Compulsive Gambling, Las Vegas, NV.
1998b An empirical examination of Jacobs' general theory of addictions: Do adolescent gamblers fit the theory? *Journal of Gambling Studies* 14(1):17-49.

Hickey, J.E., and C.A. Haertzen
1986 Simulation of gambling responses on the Addiction Research Center Inventory. *Addictive Behavior* 11:345-349.

Hill, H.E., C.A. Haertzen, A.B. Wolbach, and E.J. Miner
1963 The Addiction Research Center Inventory: Standardization of scales which evaluate subjective effects of morphine, amphetamine, pentobarbital, alcohol, LSD-25, pyrahexyl and chlorpromazine. *Psychopharmacologia* 4:167-183.

Hoffmann, E., and L. Goldstein
1981 Hemispheric quanitative EEG changes following emotional reactions in neurotic patients. *Acta Psychiatrica Scandinavica* 63(2):153-164.

Ide-Smith, S.G., and S.E. Lea
1988 Gambling in young adolescents. *Journal of Gambling Behavior* 4(2):110-118.

Indian Gaming and Regulatory Act
1988 Public Law 100-497, October 17, 1988, 102 Stat. 2467.

Jacobs, D.F.
1988 Evidence for a common dissociative-like reaction among addicts. *Journal of Gambling Behavior* 4:27-37.
1989a A general theory of addictions: Rationale for and evidence supporting a new approach for understanding and treating addictive behaviors. Pp. 35-64 in *Compulsive Gambling: Theory, Research and Practice*, H.J. Shaffer, S. Stein, B. Gambino, and T.N. Cummings, eds. Lexington, MA: Lexington Books.
1989b Illegal and undocumented: A review of teenage gambling and the plight of children of problem gamblers in America. Pp. 249-299 in *Compulsive Gambling: Theory, Research and Practice*, H.J. Shaffer, S.A. Stein, B. Gambino, and T.N. Cummings, eds. Lexington, MA: Lexington Books.
in A review of major trends in prevalence studies of juvenile gambling in
press Canada and the United States from 1984 to 1996. In *Futures at Risk: Children, Gambling, and Society*, H. Shaffer et al., eds. Boston, MA: Mosby Publishers.

Jacobs, D.F., A.R. Marston, R.D. Singer, K. Widaman, et al.
 1989 Children of problem gamblers. Special Issue: Gambling and the family. *Journal of Gambling Behavior*. 5(4)(Winter):261-268.
Jaspers, K.
 1946 *Allegemeine psychopathologie*. Berlin: Springer.
Jessor, R., and S.L. Jessor
 1977 *Problem Behavior and Psychological Development: A Longitudinal Study of Youth*. New York: Academic Press.
Kallick, M., D. Suits, T. Dielman, and J. Hybels
 1979 *A Survey of American Gambling Attitudes and Behavior*. Research report series, Survey Research Center, Institute for Social Research. Ann Arbor: University of Michigan Press.
Kennedy, H.G., and D.H. Grubin
 1990 Hot-headed or impulsive? *British Journal of Addictions* 85(5):639-643.
Kennedy, P., A. Phenjoo, and W. Shekim
 1971 Risk-taking in the lives of parasuicides. *British Journal of Psychiatry* 119:281-286.
Koella, W.P.
 1981 Electroencephalographic signs of anxiety. *Progress in Neuropsychopharmacology* 5(2):187-192.
Koepp, M.J., R.N. Gunn, A.D. Lawrence, V.J. Cunningham, A. Dagher, T. Jones, D.J. Brooks, C.J. Bench, and P.M. Grasby
 1998 Evidence for striatal dopamine release during a video game. *Nature* 393:266-268.
Kotler, M., H. Cohen, and R. Segman, et al.
 1997 Excess dopamine D_4 receptor (DRD4) exon III seven repeat allele in opioid dependent subjects. *Molecular Psychiatry* 2:251-254.
Koukkou, M., and D. Lehmann
 1976 Human EEG spectra before and during cannibis hallucinations. *Biological Psychiatry* 11(6):663-677.
Krystal, J.H., E. Webb, N. Coony, H.R. Kranzler, and D.S. Charney
 1994 Specificity of ethanollike effects elicited by serotonergic and nonadrenergic mechanisms. *Archives of General Psychiatry* 51:898-911.
Kuley, N., and D. Jacobs
 1988 The relationship between dissociative-like experiences and sensation seeking among social and problem gamblers. *Journal of Gambling Behavior* 4:197-207.
Ladouceur, R., D. Dube, and A. Bujold
 1994 Prevalence of pathological gambling and related problems among college students in the Quebec metropolitan area. *Canadian Journal of Psychiatry* 39:289-293.
Lee, M.A., and H.Y. Meltzer
 1994 Blunted oral body temperature response to MK-212 in cocaine addicts. *Drug and Alcohol Dependence* 35:217-222.

Lesieur, H.R.
1984   The Chase: Career of the Compulsive Gambler. Rochester, VT: Schenkman Books.
1987   Gambling, pathological gambling and crime. Pp. 89-110 in The Handbook of Pathological Gambling, T. Galski, ed. Springfield, IL: Charles C. Thomas.

Lesieur, H.R., and S.B. Blume
1987   The South Oaks Gambling Screen (SOGS): A new instrument for the identification of pathological gamblers. American Journal of Psychiatry 144:1184-1188.
1991   When Lady Luck loses: Women and compulsive gambling. Pp. 181-197 in Feminist Perspectives on Addictions, N. van den Bergh, ed. New York: Springer.

Lesieur, H.R., S. Blume, and R. Zoppa
1986   Alcoholism, drug abuse and gambling. Alcoholism: Clinical and Experimental Research 10:33-38.

Lesieur, H.R., J. Cross, M. Frank, M. Welch, C.M. White, G. Rubenstein, K. Moseley, and M. Mark
1991   Gambling and pathological gambling among university students. Addictive Behaviors 16:517-527.

Lesieur, H.R., and M. Heineman
1988   Pathological gambling among multiple substance abusers in a therapeutic community. British Journal of Addiction 83:765-771.

Lesieur, H.R., and R. Klein
1985   Prisoners, gambling and crime. Paper presented at the Annual Meetings of the Academy of Criminal Justice Sciences, Las Vegas, NV, April 2.
1987   Pathological gambling among high school students. Addiction Behavior 12:129-135.

Lesieur, H.R., and R.J. Rosenthal
1998   Analysis of pathological gambling. Pp 393-401 in DSM-IV Sourcebook, T.A. Widiger, A.J. Frances, H.A. Pincus, R. Ross, M.B. First, W. Davis, and M. Kline, eds. Washington DC: American Psychiatric Press.

Levison, P.K., D.R. Gerstein, and D.R. Maloff, eds.
1983   Commonalities in Substance Abuse and Habitual Behaviors. Committee on Substance Abuse and Habitual Behavior, National Research Council. Lexington, MA: Lexington Books.

Livingston, J.
1974   Compulsive Gamblers: Observations on Action and Abstinence. New York: Harper and Row.

Lukas, S.E.
1998   Brain Imaging of Altered Mood States: Implications for Understanding the Neurobiological Bases of Gambling. Paper prepared for the National Research Council, Committee on the Social and Economic Impact of Pathological Gambling. McLean Hospital, Cambridge, MA.

Lukas, S.E., R. Benedikt, and J.H. Mendelson
  1995   Electroencephalographic correlates of marihuana-induced euphoria. *Drug and Alcohol Dependence* 37:131-140.
Lukas, S.E., and J.H. Mendelson
  1988   Electroencephalographic activity and plasma ACTH during ethanol-induced euphoria. *Biological Psychiatry* 23:141-148.
Lukas, S.E., J.H. Mendelson, R.A. Benedikt, and B. Jones
  1986   EEG alpha increases during transient episodes of ethanol induced euphoria. *Pharmacology, Biochemistry and Behavior* 25(4):889-895.
Lyons, J.
  1985   Differences in sensation seeking and in depression levels between male social gamblers and male compulsive gamblers. In *The Proceedings of the Sixth National Conference on Gambling and Risk Taking*, W.R. Eadington, ed. Reno: University of Nevada, Bureau of Business and Economic Research.
Malhotra, A.K., M. Virkkunen, W. Rooney, M. Eggert, M. Linnoila, and D. Goldman
  1996   The association between the dopamine D_4 receptor (DRD4) 16 amino acid repeat polymorphisms and novelty seeking. *Molecular Psychiatry* 1:388-391.
Malkin, D., and G.J. Syme
  1986   Personality and problem gambling. *International Journal of the Addictions* 21(2):267-272.
Mark, M.E., and H.R. Lesieur
  1992   A feminist critique of problem gambling research. *British Journal of Addiction* 87:549-565.
McCormick, R.A.
  1993   Disinhibition and negative affectivity in substance abusers with and without a gambling problem. *Addictive Behaviors* 18:331-336.
McCormick, R.A., A.M. Russo, L.F. Rameriz, and J.I Taber
  1984   Affective disorders among pathological gamblers seeking treatment. *American Journal of Psychiatry* 141:215-218.
McCormick, R.A., J. Taber, N. Kruedelbach, and A. Russo
  1987   Personality profiles of hospitalized pathological gamblers: The California Personality Inventory. *Journal of Clinical Psychology* 43:521-527.
McEachern, J., L. Friedman, M. Bird, S.E. Lukas, M.H. Orzack, D.L. Katz, E.C. Dessain, B. Beake, and J.O. Cole
  1988   Self-report versus an instrumental measure in the assessment of the subjective effects of d-amphetamine. *Psychopharmacology Bulletin* 24:463-465.
Miller, W.R.
  1980   *The Addictive Behaviors*. Oxford, England: Pergamon Press.
Mok, W.P., and J. Hraba
  1991   Age and shifting gambling behavior: A decline and shifting pattern of participation. *Journal of Gambling Studies* 7(4):313-335.

Moran, E.
1969   Taking the final risk. *Mental Health* (Winter):21-22 (London).
1970   Varieties of pathological gambling. *British Journal of Psychiatry* 116:593-597.

Moravee, J.D., and P.H. Munley
1983   Psychological test findings on pathological gamblers in treatment. *International Journal of the Addictions* 18:1003-1009.

Moreno, I., J.Y. Saiz-Ruiz, and J.J. Lopez-Ibor
1991   Serotonin and gambling dependence. *Human Psychopharmacology* 6:S9-S12.

Murphy, K.L., R. Belmaker, and M.S. Buchsbaum
1997   Biogenic amine related enzymes and personality variations in normals. *Psychological Medicine* 7:149-157.

Nathan, P.
1967   *Cues, Decisions and Diagnoses.* New York: Academic Press.

Newcomb, M.D, and P.M. Bentler
1989   Substance use and abuse among children and teenagers. *American Psychologist* 44:242-248.

Novick, O., R. Ebstein, R. Umansky, B. Priel, Y. Osher, and R.H. Belmaker
1995 D_4 receptor polymorphism associated with personality variation in normals. *Psychiatric Genetics* 5:S36.

Perez de Castro, I., A. Ibanez, P. Torres, J. Saiz-Ruiz, and J. Fernandez-Piqueras
1997   Genetic association study between pathological gambling and a functional DNA polymorphism at the D4 receptor gene. *Pharmcogenetics* 7(5):345-348.

Radloff, L.
1977   The CES-D scale: A self-report depression scale for research in the general population. *Applied Psychological Measurement* 1:385-401.

Ramirez, L.F., R.A. McCormick, A.M. Russo, and J.I. Taber
1983   Patterns of substance use in pathological gamblers undergoing treatment. *Addictive Behaviors* 8:425-428.

Regier, D.A., M.E. Farmer, D. Rae, B. Locke, S.J. Keith, L.L. Judd, and F.K. Goodwin
1990   Comorbidity of mental disorders with alcohol and other drug abuse: Results from the ECA study. *Journal of the American Medical Association* 264:2511-2518.

Rose, I.
1992   The future of Indian gaming. *Journal of Gambling Studies* 8(4):383-399.

Rosenthal, R.J., and H.R. Lesieur
1992   Self-reported withdrawal symptoms and pathological gambling. *American Journal of the Addictions* 1:150-154.

Rosenthal, R.J., and V.C. Lorenz
1992   The pathological gambler as criminal offender: Comments on evaluation and treatment. *Psychiatric Clinics of North America* 15:647-660.

Roy, A., B. Ardinoff, L. Roehrich, D. Lamparski, R. Custer, V. Lorenz, et al.
    1988   Pathological gambling: A psychobiological study. *Archives of General Psychiatry* 45:369-373.
Roy, A., R. Custer, V. Lorenz, and M. Linnoila
    1989   Personality factors and pathological gambling. *Acta Psychiatrica Scandinavica* 80:37-39.
Rugle, L., and L. Melamed
    1993   Neuropsychological assessment of attention problems in pathological gamblers. *Journal of Nervous and Mental Disorders* 18(2):107-112.
Schwarz, J., and A. Linder
    1992   Inpatient treatment of male pathological gamblers in Germany. *Journal of Gambling Studies* 8(1):93-109.
Smart, R.G., and Ferris, J.
    1996   Alcohol, drugs and gambling in the Ontario adult population, 1994. *Canadian Journal of Psychiatry* 41:36-45.
Specker, S.M., G.A. Carlson, G.A. Christenson, and M. Marcotte
    1995   Impulse control disorders and attention deficit disorder in pathological gamblers. *Annals of Clinical Pschiatry* 7(4):175-179.
Specker, S.M., G.A. Carlson, K.M. Edmonson, P.E. Johnson, and M. Marcotte
    1996   Psychopathology in pathological gamblers seeking treatment. *Journal of Gambling Studies* 12:67-81.
Spunt, B., H. Lesieur, D. Hunt, and L. Cahill
    1995   Gambling among methadone patients. *International Journal of the Addictions* 30:929-962.
Steinberg, M.
    1997   *Connecticut High School Problem Gambling Surveys 1989 & 1996.* Guilford: Connecticut Council on Problem Gambling.
Steinberg, M., T. Kosten, and B. Rounsaville
    1992   Cocaine abuse and pathological gambling. *American Journal on Addictions* 1:121-132.
Stinchfield, R., and K.C. Winters
    1998   Gambling and problem gambling among youths. *Annals of the American Academy of Political and Social Science* 556:172-185.
Sugarman, A.A., L. Goldstein, H.B. Murphee, C. Pfeiffer, and E.H. Jenney
    1964   EEG and behavioral changes in schizophrenia. *Archives of General Psychiatry* 10(4):340-344.
Sullivan, S.
    1994   Why compulsive gamblers are a high suicide risk. *Community Mental Health in New Zealand* 8(2):40-47.
Tellegen, A., D.T. Lykken, T.J. Bouchard, K.J. Wilcox, N.L. Segal, and S. Rich
    1988   Personality similarity in twins reared apart and together. *Journal of Personality and Social Psychology* 54(6):1031-1039.
Templer, D.I., G. Kaiser, and K. Siscoe
    1993   Correlates of pathological gambling in prison inmates. *Comprehensive Psychiatry* 34:347-351.

Thorson, J., F. Powell, and M. Hilt
  1994   Epidemiology of gambling and depression in an adult sample. *Psychological Reports* 74:987-994.
Vilhjalmsson R., G. Kristjansdottir, and E. Sveinbjarnardottir
  1998   Factors associated with suicide ideation in adults. *Social Psychiatry and Psychiatric Epidemiology* 33:97-103.
Volavka, J., P. Crown, R. Dornbush, S. Feldstein, and M. Fink
  1973   EEG, heart rate and mood change ("high") after cannabis. *Psychopharmacologica* 32:11-25.
Volberg, R.A.
  1994   The prevalence and demographics of pathological gamblers: Implications for public health. *American Journal of Public Health* 84(2):237-241.
Volberg, R.A., and M.W. Abbott
  1997   Gambling and problem gambling among indigenous peoples. *Substance Use and Misuse* 32(11):1525-1538.
Von Knorring, L., and L. Goldstein
  1981   Quantitative hemispheric EEG differences between health volunteers and depressed patients. *Research Communications in Psychology, Psychiatry and Behavior* 7(1):57-67.
Von Knorring, L., L. Oreland, and B. Winblad
  1984   Personality traits related to monoamine oxidase activity in platelets. *Psychiatry Research* 12:11-26.
Ward, P.B., S.V. Catts, T.R. Norman, G.D. Burrows, and N. McConaghy
  1987   Low platelet monoamine oxidase and sensation seeking in males: An established relationship? *Acta Psychiatrica Scandinavica* 75:86-90.
Wiet, S.G.
  1981   The prevalence and duration of quantitative hemispheric EEG measures reflecting the affective and academic differences among a group of first year university students. *Research Communications in Psychology, Psychiatry and Behavior* 6(1):83-101.
Winokur, G., P.J. Clayton, and T. Reich
  1969   *Manic Depressive Illness.* St. Louis: C.V. Mosby.
Winters, K.C., P. Bengston, D. Dorr, and R.D. Stinchfield
  1998   Prevalence and risk factors of problem gambling among college students. *Psychology of Addictive Behaviors* 12(2):127-135.
Winters, K.C., and T. Rich
  in press   A twin study of adult gambling behavior. *Journal of Gambling Studies.*
Winters, K.C., R. Stinchfield, and J. Fulkerson
  1993a   Patterns and characteristics of adolescent gambling. *Journal of Gambling Studies* 9(4):371-386.
  1993b   Toward the development of an adolescent gambling severity scale. *Journal of Gambling Studies* 9(1):63-84.
Wray, I., and M. Dickerson
  1981   Cessation of high frequency gambling and "withdrawal" symptoms. *British Journal of Addiction* 76:401-405.

Wynne, H., G. Smith, and D. Jacobs
   1996   Adolescent Gambling and Problem Gambling in Alberta. A report prepared for the Alberta Alcohol and Drug Abuse Commission, May. Wynne Resources, Edmonton, Canada.
Zitzow, D.
   1996   Comparative study of problematic gambling behaviors between American Indian and non-Indian adolescents within and near a northern plains reservation. *American Indian and Alaska Native Mental Health Research* 7(2):14-26.

5

Social and Economic Effects

The growth of legal gambling in the United States in recent decades has been fueled largely by increasing public acceptance of gambling as a form of recreation, and by the promise of substantial economic benefits and tax revenues for the communities in which the gambling occurs. There is no question that legalized gambling has brought economic benefits to some communities; just as there is no question that problem gambling has imposed economic and social costs. The important question, from a public policy perspective, is which is larger and by how much. Clearly, to address this and related policy issues, the economic and social costs of pathological gambling need to be considered in the context of the overall impact that gambling has on society.

The benefits are borne out in reports, for example, of increased employment and income, increased tax revenues, enhanced tourism and recreational opportunities, and rising property values (e.g., Eadington, 1984; Filby and Harvey, 1988; Chadbourne et al., 1997, Oddo, 1997). American Indian communities in particular, both on and off reservations, reportedly have realized positive social and economic effects from gambling "that far outweigh the negative" (Cornell et al., 1998:iv; see also Anders, 1996; Cozzetto 1995).

Gambling has also resulted in economic and social costs to

individuals and families, as well as to communities, as discussed in this chapter. Such costs include traffic congestion, demand for more public infrastructure or services (roads, schools, police, fire protection, etc.), environmental effects, displacement of local residents, increased crime, and pathological or problem gambling. To the extent that pathological gambling contributes to bankruptcy and bad debts, these increase the cost of credit throughout the economy. We use the term "costs" to include the negative consequences of pathological gambling for gamblers, their immediate social environments, and the larger community.

As we said, the fundamental policy question is whether the benefits or the costs are larger and by how much. This can in theory be determined with benefit-cost analysis. Complicating such analysis, however, is the fact that social and economic effects can be difficult to measure. This is especially true for intangible social costs, such as emotional pain and other losses experienced by family members of a pathological gambler, and the productivity losses of employees who are pathological or problem gamblers. Beneficial effects can also be difficult to measure and, as with costs, can vary in type and magnitude across time and gambling venues, as well as type of gambling (e.g., lotteries, land-based casinos, riverboat casinos, bingo, pari-mutuel gambling, offtrack betting, sports betting).

Ideally, the fundamental benefit-versus-cost question should be asked for each form of gambling and should take into consideration such economic factors as real costs versus economic transfers, tangible and intangible effects, direct and indirect effects, present and future values (i.e., discounting), and gains and losses experienced by different groups in various settings (Gramlich, 1990:229). Moreover, the costs and benefits of pathological gambling need to be considered in the context of the overall effects that gambling has on society.[1] Unfortunately, the state of research into the benefits and costs of gambling generally, and into the costs of pathological gambling specifically, is not sufficiently advanced to allow definitive conclusions to be drawn. Few reliable

---

[1]The committee recognizes that the possibility of benefits deriving from pathological gambling are only theoretical and are neither described in the literature nor supported empirically.

economic impact analyses or benefit-cost analyses have been done, and those that exist have focused on casino gambling. Consequently, the committee is not able to shed as much light on the costs of pathological gambling as we would have preferred. We hope, however, that the chapter lays out the issues for readers and provides some guidance to researchers venturing into this area.

COSTS TO INDIVIDUALS[2]

As discussed in Chapter 2, the definition of pathological gambling includes adverse consequences to the individual, such as involvement in crime, financial difficulties, and disruptions of interpersonal relations. According to the criteria presented in the *Diagnostic and Statistical Manual of Mental Disorders* (DSM), a pathological gambler may be and often is defined by the presence of at least a few of these consequences (American Psychiatric Association, 1994). Discussions of the costs to the individual of pathological gambling would be circular if we claimed to "discover" these consequences. Instead, we focus on the magnitude and the extent to which pathological gamblers experience these adverse consequences.

The literature on individual costs of pathological gambling considers consequences for the gambler and those with whom the gambler has most frequent interactions, including family, friends, and close associates. The literature focuses primarily on crime, financial difficulties, and disruptions of interpersonal relations. Like the research on risk factors discussed in Chapter 4, because most of these studies are based on treatment populations with small samples and no controls, we urge caution when interpreting the results.

Many families of pathological gamblers suffer from a variety of financial, physical, and emotional problems (Abbott et al., 1995; Boreham et al., 1996; Lorenz and Yafee, 1986). The financial con-

---

[2]The committee expresses special thanks to Lia Nower for her synthesis and written presentation of literature pertaining to the social costs of pathological gambling to individuals, families, communities, and society.

sequences of living with a pathological gambler can range from bad credit and legal difficulties to complete bankruptcy. Lorenz and Shuttlesworth (1983) surveyed the spouses of compulsive gamblers at Gam-Anon, the family component of Gamblers Anonymous, and found that most of them had serious emotional problems and had resorted to drinking, smoking, overeating, and impulse spending. In a similar study, Lorenz and Yaffee (1988) found that the spouses of pathological gamblers suffered from chronic or severe headaches, stomach problems, dizziness, and breathing difficulties, in addition to emotional problems of anger, depression, and isolation. Jacobs and colleagues (1989) compared children who characterized their parents as compulsive gamblers with those who reported their parents as having no gambling problems. Children of compulsive gamblers were more likely to smoke, drink, and use drugs. Furthermore, they were more likely to describe their childhood as unhappy periods of their lives.

Pathological gamblers are said to distance themselves from family and friends, who are alternately neglected and manipulated for "bailouts" (Custer and Milt, 1985). The ultimate relationship costs to the gambler typically become manifest when the gambler reaches a stage of desperation or hopelessness. Lesieur and Rothschild (1989) found that children of pathological gamblers frequently reported feelings of anger, sadness, and depression. Bland and colleagues (1993) estimated that 23 percent of the spouses and 17 percent of the children of pathological gamblers were physically and verbally abused. These percentages vary somewhat across studies. Lorenz and Shuttlesworth (1993) estimated that 50 percent of spouses and 10 percent of children experienced physical abuse from the pathological gambler.

Research has not examined the nature and extent of the gambler's retrospective perception of losses with regard to children, friends, and family members. However, Frank and colleagues (1991) have suggested that dysfunctional family relationships bear on a pathological gambler's tendency toward self-harm. As discussed earlier, as gambling progresses toward a pathological state, there is frequently a corresponding increase in depression, shame, and guilt. Research suggests that as many as 20 percent of persons in treatment for or diagnosed with pathological gambling may attempt suicide (Moran, 1969; Livingston,

1974; Custer and Custer, 1978; McCormick et al., 1984; Lesieur and Blume, 1991; Thompson et al., 1996). In a national survey of 500 Gamblers Anonymous members, those assessed as being at highest risk for suicide were more likely to be separated or divorced (24 percent) and to have relatives who gambled or were alcoholic (60 percent). About 17 percent of gamblers who considered suicide, and 13 percent of those who had attempted it, had children with some type of addiction.

FINANCIAL PROBLEMS AND CRIME

Financial losses pose the most immediate and compelling cost to the gambler in the throes of his or her disorder. As access to money becomes more limited, gamblers often resort to crime in order to pay debts, appease bookies, maintain appearances, and garner more money to gamble (Lesieur, 1987; Meyer and Fabian, 1992). Several descriptive studies have reported widely ranging estimates of the proportion of pathological gamblers who commit offenses and serve prison terms for such offenses as fraud, stealing, embezzlement, forgery, robbery, and blackmail (Bergh and Kuhlhorn, 1994; Blaszczynsi and McConaghy, 1994a, 1994b; Lesieur and Anderson, 1995; Schwarz and Linder, 1992; Thompson et al., 1996a, 1996b). Still, when gambling establishments come to economically depressed communities with high rates of unemployment, as is the case with riverboat casinos in Indiana, there may be, in addition to the costs, social benefits to providing job training and jobs to the previously unemployed.

Blaszczynski and Silove (1996) noted that criminal behaviors among adolescent gamblers may be more prevalent than among adult gamblers, in part because youths have few options for obtaining funds and greater susceptibility to social pressure among gambling peers. In the United Kingdom, Fisher (1991) reported that 46 percent of adolescents surveyed stole from their family, 12 percent stole from others, 31 percent sold their possessions, and 39 percent gambled with their school lunch or travel money.

Two studies attempted to assess theft by problem gamblers, one in Wisconsin (Thompson et al., 1996a) and one in Illinois (Lesieur and Anderson, 1995; cited in Lesieur, 1998). These studies came to widely differing estimates of the magnitude of theft, probably because of methodological differences. In an Australian study (Blaszczynski and McConaghy, 1994a), most of the gamblers reported using their wages to finance gambling, supplemented by credit cards (38.7 percent), borrowing from friends and relatives (32.9 percent), and loans from banks and financial institutions (29.8 percent). This study did not provide a comparison, however, of differences between the financing of gambling and other household expenditures. In Canada, Ladouceur et al. (1994) found that, on average, the pathological gambler spent between $1,000 and $5,000 a month on gambling and used family savings (90 percent), borrowed money (83 percent), or both.

Another cost to the pathological gambler is loss of employment. Roughly one-fourth to one-third of gamblers in treatment in Gamblers Anonymous report the loss of their jobs due to gambling (Ladouceur et al., 1994; Lesieur, 1998; Thompson et al., 1996b). One study estimated that more than 60 percent of those surveyed lost, on average, more than seven hours of work per month (Thompson et al., 1996b). In addition, the authors found that the average gambler costs employers more than $1,300 a month, and lost labor costs due to the unemployment totaled about $1,300 per gambler yearly.

Bankruptcy presents yet another adverse consequence of excessive gambling. In one of the few studies to address bankruptcy, Ladouceur et al. (1994) found that 28 percent of the 60 pathological gamblers attending Gamblers Anonymous either reported that they had filed for bankruptcy or reported debts of $75,000 to $150,000.

Published news accounts, bankruptcy court opinions, and bankruptcy attorneys serve as the primary reporters of the effects of gambling on bankruptcy. These accounts, however, are often region-specific, anecdotal, and poorly documented. In one such study (Ison, 1995a), the records examined suggested that 20 percent of all bankruptcies filed were gambling-related; of 105 gambling filers, the average gambler owed more than $40,000 in unsecured debt and possessed an average of eight credit cards with balances of $5,000 to $10,000 each; in total, the group owed about $1.1 million, exclusive of delinquent mortgages and car and income tax payments. Ison (1995b) reported that these gamblers cost one state (Minnesota) about $228 million annually.

In summary, although the research in this area is sparse, it suggests that the magnitude and extent of personal consequences on the pathological gambler and his or her family may be severe. These destructive behaviors contribute to the concern about pathological gambling, and the need for more research to understand its social cost to individuals, families, and communities.

ISSUES AND CHALLENGES IN
BENEFIT-COST ANALYSES OF GAMBLING[3]

A wide variety of economic techniques is available to assess the effects of new or expanded gambling activities. What seems to be a straightforward task of identifying benefits and costs associated with legalized gambling and with pathological and problem gambling is really more difficult than it first appears. Not surprisingly, most reported economic analysis in the literature is methodologically weak. In their most rudimentary form, such studies are little more than a crude accounting, bringing together readily available numbers from a variety of disparate sources. Among studies of the overall effects of gambling, such rough-and-ready analyses are common. In the area of gambling, pathological gambling, and problem gambling, systematic data are rarely to be found, despite considerable pressure for information. The consequence has been a plethora of studies with implicit but untested assumptions underlying the analysis that often are either unacknowledged by those performing the analysis, or likely to be misunderstood by those relying on the results. Not surprisingly, the findings of rudimentary economic impact analyses can be misused by those who are not aware of their limitations.

When properly done, however, economic impact and benefit-cost analyses can be powerful policymaking tools. However, it requires an investment of time and money to operationalize, identify, measure, and analyze both benefits and costs. Many studies have identified the categories of benefits and costs associated with legalized gambling (e.g., Eadington, 1984;

---

[3]The committee thanks Kurt Zorn for his written synthesis, analysis, and presentation of the literature in the remainder of this chapter.

Chadbourne et al., 1997; Oddo, 1997). But most studies have focused on the benefits and costs to the community rather than those that accrue to individual gamblers and their families, or to other individual members or groups in the community. In fairness, this is probably attributable to the difficulty of measuring benefits and costs in complex areas like pathological and problem gambling. Analytic factors contributing to this difficulty are described below in general and later described in specific examples taken from the literature.

Real Versus Transfer Effects

One of the biggest stumbling blocks in economic impact analysis is determining which effects are real and which are merely transfers.[4] What appears to be a cost may in fact be a transfer from one person or entity in society to another. For example, when a person borrows money to take a trip involving social or recreational gambling, the money borrowed is not a cost to society. Rather, the person is transferring consumption from the future, when the debt will be repaid, to the present, in much the same way as when he or she borrows money to purchase a new car. Thus, money is transferred from the future to the present through a lender, who is willing to forgo present consumption when the loan is made, in exchange for future consumption when the loan is repaid with interest.

Conversely, there may be situations in which what appears to be a benefit is also a transfer. For example, the money spent by recreational gamblers at a casino is an indication of income generated in the community as a result of the casino. To the extent that the money comes from recreational gamblers who live in other communities, such money represents a real benefit to the casino and the community in which the gambling occurred. However, some of the money spent in the casino by local residents is not an economic benefit, but merely a transfer within the community. Had the casino not been in their community, some of the money

---

[4]The category of transfer is often referred to as pecuniary in the economics literature.

local residents spend on gambling would probably have been spent on other locally available entertainment or recreation (e.g., going to movies or buying new sporting goods equipment) instead. In addition, some of the money spent on gambling may be paid to suppliers, as well as gambling establishment owners or investors from outside the community, in which case the benefits "leak" into other communities.

Transfer effects are notoriously difficult to identify. McMillen (1991), for example, provides an excellent discussion of some of the challenges associated with the identification and valuation of benefits and costs associated with casino gambling in Australia. McMillen points out that economic impact studies often fail to explain the potential for one expenditure to displace another. Construction and gambling expenditures often are treated as net additions to the community, but this is too simplistic an approach. The real question is what else might have been done with the resources used to construct the casino. If, for example, the construction dollars would have been spent elsewhere in the community had the casino not been built, then the construction expenditure is merely a transfer and not an influx of new dollars into the community.

McMillen further argues that the economic impact of a casino should be evaluated as one would evaluate a question of foreign trade. A casino may at first glance appear to benefit its community. But if it imports most of its supplies from outside the region and also sends its profits to owners outside the region, then there will be less benefit to the region than if suppliers and owners are local. McMillen (1991:88) also underscores the difficulty associated with identifying the direct costs and benefits of casinos. He contends that "the impact of the casinos on crime is impossible to disentangle from other factors which also may have affected changes in local criminal patterns (e.g., changing economic conditions, social attitudes, policing and judicial practices, unemployment, cut-backs in social services). The committee's review of gambling research found that these complex cause-and-effect relationships have not yet been sorted out adequately in the empirical literature.

Direct and Indirect Effects

A casino will have both direct and indirect effects on an area's income and jobs. The direct effect represents a net addition to the community's resources. The direct effect of a casino, for example, is the income and employment associated with providing goods and services to its patrons—the wages casino employees earn are direct effects of the casino. Indirect effects refer to the secondary effects that casinos have on the community. For example, visitors to the casino may purchase gasoline from a local gas station, causing the station to hire another attendant. Casino employees will spend their paychecks in the local community, causing more business and more employment for grocery stores, clothing stores, and so forth. Both these direct and indirect effects, or primary and secondary effects as they are sometimes called, are appropriate to consider as benefits.

The most common approach to estimating indirect effects is by using an input-output model. These models are used to evaluate the economic development effects of many kinds of investments. By measuring the indirect ripple effect of a change in a regional economy, an input-output model recognizes that the outputs of one industry are often inputs to other industries, and that the wages that employees of one industry earn are spent on a variety of goods produced by other industries. Thus, changes in the activity of one industry, like a casino, affect both the casino's suppliers and its customers. Through this accounting-type framework, a change in the output, earnings, or employment level of an industry can be traced through the regional economy to determine its secondary effects. Input-output models are flexible enough to assess the effects of facility expansions, contractions, and closings (Richardson, 1972).

An input-output model works through the development of multipliers, which are a convenient way of summarizing these ripple effects throughout the economy. An employment multiplier, for example, captures all of the direct effects of the addition of a job to a particular industry in the local economy. Perhaps the most widely used input-output model was developed by the U.S. Department of Commerce's Bureau of Economic Analysis (BEA). The BEA developed the Regional Input-Output Modeling System

(RIMS) model in the mid-1970s. In the mid-1980s, a major enhancement of the model was completed and the new model was designated as RIMS II. The RIMS II model is periodically updated (U.S. Department of Commerce, 1992). The multipliers supplied to the model by the BEA are created from extensive data on national and regional economies. Multipliers can be developed for the entire country, an individual state, an individual county, or a region comprised of a group of counties.

Input-output models have been used to evaluate the economic effects of new casino gambling facilities in a community and a state.[5] Three potential problems are often encountered when using these models to analyze gambling. First, because the expansion of casino gambling is so recent, the RIMS II model does not have casino gambling multipliers to apply to regions in which gambling is being introduced. This forces researchers to use other multipliers as proxies for gambling. Second, input-output analysis is best suited for modest changes to a community's economic structure. When a casino is introduced into a small community, as has often been the case, it may bring major changes to the whole structure of economic activity in the community. When the change to a community's economic structure is significant, input-output models do not predict indirect effects well (Oster et al., 1997). Third, the model's estimate of indirect effects is based on the measurement of direct effects. If direct effects have not been measured properly, then those measurement errors will carry over to the estimate of indirect effects as well.

Tangible and Intangible Effects

Both the direct and the indirect effects mentioned above are tangible, because they result in measurably more jobs and additional income being generated in the local economy. As mentioned at the beginning of this chapter, intangible benefits and costs are identifiable effects that are difficult or impossible to measure or to quantify in dollar terms. Intangible benefits and costs

---

[5]The Indiana Gaming Commission used input-output models to compare and evaluate the competing applications for riverboat gambling licenses.

are usually omitted from consideration in gambling-related economic analysis studies—a clear shortcoming. However, as with many effects that have traditionally been considered intangible, such as various environmental effects, considerable progress has been made toward making them tangible. For example, construction of the casino facility may destroy a wetland. Under current federal law, this would require creating or expanding a wetland somewhere else in compensation. But, in many instances, the new wetland may not provide all of the functional benefits that the old wetland did and thus does not completely compensate for the loss. In the past, this would have been considered an intangible cost. Recently, however, the ability to measure and value wetland functions has improved, so this would now be a tangible cost. Improvements in the ability to measure benefits and costs formerly thought to be intangible have reduced the problem of including all of the costs and benefits, but they have not eliminated it. There remain intangible costs and benefits that still defy measurement.

Defining the Frame of Reference

A central issue critical to all economic impact studies is the frame of reference for the analysis (McMillen, 1991). Proper classification of benefits and costs as real or as transfers is contingent on defining what the community is—city, region, state, or nation. Consider, for example, a riverboat casino on Lake Michigan in northwest Indiana. As discussed earlier, the business of social and recreational gamblers coming to the riverboat from outside the community can be considered a benefit to the community. But what about social and recreational gamblers who live elsewhere in Indiana? The impact of their business can be considered a benefit to the community with the casino but not to the state. The state does not benefit from having less money spent in one community and more spent in another. A similar question can be raised about social and recreational gamblers who come to the Indiana riverboat from Illinois. Their business is a benefit to the riverboat's community and the state of Indiana, but from a national perspective it is simply a transfer from one state to another. Thus, what the analyst considers a benefit (or cost) and what is considered a transfer depends on the geographic region chosen for the analysis.

Identifying and Measuring Costs:
An Example of Unpaid Debt

When one measures the economic effects of pathological and problem gambling (Lesieur, 1989, 1992, 1998), financial costs such as debt, insurance, medical, work-related, and criminal justice costs are fairly easy to measure. However, measuring intangibles, such as the effects of pathological or problem gambling on children and the family structure, poses more difficult challenges. In addition, the consequences of pathological gambling may be caused by other, less harmful forms of gambling (e.g., problem gambling). Correctly identifying and measuring even the tangible costs is an involved process, one that many do not fully appreciate.

Consider, for example, the treatment of gambling debt. Lesieur relates that the debt incurred by problem gamblers in New Jersey has been estimated to be over $500 million dollars per year (Lesieur, 1992). This estimate is based on the assumption that the average debt incurred by problem gamblers in treatment is the same as the average debt of those not in treatment. This average debt is then multiplied by the estimated number of problem gamblers in New Jersey, which is, in turn, based on estimates of the prevalence rate of problem gambling among adults in the state multiplied by an estimate of the number of adults in New Jersey.

Three problems appear in this analysis. First, the assumption that the debt of those in treatment is the same as those not in treatment is a strong assumption that has not been tested empirically. It seems possible, even likely, that this assumption will bias the overall estimate upward. Notwithstanding the fact that some pathological gamblers seek treatment even while winning, it can be argued that those who seek treatment generally are worse off financially and therefore have amassed larger debts than those not in treatment. A counterargument might be made that the total debt does not include all the transaction costs associated with indebtedness and bankruptcy and thus the estimate is understated. But this is really an argument for a more complete measurement of debt, rather than an argument for the doubtful proposition that the best way to compensate for one bias of unknown magnitude is to introduce another bias of unknown magnitude in the opposite direction. And, of course, the total indebtedness estimate is only as good as the underlying estimate of the statewide prevalence rate. All too often, studies use prevalence estimates that have been taken from other studies and do not represent prevalence rates directly estimated for the state or community under study.

The second problem is that this indebtedness estimate is the total debt that pathological gamblers incur rather than the incremental or additional debt incurred by such gamblers relative to the rest of the population. Even if the $500 million estimate indeed is a sound estimate of the total, it is not the right number to use in the analysis. People who do not gamble have debts as well. This means that the analyst needs to know the average indebtedness for those who are not pathological gamblers as well as for those who are. This estimate for nongamblers then needs to be multiplied by the number of pathological gamblers in the state to determine the total amount of debt that could be expected under typical circumstances for this group if they were not pathological gamblers. Finally, the estimate of total indebtedness for pathological gamblers minus the total indebtedness that could be expected from the same size population that is demographically similar but is not pathological gamblers will provide an estimate of the incremental or additional debt that is due to pathological gambling. The issue is how much more debt is incurred because of pathological gambling, not how much debt pathological gamblers incur.

The third problem is the transfer issue. As discussed earlier, consumer debt is a means of transferring consumption from the future to the present. There is no cost to society if a consumer borrows $100 one month and pays it back in the next. People do this all the time when they borrow money to purchase cars or take vacations and then do not to pay off their bills in full at then end of the month. As with other consumption activities, so with gambling. Does the additional debt incurred because of pathological gambling represent a real cost to society, or is it merely a transfer, a temporary redistribution of money from one group in society (lenders) to another (borrowers), which in due time will be undone by repayment of the debt? In economic impact analysis, only that portion of the incremental debt that is unrecoverable due to bankruptcy or nonpayment should be considered a real cost to society (along with the transaction costs associated with the indebtedness, such as bankruptcy proceedings, civil court actions, and the like). Even then, all of that debt may not be attributable to pathological gambling. It is likely that some pathological gamblers would have defaulted on their debts even if they had not been pathological gamblers.

Many of the criticisms leveled at research on the identification and measurement of total debt for pathological gamblers can be leveled at research on other costs associated with pathological gambling. First, it is not sufficient to describe the characteristics of pathological gamblers under treatment and assume they are representative of the entire population of pathological gamblers. More effort must be made to determine whether the chosen subsample is representative. Second, a control group of people who are not pathological gamblers but who have similar demographic characteristics must be identified, and similar costs estimated for the control group to assist in the determination of the incremental or additional cost introduced by pathological gambling. Without this control group and the associated estimate of their costs, the estimated costs for the pathological gamblers represent the gross attributes of the pathological gambler population, rather than the incremental effect of pathological gambling.

Finally, a very difficult problem arises when assessing the costs of pathological gambling. Lesieur and others point out that there is a strong correlation between pathological gambling and other addictive behavior, such as alcohol and substance abuse (Lesieur, 1992). Thus, some of the problems observed in pathological gamblers may be caused not by pathological gambling but by (for example) alcoholism. Pathological gambling may be a symptom of other underlying disorders that would show up in other ways if legalized gambling were not available. A relevant question to ask is whether, in the absence of legalized gambling, a pathological gambler would have engaged in some similarly destructive and costly addiction, such as alcoholism. To the extent that the answer is yes, the costs associated with that individual's gambling problem are not additional costs to society. They represent transfers of costs from one problem category to another.

Clearly the task of identifying and measuring the costs of pathological gambling is far from a straightforward exercise. Even those effects that appear, at first glance, to be direct and tangible costs may, on closer investigation, be overstated or merely transfers. The need to engage in much more research in the area of identifying and estimating the impacts of pathological gambling should come as no surprise. There appears to be a dearth of literature dealing with the careful study of the economic and social effects of both casino gambling and gambling in general (Federal Reserve Bank of Boston, 1995).

ASSESSMENT OF STUDIES MEASURING THE COSTS AND BENEFITS OF GAMBLING[6]

Although there are studies that purport to investigate the economic effects of gambling, few show the careful, thorough efforts that are needed to estimate the actual net effects of gambling on society, and therefore few have made a real contribution to understanding these issues (e.g., Ricardo, 1998). In general, economic impact studies fall into three groups. The first group of studies, gross impact studies, tends to focus on only one aspect of the issue (e.g., positive economic effects) and therefore fails to provide a balanced perspective. A second group, descriptive studies, provides little more than descriptions that suggest what needs to be done to identify benefits and costs. A third group of studies, balanced measurement studies, attempts to provide a balanced analysis of the net effects of gambling. Studies in these groups range in quality and contribution, demonstrating an evolutionary developmental path, especially in their attention to the costs of pathological and problem gambling. Earlier studies tend to rely heavily on third-party calculations to arrive at their estimates of the costs of problem gambling. Later studies actually

[6]The committee thanks Rina Gupta for her investigation and written summary of state-level lottery and gambling commission reports.

build such estimates from scratch. Each group of studies is examined in more detail below.

Gross Impact Studies

Gross impact studies focus on a single aspect of economic effect. They generally do not pretend to provide a balanced perspective of gambling's effects. Typically, most emphasis is placed on identifying and quantifying economic benefits, with little effort placed on the identification of costs. In their most basic form, this kind of study provides a simple accounting of the aggregate effects of gambling, covering items such as casino revenues and expenditures, number of jobs created, and taxes paid. They do not try to consider expenditure substitution effects or to be explicit about the geographic scope of the analysis. They also typically ignore the distinction between direct and indirect effects, tangible and intangible effects, and real and transfer effects (Fahrenkopf, 1995; Meyer-Arendt 1995).

A slightly more sophisticated form of gross impact analysis involves the use of input-output analysis to capture both the direct and the indirect effects associated with gambling. The first step involved in capturing direct and indirect effects is to measure the final demand for the gambling industry. In the case of casino gambling, final demand is determined by examining the casino's employment expenditures, its capital investment outlays, the goods and services it purchases in order to operate, and the taxes it pays. In essence, final demand is the flow of dollars from the casino business to households, other businesses, and government (Illinois Gaming Board, 1996). Multipliers derived from input-output models are then used to estimate the ripple effects of the casino's expenditures through the community.[7] However, if the study fails to consider substitution of expenditures and leakage outside the local economy, use of the input-output technique

---

[7]Because there is no specific multiplier for the gambling industry, the entertainment and recreation sector multiplier often is used as a proxy because gambling is contained in this Census Bureau category.

can overstate the economic impact (Anders, 1997; Hewings et al., 1995, 1998).[8]

The most sophisticated gross impact studies painstakingly attempt to measure the net positive economic effects of casino gambling without considering the full range of costs. These studies estimate the substitution of expenditures and the leakage of direct gambling expenditures that occur in an economy, along with the ripple effect that these expenditures have on the economy. An excellent example of this type of analysis is a study that looked at the economic effects that casinos have had in Illinois and Wisconsin (Thompson et al., 1996b). The authors constructed what they refer to as a monetary impact model using a detailed input-output analysis of each gambling jurisdiction in the two states. Not only did the researchers collect gambling operation expenditures and revenues, but they also determined the locations of the recipients of the gambling expenditures, which allowed them to ascertain what portion of the monetary flows came from and went to the local area, to other areas of the state, and out of state. The result was a set of estimates of the positive and negative monetary effects of casino gambling in both Illinois and Wisconsin. This, in turn, provided a good estimate of the positive effects of casinos in the two states.[9]

Descriptive Studies

A second set of studies generally emphasizes description over analysis. The emphasis in these studies tends to be on simple identification of benefits and costs associated with gambling, with limited emphasis on estimating their value (Aasved and Laundergan, 1993; Aasved, 1995; Stokowski, 1996). When an attempt is made to discuss economic effects, especially the social costs associated with problem gambling, the estimates are taken directly from other studies, without any independent analysis or attempts to

---

[8]Hewings et al. (1996) acknowledge that these are analyses of the gross impacts and do not attempt to consider those things that would reduce the gross impact.

[9]The authors were careful to point out that their analysis dealt only with the benefit side of the equation.

determine whether the results of other studies are applicable in the situation under investigation (Grinols, 1995).

Balanced Measurement Studies

Balanced measurement studies encompass a variety of economic impact analysis studies. Although these studies differ in their approaches and vary in their contributions to advancing gambling-related economic impact analysis, they all emphasize the identification and measurement of costs, including costs related to pathological and problem gambling. They also reflect a discernible evolution in the methodology used to arrive at impact estimates, beginning with a heavy reliance on earlier work and slowly moving to a more innovative approach. The strength of these studies precludes them from being relied on for policymaking, but it may not be long before useful studies are available. The six studies described exemplify the application of methodological considerations described above, as well as the progression of economic impact analysis in the field of pathological gambling.

Chicago Study

This study assessed the effects that additional pathological gamblers would have on Chicago with the introduction of casino gambling. Whenever possible, the authors assigned monetary values; when they could not, they at least discussed the costs that they could not quantify. Rather than building their cost estimates from scratch, the authors relied on previously published estimates of prevalence rates and gambling costs from other sites to estimate likely costs for Chicago (Politzer et al., 1981).

There is nothing inherently wrong with relying on estimates derived from other studies, as long as the estimates are appropriate for the task at hand. The analysts must understand the size, structure, and the composition of the sample that was used to arrive at the estimate; they must clarify the assumptions underlying the calculations, along with the influences the assumptions may have on the estimates; and they must determine if the characteristics of the source community are sufficiently similar to that of the subject community to allow the use of the estimates without reservations or adjustments. Unless these conditions are satisfied, the resultant estimates may be of questionable value. There is no evidence that the Chicago study attempted to consider whether the estimated costs and prevalence rates borrowed from other studies were appropriate to Chicago. In addition, the authors do not appear to have tried to separate real costs from transfer costs, nor did they try to estimate aggregate pathological gambling costs rather than incremental costs due to pathological gambling.

U.S. National Assessment

In a study that strays from traditional economic impact analysis, Grinols and Omorov (1995) attempted to determine, using benefit-cost analysis, whether improved access to casino gambling offsets the externality (or spillover) costs associated with pathological gambling. Their study takes a unique approach to the estimation of the net economic effects of gambling. Instead of focusing on a particular geographic area, as most economic impact studies do, they attempted to estimate the effect of increasing gambling accessibility nationwide. They define externality costs as criminal justice system costs, social service costs, and costs due to lost productivity. In order to estimate the per capita social costs due to pathological gambling, they relied on the annual cost estimates per pathological gambler and prevalence rates for pathological gambling computed in earlier studies (Goodman, 1994; Lorenz et al., 1990; Politzer et al., 1981). They do not, however, further the understanding of what constitutes the costs of pathological gambling or the magnitude of these costs. Instead, Grinols and Omorov relied on the work done by others to assign dollar values to the externalities and used these estimates without any attempt to determine whether the estimates were appropriate for the task at hand.

South Dakota Study

In a study that attempted to identify the benefits and costs associated with gambling, Madden (1991) looked at the socioeconomic costs of gambling in South Dakota. The analysis—a simple time series analysis of data for identified benefits and costs—represents one of the first attempts to determine whether some of the alleged costs associated with pathological and problem gambling were appearing in communities that were adopting or expanding legalized gambling. Madden does not specifically consider the costs of pathological and problem gambling but does analyze trends in factors that often are cited as being affected by such gambling, including the number of recipients of Aid to Families with Dependent Children, the number of families receiving food stamps, the number of child abuse and neglect cases, the number of child support cases, the number of divorce filings, the percentage of property taxes that are not collected, the number of bankruptcy filings, the number of small claims filings, and the number of real estate foreclosures.[10] He concluded that there does not appear to be any correlation between the increased availability of gambling and these socioeconomic indicators.

This study raises another potentially difficult problem with gambling studies. When gambling is introduced to an area, there is a natural temptation to do simple before-and-after comparisons and to attribute (positive or negative) differences to the introduction of gambling. In other words, the effects of gambling are deemed to be any changes that have occurred since gambling was introduced. But this is not necessarily true. For example, if per capita income is found to be higher after gambling was introduced, is the rise in income attributable to gambling? Perhaps it is, but perhaps not. Per capita incomes have typically been rising in the United States, so perhaps some of the gain is due simply to general economic growth. Perhaps other things happened in the community that would increase per capita income. During the same period in which per capita incomes were found to rise in the community in which gambling was introduced, per capita incomes may well have also risen in communities in which gam-

---

[10]Problem gambling has been linked to these factors, and one would expect problem gambling to be on the rise in South Dakota due to the spread of legalized gambling. Therefore a worsening in one or more of these factors may suggest that at least part of the costs are due to problem gambling.

bling was not introduced. Similarly, if personal bankruptcies increased following the introduction of gambling, the analyst would also need to know what the trend in personal bankruptcies was elsewhere and during the same time period before attributing the increase to increased gambling availability.

Florida Study

A Florida study of the effects of casino gambling represents an improvement in the identification and estimation of the benefits and costs of pathological and problem gambling (Florida Office of Planning and Budgeting, 1994). Its derivation of the net positive benefits considered the direct and indirect effects that casinos will have on the state economy, carefully considering expenditure substitution and leakage to ensure that the focus is on additional spending associated with the casino and not some measure of gross economic activity.

To estimate the costs associated with pathological and problem gambling, the study relied on an estimate calculated by Volberg (1994) of $13,600 on average per pathological or problem gambler. Rather than accept the Volberg estimate without question, the researchers examined circumstances specific to Florida to ensure that the estimates were appropriate. This was accomplished by estimating the incarceration, supervision, and new prison construction costs that would be attributable to problem gambler criminal incidents, using Florida Department of Corrections data. These estimates indicated that Volberg's annual societal cost figures were reasonable to use for estimating potential impacts in Florida.

In order to determine the increase in pathological and problem gamblers that would result from casino gambling, the study also relied on estimates generated from three different sources, rather than adopting without question a prevalence rate generated for a different single community. The three estimates are based on: (1) the projected market share that casinos would command in the legalized gambling market in the state, (2) a number derived from experiential data provided by the Florida Council on Compulsive Gambling, and (3) a figure based on information provided by the National Council on Compulsive Gambling. The estimates for increased numbers of pathological and problem gamblers were multiplied by the estimated social cost per such gambler to arrive at total net cost estimates of $3.8 billion, $3.22 billion, and $2.72 billion. Subtracting the estimated net positive effect of casino gambling— $536 million—the study concluded that the net cost of casinos in Florida would range from $2.16 billion to $3.25 billion.

The Florida study cost estimation methodology is noteworthy because, although the study relied on per gambler estimates calculated for another jurisdiction, it first assessed the appropriateness of applying that estimate to Florida. In addition, the study used three prevalence estimates derived from three communities rather than relying on a single generic estimated prevalence rate. Taken together, the per pathological gambler cost estimate and the three prevalence estimates enabled the analysts to provide a range of costs attributable to pathological gamblers if casinos were approved in Florida.

Unfortunately, the study was based on several key but untested assumptions that may have had the effect of overestimating costs associated with pathological and problem gambling and minimizing the benefits of casino gambling. Specifically, the researchers advance a conservative estimate of new tourism and also assumed that Florida would experience substantial substitution effects in the food and recreation industries if casino gambling were approved. Closer examination also reveals that, in relying on the Volberg (1994) cost to society estimate per pathological or problem gambler, the state adopted her reliance on the estimate by Lesieur and Klien (1985) that two out of three pathological or problem gamblers become incarcerated or otherwise impose substantial criminal justice costs—an assumption not independently tested.

Australian Study

A significant improvement in the methodology used to identify and estimate the social costs of gambling, and specifically pathological and problem gambling, is found in a study conducted in Australia (Dickerson et al., 1995). This study apparently is one of the first studies to perform a comprehensive and carefully thought-out economic impact analysis of gambling.[11] The study is based on what is referred to as a doorknock, or house-to-house, survey. The survey provides extensive information about patterns of gambling in New South Wales, attitudes toward gambling, gambling preferences, and information relating to the negative effects associated with problem gambling, among other things. The study details the approach taken to estimate the prevalence of problem gambling. Clearly, the researchers carefully considered the appropriateness of their estimate for the subject community, not choosing to rely on estimates developed elsewhere. To identify the costs associated with problem gambling, the researchers used information from their survey and from their own clinical databases. Once the identification phase was completed, they used the following methodology to place a dollar value on as many of the costs as they could (pp. 57-58):

- "the cost of impacts is undertaken from a community perspective. Personal costs, which involve a transfer of money between different sectors of the economy, without impinging on economic activity (such as the stock of debts owed by gamblers), are not included

- prevalence was estimated either from the survey results or, where more appropriate, from the clinical databases available

- responses to survey questions were grouped and directly linked to impacts where appropriate

- the team's professional judgment was used to decide whether the survey results or incidence from clinical databases were used as the basis for costings

---

[11]The reason for a lack of precision regarding whether this indeed is the first study of its type is attributable to information provided in another study, Study Concerning the Effects of Legalized Gambling on the Citizens of the State of Connecticut (report prepared for the Division of Special Revenue, Department of Revenue Services, State of Connecticut, June 1997). This study refers to five noteworthy studies that have been conducted in this area: a 1994 study in Quebec, a 1995 study in Germany, a 1995 study in Illinois, a 1995 study in Australia, and a 1996 study in Wisconsin. Only the last two studies were obtained by the committee, leading to uncertainty as to whether the Australian study is the first or one of the first studies to undertake this approach to the estimation of pathological gambling costs.

- the incidence of each impact was converted to annual cases per annum for the [New South Wales] adult population . . .
- costing assumptions were then sourced or estimated for each impact and applied to the prevalence data. . . . It should be added that we have been conservative in our costing assumptions, where data on which to base assumptions [have] not been readily available."

The study was able to "cost out" a number of factors associated with pathological gambling. The effects of gambling on employment, consisting of job change costs, unemployment, and productivity loss, were estimated at A$27.8 million annually.[12] The largest component of this estimate was productivity loss, accounting for almost A$20 million, followed by A$5.2 million for job change and A$2.7 million for unemployment.

The process used to arrive at the productivity loss estimate shows the care the researchers used as they developed their cost estimates. They looked at data from both the survey and the clinics to identify employment-related costs and the extent to which problem gamblers were affected. On the basis of these data, the productivity loss estimate was derived using an assumption that one hour per week was lost per problem gambler, an estimate of the number of problem gamblers affected, the average earnings earned, and the percentage of individuals in the workplace versus the home. The authors also were careful to underscore how sensitive the estimate is to the assumption regarding average time lost at work.

A second factor associated with problem gambling in the study is legal costs. Legal costs were separated into court costs, estimated at an annual cost of A$5.6 million; prison costs, estimated at an annual cost of approximately A$9 million; and police costs, estimated at an annual cost of A$2.6 million. The total estimate of legal costs emanating from problem gambling in New South Wales was approximately A$17.2 million.

Although an estimate is included for family and individual

---

[12]Because this study was conducted in Australia, the monetary amounts presumably are in Australian dollars.

costs, the researchers note that many of the family-related effects identified do not lend themselves to quantification because it would involve a very subjective process. As a result, only two family and individual effects are given a dollar value: the costs of divorce proceedings and acute treatment costs.[13] Total family and individual costs amounted to A$0.7 million, with A$300,000 coming from divorce proceedings and A$455,000 from acute treatment. Financial impacts on the family and the individual due to problem gambling are estimated by determining the dollar amount of business and personal bankruptcies, estimated at A$65,000. Finally, the researchers costed out the value of existing services that are provided for problem gamblers and their families, which are estimated at slightly less than A$2.3 million per year.[14]

The total cost associated with pathological and problem gambling was estimated at A$48.1 million per year, or A$9.70 per capita among the adult population in New South Wales. This estimate is compared with the A$2.9 billion in net benefit introduced by gambling in New South Wales. The methodology used by the researchers to reach this estimate of net positive effect involved the use of input-output multipliers, carefully adjusted for substitution of expenditures and leakage. It is noted that the costs amount to 1.6 percent of the estimated positive effects. However, the authors are quick to note that they use conservative costing assumptions and that a number of the effects identified are not assigned dollar values. The net economic benefit is therefore likely to be overstated.

Wisconsin Study

A second study that makes a significant contribution to the literature on the economic impacts of gambling is one that identi-

---

[13]The acute treatment incidence was based on reported suicide attempts, taken from the clinical database.

[14]The authors are quick to note that this estimate does not include any additional costs that may be incurred due to the need for additional services in the future.

fies and quantifies the social costs of gambling in the state of Wisconsin (Thompson et al., 1996a). The authors point out that there is little objective information about the benefits and costs associated with gambling, much less the costs of pathological and problem gambling, but that many studies have offered opinions about the effects such gambling has on society. "However, for the most part, we have only seen attempts either to list all the cost factors without analysis, and without totaling up the effects, or we have seen concluding numbers without any indication of how the numbers were determined" (Thompson et al., 1996a:13).

The approach taken by these researchers to arrive at estimates of the costs of pathological and problem gambling involved using a survey instrument to get information from serious problem gamblers in Wisconsin (Thompson et al., 1996a). They distributed questionnaires to members of Gamblers Anonymous chapters and received 98 completed surveys. The questionnaires provided the researchers with demographic data on the respondents, gambling histories, information about some of the games they played, volume of gambling activity and the source of funds, and the consequences of gambling. The authors used the information obtained from the survey to attempt to answer the following questions: (1) How much does one serious problem gambler cost society? (2) How much do the serious problem gamblers of Wisconsin cost Wisconsin society? (3) What are the societal costs of having casinos in Wisconsin?

To answer these questions, they used information from their survey as well as information provided by earlier research on the costs of problem gambling. They chose to focus on employment costs, bad debts and civil court costs, thefts and criminal justice system costs, therapy costs, and welfare costs. They calculated the costs for all problem gamblers in the state and for a subset of problem gamblers who could be associated with the state's American Indian casinos. Employment costs included both the annual cost of working hours lost due to gambling plus the unemployment compensation attributable to gambling. It was estimated that the annual cost of lost working hours amounted to $1,330 per problem gambler for all problem gamblers in the state, and $1,390 per problem gambler for those who gambled at American Indian casinos. Annual unemployment compensation costs were calculated as $210 for all problem gamblers and $120 for the casino gamblers.

Estimates of the loss in productivity due to gambling were based on how many hours of work the gambler lost due to unemployment. The researchers chose to use this measure rather than attempt to estimate the loss of productivity on the job, which they thought involved too much subjectivity. The estimates for annual loss in productivity amounted to $1,400 for all gamblers and $1,330 for casino gamblers. Adding these estimates together provides a total employment cost estimate of $2,940 for all gamblers and $2,840 for casino gamblers. Bad debts were calculated by focusing on the debt burden of the problem gamblers in the study who were involved in bankruptcy court proceedings. These individuals had an average debt of $8,910. It was assumed that society lost half of these debts, with an annualized value of $1,490 for all gamblers and $2,130 for casino gamblers. Thompson et al. (1996a) note that these are very conservative estimates because they looked only at those who declared bankruptcy and accounted for only half of their debt. In reality, it is likely that many problem gamblers will ultimately pay little of their debts.

Annual criminal justice costs include a number of factors, including bankruptcy court costs, estimated at $330 for all gamblers and $510 for casino gamblers; the cost of civil cases, estimated at $510 for all gamblers and $530 for casino gamblers; the cost of criminal cases, estimated at $370 for all gamblers and $510 for casino gamblers; the cost of probation, estimated at $190 for all gamblers and $190 for casino gamblers; the cost of imprisonment, estimated at $1,160 for all gamblers and $760 for casino gamblers; and the cost of arrests, estimated at $50 for all gamblers and $40 for casino gamblers. Summing the estimates for these factors led to estimates of $2,610 for all gamblers and $2,550 for casino gamblers for annual total police and judicial costs. An additional criminal justice cost, the cost of thefts, was estimated at $1,730 for all gamblers and $1,670 for casino gamblers. These estimates were combined with the bad debt estimates to provide the estimates for the annual total bad debt and theft-related costs per gambler.

Thompson et al. (1996a) estimated therapy costs as $360 for all gamblers and $440 for casino gamblers based on the assumption that half of the costs were individual and half would be borne by society. Estimates for additional costs due to gambling amounted to, for food stamps, $100 for all gamblers and $140 for casino gamblers and, for Aid for Families with Dependent Children, to $230 for all gamblers and $360 for casino gamblers. Total health and welfare-related costs therefore amounted to $700 for all gamblers and $920 for casino gamblers. Even this study, however, is not without serious flaws and often counts as benefits things that would properly have been considered transfers. Nevertheless, this study is an important improvement over many previous ones.

The researchers compare their estimates of the annual total social costs for the state of Wisconsin due to problem gambling— $307 million for all gamblers including $138 million for casino gamblers to estimates of the net positive effects of gambling activities estimated in an earlier study (Thompson et al., 1995). That study determined that the state of Wisconsin experienced an annual economic gain of $326 million from gambling activities and related expenditures at or near the 17 casino sites. Combining the two estimates for the positive impact and the negative impact associated with casino gambling ($326 million and $138 million, respectively), social costs represent about 42 percent of the economic gain, and the net economic impact on the Wisconsin economy due to casinos is approximately $188 million.

Thompson et al. argue that their estimates of the social costs of problem gambling are conservative but realistic, although others have suggested the estimates are too high (see Walker and Barnett, 1997). Thompson et al. point out that the calculations are based on information obtained from the survey of problem gamblers and other outside sources. In addition, they are careful to identify the assumptions and methodology used in the calculations, something most previous studies failed to do. The researchers underscore the intentional conservatism of their analysis (Thompson et al., 1996a:26):

> We wish the information we present to be useful for policy makers, so we have carefully avoided adding numbers into the formula where we felt that we could not reasonably make good assumptions and good estimates of the costs. Nonetheless, we suspect that the areas not considered do represent social costs, and these may be

revealed in more refined studies in the future. Some areas where costs must exist, but were not considered, include the lower productivity on the job, family disorganization, and bad debts by those who do not declare bankruptcy.

Thompson et al. (1996a) acknowledge the estimate of productivity loss used in the Chicago study by Politzer et al. (1981) but do not use it because they found it unreasonable. Because they did not have sufficient information themselves to make a reasonable estimate, they chose to not make one.

CONCLUSIONS

Despite the recent improvements made in the estimation of the benefits and costs of gambling, this area of inquiry is still in its infancy. A very few studies have recently made large strides over the contributions of earlier studies, which generally focused only on the positive economic benefits or provided descriptions of the cost factors associated with pathological and problem gambling, but did not attempt to estimate the costs of gambling, much less the costs of pathological and problem gambling. Still, benefit-cost analysis of pathological and problem gambling remains undeveloped.

In most of the impact analyses of gambling and of pathological and problem gambling, the methods used are so inadequate as to invalidate the conclusions. Researchers in this area have struggled with the absence of systematic data that could inform their analysis and consequently have substituted assumptions for the missing data. The assumptions adopted for specific studies were rarely examined or tested to ensure they were appropriate for the specific research being conducted. There is always the risk that such assumptions and resulting estimates may reflect the bias of the analyst rather than the best-informed judgment. Critical estimates have been frequently taken from one study and haphazardly applied in different circumstances. Often, the costs and benefits were not properly identified so that things that should have been counted as costs or benefits were omitted and other things that should have been omitted were counted. Even when these limitations were recognized by the authors, they were rarely acknowledged.

Clearly there continues to be a need for more objective and extensive analysis of the economic impact that gambling has on the economy. Although the methodology to estimate the net positive effects is fairly well developed, substantial work needs to be done on the cost side. It is especially important to focus on the effects that are associated with problem gambling. The task will not be easy and the effort will be costly and time-consuming. The Australian and Wisconsin research studies have set the stage for others by outlining the process that needs to be followed and by showing how such studies should proceed. These studies do have their limitations, however. For example, more attention could have been focused on ensuring that the costs being estimated are real costs and not just transfers. But they provide a framework so that others can replicate their findings and to advance knowledge about the costs of problem gambling.

Other important issues remain unexplored. One issue is the question of how important the problem gambler is to the gambling industry's financial health. A casual look at the casino industry suggests that this is an industry with high fixed costs and very low marginal costs to serve an additional patron. If that is indeed the industry's cost structure, then very little additional revenue can result in substantial increases in profits. By the same token, a small decrease in revenue can result in a substantial decrease in profits. Thus, even if problem gambling proves not to be very prevalent in aggregate terms, it could still have a substantial influence on industry profits. Another unexplored issue is to what degree the findings on the economic impact of casino gambling apply to other forms of gambling. As this chapter indicates, most of the research deals with casinos. We know little about the economic impact of other forms of gambling. Finally, few of the studies on the economic impact of gambling to date have appeared in peer-reviewed publications. Most have appeared as reports, chapters in books, or proceedings at conferences, and those few that have been subject to peer review have, for the most part, been descriptive pieces. As this research evolves, it should be subjected to peer review to help ensure that it indeed is advancing the body of knowledge.

REFERENCES

Aasved, M.J.
1995 Legalized gambling and its impacts in a central Minnesota vacation community: A case study. *Journal of Gambling Studies* 11(2):137-163.

Aasved, M.J., and J.C. Laundergan
1993 Gambling and its impacts in a Northeastern Minnesota commmunity: An exploratory study. *Journal of Gambling Studies* 9(4):301-319.

Abbott, D.A., S.L. Cramer, and S.D. Sherrets
1995 Pathological gambling and the family: Practice implications. *Families in Society* 76(4):213-219.

American Psychiatric Association
1994 *DSM-IV: Diagnostic and Statistical Manual of Mental Disorders,* 4th ed. Washington, DC: American Psychiatric Association.

Anders, G.C.
1996 The Indian Gaming Regulatory Act and Native American development. *International Policy Review* 6(1):84-90.
1997 *Estimating the Economic Impact of Indian Casino Gambling: A Case Study of the Fort McDowell Reservation.* Reno: Institute for the Study of Gambling and Commercial Gaming, University of Nevada.

Bergh, C., and E. Kuhlhorn
1994 Social, psychological and physical consequences of pathological gambling in Sweden. *Journal of Gambling Studies* 10(3):275-285.

Bland, R.C., S.C. Newman, H. Orn, and G. Stebelsky
1993 Epidemiology of pathological gambling in Edmonton. *Canadian Journal of Psychology* 38:108-112.

Blaszczysnki, A.P., and N. McConaghy
1994a Antisocial personality disorder and pathological gambling. *Journal of Gambling Studies* 10(2):129-145.
1994b Criminal offenses in Gamblers Anonymous and hospital treated pathological gamblers. *Journal of Gambling Studies* 10(2):99-127.

Blaszczynski, A.P., and D. Silove
1996 Pathological gambling: Forensic issues. *Australian and New Zealand Journal of Psychiatry* 30(3):358-369.

Boreham, P., M. Dickerson, and B. Harley
1996 What are the social costs of gambling? The case of the Queensland machine gaming industry. *Australian Journal of Social Issues* 31(4):425-442.

Chadbourne, C., P. Walker, and M. Wolfe
1997 *Gambling, Economic Development, and Historic Preservation.* Chicago: American Planning Association.

Cornell, S., J. Kalt, M. Krepps, and J. Taylor
1998 *American Indian Gambling Policy and Its Socioeconomic Effects: A Report to the National Gambling Impact Study Commission.* Cambridge, MA: The Economics Resource Group, Inc.

Cozzetto, D.A.
1995   The economic and social implications of Indian gambling: The case of Minnesota. *American Indian Culture and Research Journal* 19(1):119-131.

Custer, R.L., and L.F. Custer
1978   Characteristics of the Recovering Compulsive Gambler: A Survey of 150 Members of Gamblers Anonymous. Paper presented at the Fourth Annual Conference on Gambling, Reno, NV, December.

Custer, R.L., and H. Milt
1985   *When Luck Runs Out.* New York: Facts on File Publications.

Dickerson, M., C. Allcock, A. Blaszczynski, B. Nicholls, J. Williams, and R. Maddern
1995   *An Examination of the Socioeconomic Effects of Gambling on Individuals, Families, and the Community Including Research into the Costs of Problem Gambling to New South Wales.* Sydney: Australian Institute for Gambling Research.

Eadington, W.R.
1984   The casino gaming industry: A study of political economy. *Annals of the American Academy of Political and Social Science* 474:23-35.

Fahrenkopf, F.J., Jr.
1995   Testimony. *Hearing on the Gambling Impact Study Commission,* Committee on Governmental Affairs, U.S. Senate, November 2. Washington, DC: U.S. Government Printing Office.

Federal Reserve Bank of Boston
1995   Casino Development: How Would Casinos Affect New England's Economy? Proceedings of a Symposium Sponsored by the Federal Bank of Boston, June 1.

Filby, M.P., and L. Harvey
1988   Recreational betting: Everyday activity and strategies. *Leisure Studies* 7(2)(May):159-172.

Fisher, S.
1991   Governmental response to juvenile fruit machine gambling in the U.K.: Where do we go from here? *Journal of Gambling Studies* 7(3):217-247.

Florida Office of Planning and Budgeting
1994   *The Anticipated Impact of Casino Gambling in Florida.* Florida Bureau of Economic Analysis, Department of Commerce. Tallahassee, FL: The Executive Office of the Governor.

Frank, M.L., D. Lester, and A. Wexler
1991   Suicidal behavior among members of Gamblers Anonymous. *Journal of Gambling Studies* 7:249-254.

Goodman, R.
1994   *Legalized Gambling as a Strategy for Economic Development.* Northampton, MA: United States Gambling Study.

Gramlich, E.M.
1990   The fundamental principle of benefit-cost analysis. Chapter 3. In *A Guide to Benefit-Cost Analysis, Second Edition.* Englewood Cliffs, NJ: Prentice Hall, Inc.

Grinols, E.L.
   1995   Incentives explain gambling's growth. *Forum for Applied Research and Public Policy* 11(Summer):119-124.

Grinols, E. L., and J.D. Omorov
   1995   Development or dreamfield illusions: Assessing casino gambling's costs and benefits. Pp. 384-405 in *Hearing on the Gambling Impact Study Commission*, Committee on Governmental Affairs, U.S. Senate, November 2. Washington, DC: U.S. Government Printing Office.

Hewings, G.J.D., and M. Madden, eds.
   1995   *Social and Demographic Accounting.* New York: Cambridge University Press.

Hewings, G.J.D., G.R. Schindler, D. Anderson, and Y. Okuyama
   1998   *The Impact of Riverboat Casino Gambling on the Illinois Economy 1995.* Report prepared for the Illinois Gaming Board. Champaign: University of Illinois.

Illinois Gaming Board
   1996   *The Economic and Fiscal Impacts of Riverboat Casino Gambling in Illinois. Phase One: Direct Impact Data, 1991-1995,* J.T. Johnson, M.A. Belletire, and D.S. O'Brien, authors. Springfield: Illinois Gaming Board.

Ison, C.
   1995a Dead broke. *Star Tribune,* December 5, 1995. News section.
   1995b Dead broke. *Star Tribune,* December 3, 1995. News section.

Jacobs, D.F., A.R. Marston, R.D. Singer, K. Widaman, et al.
   1989   Children of problem gamblers. Special Issue: Gambling and the Family. *Journal of Gambling Behavior* 5(4)(Winter):261-268.

Ladouceur, R., J.M. Boisvert, M. Pepin, M. Loranger, and C. Sylvain
   1994   Social costs of pathological gambling. *Journal of Gambling Studies* 10:399-409.

Lesieur, H.R.
   1987   Gambling, pathological gambling and crime. In *The Handbook of Pathological Gambling*, Thomas Galski, ed. Springfield, IL: Charles C. Thomas.
   1989   Experience of employee assistance programs with pathological gamblers. *Journal of Drug Issues* 19(4):425-436.
   1992   Compulsive gambling. *Society* 29(4):43-50.
   1998   Costs and treatment of pathological gambling. *Annals of the American Academy* 556:153-171.

Lesieur, H.R., and C. Anderson
   1995   Results of a Survey of Gamblers Anonymous Members in Illinois. Illinois Council on Problem and Compulsive Gambling.

Lesieur, H.R., and S.B. Blume
   1991   Evaluation of patients treated for pathological gambling in a combined alcohol, substance abuse, and pathological gambling treatment unit using the Addiction Severity Index. *British Journal of Addiction* 86:1017-1028.

Lesieur, H.R., and R. Klein
  1985   Prisoners, gambling and crime. Paper presented at the Annual Meeting of the Academy of Criminal Justice Sciences, Las Vegas, NV, April 2. Institute for Problem Gambling, Middletown, CT.
Lesieur, H.R., and J. Rothschild
  1989   Children of Gamblers Anonymous members. *Journal of Gambling Behavior* 5:269-281.
Livingston, J.
  1974   *Compulsive Gamblers: Observations on Action and Abstinence.* New York: Harper Torchbooks.
Lorenz, V.C., R.M. Politzer, and R.A. Yaffee
  1990   Final Report of the Maryland Task Force on Gambling Addiction.
Lorenz, V.C., and D.E. Shuttlesworth
  1983   The impact of pathological gambling on the spouse of the gambler. *Journal of Community Psychology* 11:67-76.
Lorenz, V.C., and R.A. Yaffee
  1986   Pathological gambling: Psychosomatic, emotional and marital difficulties as reported by the gambler. *Journal of Gambling Behavior* 2(1):40-49.
  1988   Pathological gambling: Psychosomatic, emotional, and marital difficulties as reported by the spouse. *Journal of Gambling Behavior* 4:13-26.
Madden, M.K.
  1991   *Economic and Fiscal Impacts Associated with the First Year of Gaming: Deadwood, South Dakota.* Pierre: South Dakota Commission on Gaming.
McCormick, R.A., A.M. Russo, L.F. Ramirez, and J.I. Taber
  1984   Affective disorders among pathological gamblers seeking treatment. *American Journal of Psychiatry* 141:215-218.
McMillen, J.
  1991   The impact of casinos in Australian cities. Pp. 87-102 in *Gambling and Public Policy: International Perspectives,* William R. Eadington and Judy A. Cornelius, eds. Reno: Institute for the Study of Gambling and Commercial Gaming, University of Nevada.
Meyer, G., and T. Fabian
  1992   Delinquency among pathological gamblers: A causal approach. *Journal of Gambling Studies* 8(1):61-77.
Meyer-Arendt, K.J.
  1995   Casino gaming in Mississippi: Location, location, location. *Economic Development Review* 13(4):27-33.
Moran, E.
  1969   Taking the final risk. *Mental Health* 3(Winter):21-22 (London).
Oddo, A.R.
  1997   The economics and ethics of casino gambling. *Review of Business* 18(3):4-8.

Oster, C.V., B.M. Rubin, and J.S. Strong
1997 Economic impacts of transportation investments: The case of Federal Express. *Transportation Journal* 37(2):34-44.

Politzer, R.M., J.S. Morrow, and S. Leavy
1981 Report on the societal cost of pathological gambling and the cost benefit/effectiveness of treatment. *Proceedings of the 1981 Conference on Gambling.* Reno: University of Nevada.

Ricardo, G.
1998 The economic impacts of casino gambling at the state and local levels. *Annals of the American Academy of Political and Social Science* 556(March):66-84.

Richardson, H.W.
1972 *Input-Output and Regional Economics.* New York: John Wiley.

Schwarz, J., and A. Lindner
1992 Inpatient treatment of male pathological gamblers in Germany. *Journal of Gambling Studies* 8:93-109.

Stokowski, P.A.
1996 *Riches and Regrets: Betting on Gambling in Two Colorado Mountain Towns.* Niwot: University Press of Colorado.

Thompson, W.N., R. Gazel, and D. Rickman
1995 *The Economic Impact of Native American Gaming in Wisconsin.* Milwaukee: Wisconsin Policy Research Institute.
1996a *Casinos and Crime in Wisconsin: What's the Connection?* Thiensville: Wisconsin Policy Research Institute Inc.
1996b The social costs of gambling in Wisconsin. *Wisconsin Policy Research Institute Report* 9(6):1-44.

U.S. Department of Commerce
1992 *Regional Multipliers: A User Handbook for the Regional Input-Output Modeling System (RIMS II).* Washington, DC: U.S. Department of Commerce.

Volberg, R.A.
1994 The prevalence and demographics of pathological gamblers: Implications for public health. *American Journal of Public Health* 84:237-241.

Walker, Douglas M., and A.H. Barnett
1997 The Social Costs of Legalized Gambling Reconsidered. Unpublished manuscript, Department of Economics, Auburn University, May.

6

Treatment of Pathological Gamblers

The treatments and interventions for pathological gambling that have been developed and reported in the literature are quite similar to methods of treating other disorders or addictions. Substantial progress has not been made in understanding the treatment of this disorder or the characteristics of those seeking help for it, nor is there research basis for matching clients to treatments. Most published investigations are case studies or studies with small samples of clients whose circumstances may not be generalizable to larger populations (Knapp and Lech, 1987; Murray, 1993). Moreover, treatment approaches have not been subjected to rigorous and detailed empirical research (Blaszczynski and Silove, 1995). Given the lack of national attention to the treatment of pathological gambling, it is difficult to estimate the scope of intervention services available in the United States.

We begin with a discussion of the definition of treatment and challenges in treating such disorders as pathological gambling. We then discuss what is known about the characteristics of those who seek treatment for pathological gambling. We then turn to treatment models that have been applied for helping pathological gamblers, what is known about treatment effectiveness, whether treatment is warranted, and issues related to treatment availability, utilization, funding, and treatment providers in the United

States. We also identify priorities for further research, including treatment effectiveness, cost-effectiveness, how patients should be matched to treatments, and prevention strategies.

DEFINING TREATMENT AND CHALLENGES TO TREATMENT

In the committee's view, the definition of treatment needs to be a broad one. We define treatment as: (1) activities directed at individuals for the purpose of reducing problems associated with problem or pathological gambling and (2) activities aimed at groups of individuals (e.g., communities) to prevent gambling problems from arising in the first place. Comprehensive treatments move through three stages: acute intervention, followed by rehabilitation, and ending with maintenance. These three stages can vary according to the philosophy of the providers, the settings in which treatment takes place, and the specific approaches employed. No systematic compilation of treatment services for pathological gambling has been made in the United States. Treatment is provided in many ways and in many settings, although outpatient treatment is probably the most common; no single treatment approach dominates the field. In fact, it appears to be common for approaches to be combined in most clinical settings. It is important, as well, to recognize that recovery from pathological gambling can take place without formal treatment. Such individuals have been classified by various descriptors, for example, so-called spontaneous recovery and natural recovery (Wynne, personal communication, 1998). Although the subject of natural recovery from psychoactive substances, such as alcohol and opiates, has received some attention in the professional literature (McCartney, 1996), no such attention has been given to gambling.

Functionality of Addictive Behaviors

All addictions, by their nature, pose special problems to treatment providers. Like other purposive human behavior, addictive behaviors have adaptive or functional value, with the result that efforts to change these behaviors often fail.

Ambivalence is at the core of addiction (Shaffer, 1997). Those who are addicted and thinking about change want to free themselves from their addiction. At the same time, they crave the satisfactions that their addiction provides. As they become aware of the harm their addiction is doing, they begin to say that they want to quit. Of course, wishing or expressing a desire to quit a behavior is not the same as doing it. Despite the obvious harmful consequences, people in the throes of addiction cling to the part of the experience that they like: the part that was adaptive originally and may have even produced positive consequences, such as relief from painful emotions (Khantzian et al., 1990). The key to change comes when those addicted begin to realize that the costs of their addiction exceed the benefits, as when pathological gamblers identify gambling as a destructive agent in their life. It is at this point that addicted people often ask those who they trust to help them stop, and they take the first steps to seek professional help. This turning point is but the first step of a complex dynamic process, including the possibility that bouts of abstinence and relapse may occur for some time (Marlatt and Gordon, 1985).

Preventing Relapse

A challenge in the treatment of pathological gambling is preventing relapse. For example, few people who stop using drugs remain abstinent thereafter. Marlatt and Gordon examined how slips, that is, single episodes of drug use, can lead to a full-blown relapse (Marlatt and Gordon, 1985). Many personal and environmental factors interact to influence the risk of relapse for any individual trying to recover from an addiction. Successful recovery also involves the development of new skills and lifestyle patterns that promote positive patterns of behavior. The integration of these behaviors into day-to-day activities is the essence of relapse prevention (Brownell et al., 1986). Successful quitters substitute a variety of behavior patterns for their old drug-using lifestyle. For example, many take up some form of exercise. Spiritual conversions sustain others. In some patients, new behavior can become excessive, almost another addiction. We do not know whether the same substitute behaviors occur in pathological gamblers determined to quit.

CHARACTERISTICS OF TREATMENT SEEKERS[1]

Understanding the characteristics of those who seek help for a given disorder can assist in developing effective treatments. As already noted, most clinical investigations in this field are case studies or studies with small samples of clients whose data may not be generalizable to larger populations. Thus, establishing an accurate profile of those seeking treatment is difficult. We can say a few things, however.

Demographics

Treatment seekers tend to be white middle-aged men (Blackman et al., 1989; Ciarrocchi and Richardson, 1989; Volberg, 1994; Volberg and Steadman, 1988), although more recent investigations suggest that admissions of women are increasing (Moore, 1998; Stinchfield and Winters, 1996). The majority tend to be in their 30s and 40s and have graduated from high school and attended some college (Blackman et al., 1989; Moore, 1998; Yaffee et al., 1993; Stinchfield and Winters, 1996).

Gambling Severity

Most clinical studies indicate that, before pathological gamblers come in for treatment, they gamble either every day or every week (Moore, 1998; Stinchfield and Winters, 1996). Little is known at this time about their preferences for types of gambling. One factor that may influence preference is proximity of certain games to gamblers; for example, one study showed that the preferred game of gamblers in Maryland was horse racing at Maryland tracks (Yaffee et al., 1993), and for Oregon clients, it was the video poker that is widely available there (Moore, 1998). Game availability does not simply translate to preference. Minnesota gamblers have been shown to prefer to gamble in casinos, which may be far from their homes, over purchasing lottery tickets,

---

[1]The committee thanks Randy Stinchfield for his written summary and presentation of the literature in this section.

which can be bought almost everywhere in the state (Stinchfield and Winters, 1996).

Legal and Financial Consequences

Although clients may be reluctant to fully disclose their legal entanglements, most clinical studies indicate that a sizable percentage reports having criminal charges pending as a result of engaging in illegal activity to fund their gambling or pay off their debts (Yaffee et al., 1993; Stinchfield and Winters, 1996; Taber et al., 1987). Some reports indicate that from half to two-thirds of pathological gamblers have committed an illegal act to get money to gamble (Dickerson, 1989; Dickerson et al., 1990; Lesieur et al., 1986). Large debts, most often in the tens of thousands of dollars, are also part of the picture (Blackman et al., 1989; Moore, 1998; Stinchfield and Winters, 1996). One study reported that 10 percent of 128 gamblers ages 20 to 68 treated as outpatients at a gamblers' treatment clinic had debts in excess of $100,000 (Blackman et al., 1989).

Other Characteristics

Additional personal and social consequences reported by those seeking treatment include work absenteeism and lost productivity on the job, presumably because they either skip work in order to gamble or are involved in gambling-related activities while at work; and marital discord and family estrangement, due to the deception, lying, and stealing associated with their gambling (Ciarrocchi and Richardson, 1989; Ladouceur et al., 1994; Lorenz and Yaffee, 1988; Stinchfield and Winters, 1996).

Comorbidity

As discussed in Chapter 4, a number of studies have found significant rates of cooccurring mental disorders and psychiatric symptoms among pathological gamblers. Studies have indicated evidence of pathological gambling cooccurring with substance use disorders, depression, suicidal thoughts and attempts, and various personality disorders.

TREATMENT APPROACHES AND EFFECTIVENESS

Methods for treating pathological gambling include approaches that are psychoanalytic, psychodynamic, behavioral, cognitive, pharmacological, addiction-based and multimodal, and self-help. Often these approaches are combined to varying degrees in most treatment programs or counseling settings. The discussion below briefly describes each method and summarizes what is known from the empirical research about its effectiveness. In doing so, the discussion expands on the other literature reviews of treatment outcome (e.g., Blaszczynski and Silove, 1995; DeCaria et al., 1996; Lesieur, 1998; Murray, 1993; Walker, 1993; Lopez Viets and Miller, 1997; R.W. Wildman, personal communication to the committee, 1998). A table summarizing the literature on treatment outcome studies reviewed by the committee appears in Appendix D.

Psychoanalytic/Psychodynamic

Psychoanalysts seek to understand the basis of all human behaviors by considering the motivational forces that derive from unconscious mental processes (Wong, 1989). Psychodynamics refers to the "science of the mind, its mental processes, and affective components that influence human behavior and motivations (Freedman et al., 1975:2601) and how these potentially opposing forces of cognition and emotion are translated into behavior. During the first half of the twentieth century, psychoanalysts provided the first systematic attempts to understand and treat gamblers (Rabow et al., 1984; Rosenthal, 1987).

Psychoanalytic and psychodynamic treatment approaches have not been proven effective through evaluation research. They are briefly described here because they are the most common forms of treatment for pathological gambling at this time. These approaches are based on the principle that all human behavior has meaning and is functional. Even the most self-destructive behaviors can serve a defensive or adaptive purpose. This perspective suggests that pathological gambling is a symptom or expression of an underlying psychological condition. This approach takes the view that, although some individuals don't need to understand why they gamble in order to stop, there are many others whose lives do not improve with abstinence, which is experienced as futile and hopeless (Rosenthal and Rugle, 1994). They then develop a major depression, turn back to gambling, or seek out some other addictive or self-destructive behavior with which to distract themselves.

Psychoanalytic and psychodynamic therapy attempts to help pathological gamblers to understand the underlying source of their distress and confront it. Clinicians have considered psycho-dynamically oriented psychotherapy useful in treating some of the comorbid disorders and character pathology observed among pathological gamblers, perhaps especially the narcissistic and masochistic subtypes. Although several others have noted the value of psychodynamic treatment for addictive behaviors (Boyd and Bolen, 1970; Kaufman, 1994; Khantzian, 1981; Shaffer, 1995; Wurmser, 1978), there have been no controlled or randomized studies exploring the effectiveness of this approach for treating pathological gamblers.

The psychoanalytic understanding of gambling problems rests on the foundation formulated by Freud (1928), who thought that it was not for money that the gambler gambled, but for the excitement. In fact, Freud speculated that some people gamble to lose. He thought this tendency was rooted in a need for self-punishment, to expiate guilt, and, for the male gambler, because of ambivalence toward the father. Bergler (1936, 1943, 1958) expanded on this concept of masochism, emphasizing the pathological gambler's rebellion against the authority of the parents and specifically the reality principle they represent.

A number of early psychoanalysts, dating back to Simmel in 1920, emphasized narcissistic fantasies and a sense of entitlement, pseudo-independence, and the need to deny feelings of smallness and helplessness. Other analysts (Greenson, 1947; Galdston, 1960) described early parental deprivation, with the gambler then turning to Fate or to Lady Luck for the love, acceptance, and approval he or she had been denied. Several analysts (Greenson, 1947; Comess, 1960; Niederland, 1967) saw compulsive gambling as an attempt to ward off an impending depression. Boyd and Bolen (1970) viewed it as a manic defense against helplessness and depression secondary to loss. Still others have emphasized the eroticization of tension and fear (Von Hattingberg, 1914), the central role of omnipotence (Simmel, 1920; Bergler, 1936; Greenson, 1947; Lindner, 1950), and problems identifying with parents (Weissman, 1963). More recently, analysts have been investigating deficiencies in self-regulation as they pertain to gambling and other addictive disorders (Krystal and Raskin, 1970; Wurmser, 1974; Khantzian, 1981; Schore, 1994; Ulman and Paul, 1998).

The psychoanalytic literature provides individual case histories of gamblers treated successfully (Lindner, 1950; Harkavy, 1954; Reider, 1960; Comess, 1960; Harris, 1964; Laufer, 1966). The only analyst to present information about a series of treated gamblers was Bergler (1958). In his account of 200 referrals, 80 appeared to be severe cases and, of those, 60 remained in treatment. A critique of his treatment appears in Rosenthal (1986). According to Bergler, 45 were cured and 15 experienced symptom removal. By a cure, he meant not only that they stopped gambling, but also that they addressed core conflicts and gave up their pattern of self-destructiveness. There is no information on whether "cured" patients were followed up after treatment.

There is a significant need, not only for randomized treatment outcome studies, but also for clinical vignettes and case histories that discuss what it is that clinicians who use these treatments actually do. It is necessary to deconstruct psychoanalytically and psychodynamically oriented interventions and techniques to see what specific components contribute to favorable treatment outcomes. And of course there are differences between one therapist and another with regard to their capacities for empathy, timing, tact, role-modeling, and support—which can complicate research on treatment effectiveness in general and psychodynamic treatment in particular.

Behavioral

Behavioral treatment methods actively seek to modify pathological gambling behavior on the basis of principles of classical conditioning or operant theory. Several variations of behavioral treatment methods are used today, often in combination. Aversion treatment consists of applying an unpleasant stimulus, such as a small electric shock, while the patient reads phrases that describe gambling behavior. During the procedure's final phrase, the patient reads about an alternative activity to gambling, such as returning home, but receives no shock (McConaghy et al., 1991). Imaginal desensitization consists of two steps. Patients first engage in a procedure to relax. Then they are asked to imagine a series of scenes related to gambling that they find arousing. They learn from this procedure to relax when they encounter opportunities to gamble, rather than to submit to their cravings. An extension of imaginal desensitization is in vivo exposure, in which relaxation techniques are applied while the patient is actually experiencing a gambling situation.

Behavioral counseling has been used in both individual and group treatment settings. Subjects receive reinforcement for desired gambling behaviors, such as gambling at a reduced level, betting less money, and so on. Specific treatment goals can be more formalized in the form of contingency contracting, in which specific aspects of behavior are rewarded or punished. Other behavioral techniques have been reported in the gambling treatment literature. Two of them, behavioral counseling, in which the gambler is given verbal reinforcement for desired outcome behaviors, and in vivo exposure, in which the gambler is exposed to gambling behaviors but is not allowed to gamble, are mentioned in the literature but have not been empirically tested.

Although behavioral treatment methods have been used and evaluated, such studies typically have had small sample sizes and no control groups. Case studies using various combinations of behavior treatments are common (e.g., Dickerson and Weeks, 1979; Cotler, 1971; McConaghy, 1991; Rankin, 1982; Greenberg and Marks, 1982; Greenberg and Rankin, 1982). However, findings from these limited studies are not consistent enough to reach conclusions about treatment effectiveness. Early studies of effectiveness on behavioral forms of treatment for pathological gamblers focused on aversion treatment. The studies involved single patients and provided minimal evidence of treatment success (e.g., Barker and Miller, 1966; Goorney, 1968). Subsequent research on aversion treatment using electric shock for pathological gamblers had only slightly larger samples (e.g., Seager, 1970; Koller, 1972;

Seager et al., 1966; Salzman, 1982) and produced equally questionable findings.

Larger outcome studies have been undertaken and provide more evidence for treatment effectiveness. In a study of 110 German pathological gamblers, Iver Hand (1998) described a behavioral treatment that begins with an extensive assessment of the client's motivation for treatment, symptoms, the consequences of his or her gambling, and social competence. This assessment is followed by client training in emotional awareness, coping with negative emotions, and social and problem-solving skills. An uncontrolled evaluation of this approach revealed favorable treatment results (Hand, 1998).

The most rigorous work on behavior treatments with pathological gamblers has been published in a series of study reports by McConaghy, Blaszczynski, and colleagues (McConaghy et al., 1983, 1991; Blaszczynski et al., 1991). The earlier studies by this group compared imaginal desensitization with either aversion treatment or behavioral approaches. In a 1988 study (McConaghy et al., 1988), the effectiveness of imaginal desensitization was compared with imaginal relaxation (teaching the client general relaxation techniques). Although the early studies by this group had relatively small sample sizes, otherwise strong methodologies revealed that treatment techniques were successful at one month and also at one year following treatment.

Using a large sample and expanding the comparisons of behavioral approaches, McConaghy et al. (1991) randomly allocated 120 participants to one of four techniques: aversion treatment, imaginal desensitization, imaginal relaxation, or in vivo exposure. A total of 63 clients were recontacted two to nine years later (a 53 percent follow-up response rate). The group that received imaginal desensitization benefited more than those receiving the other three behavioral approaches when abstinence and controlled gambling were combined as the outcome variable. (The authors defined controlled gambling as gambling in the absence of the subjective sense of impaired control and adverse financial consequences, based on self-rating and confirmation from a spouse or significant other). If just abstinence was considered, imaginal desensitization was equivalent to the other treatments' combined rate of abstinence (30 percent and 27 percent, respectively).

In a further investigation of this sample, Blaszczynski and colleagues (1991) found that the abstainers and controlled gamblers showed a significant reduction in arousal levels, anxiety, and depression during the follow-up period compared with those who could not control their gambling. Also of significance are the study's findings pertaining to the controlled gamblers. The pattern of gambling suggested that controlled gambling is not necessary a temporary response followed by a relapse to heavier gambling (Blaszczynski et al., 1991:299). Because the sample sizes of the McConaghy and Blaszczynski studies are relatively small and because only about half of the original sample was contacted for follow-up (although the long follow-up periods used were laudable), these results should be interpreted with caution.

Cognitive and Cognitive-Behavioral

Several clinicians and researchers have convincingly argued (see Blaszczynski and Silove, 1995; Walker, 1992; Gaboury and Ladouceur, 1989) that pathological and problem gamblers share irrational core beliefs about gambling risks, an illusion of control, biased evaluations of gambling outcomes, and a belief that gambling is a solution to their financial problems (Ladouceur et al., 1994; Toneatto, personal communication to the committee, 1998). Cognitive treatment aims to counteract underlying irrational beliefs and attitudes about gambling that are believed to initiate and maintain the undesirable behavior (Gaboury and Ladouceur, 1989). Treatment typically involves teaching clients strategies to correct their erroneous thinking. Many, for example, do not understand the concepts of probability and randomness, believing that they can exert some control over whether they win or lose.

The effectiveness of cognitive treatments has received limited attention by researchers and, as for other studies of treatment success, most have small sample sizes and no control groups (e.g., Gaboury and Ladouceur, 1989; Sylvain and Ladouceur, 1992), from which little can therefore be concluded. However, a push for more comprehensive models to explain the origins of problem gambling (Sharpe and Tarrier, 1993) has elicited investigations of the efficacy of combining cognitive and behavioral approaches. Investigations combining these treatments include case studies

(Bannister, 1977; Sharpe and Tarrier, 1992), small and uncontrolled studies (Arribas and Martinez, 1991), and controlled studies with larger samples (Echeburura et al., 1994). Combined cognitive-behavioral approaches have been successful for both adolescent problem gamblers (Ladouceur et al., 1994) and adult pathological gamblers (Bujold et al., 1994; Sylvain et al., 1997). The Sylvain study (1997) is noteworthy in that it expanded the cognitive-behavior treatment to include a waiting-list control group. The study found that the cognitive behavioral group improved vastly more than the control group. However, 11 of the original 40 individuals dropped out of the study and the follow-up data suffered from appreciable attrition.

Another cognitive-behavioral controlled investigation with a waiting-list control group was done by Echeburura and his colleagues (1994). They compared the effectiveness of cognitive and behavioral techniques in a Spanish sample of 64 men and women who met DSM-III-R criteria for pathological gambling. Participants were randomly assigned to one of four treatments: individual stimulus control and in vivo exposure with response prevention; group cognitive restructuring; a combination of the first two; and a waiting-list control group. At six-month follow-up, the outcome data indicated that the most favorable outcome was associated with the first two groups; these groups significantly outperformed the control group and reported therapeutic success rates (abstinence or 1 or 2 gambling episodes in which the amount gambled did not exceed the amount gambled in the week prior to treatment) of 75 percent and 63 percent, respectively. However, the combined individual and group treatment condition showed significantly poorer results compared with the other treatment groups.

Pharmacological

Pharmacotherapy is a relatively new approach to the treatment of pathological gambling. There are only a few studies and reports in the literature. In 1980, just prior to the introduction of DSM-III, Moskowitz (1980) described the treatment of three compulsive gamblers with lithium carbonate. Significant abstinence was achieved in all three cases, with improvement documented by long-term follow-up. However, two of the three were clearly manic depressive, and the third had a bipolar spectrum disorder. Twelve years later, Hollander et al. (1992) described the treatment of a single patient with clomipramine. When the patient entered the study, she had been gambling consistently 2 to 3 times per week for the previous 6.5 years, although she had periods of abstinence in the past. The study's design was double-blind, placebo controlled, 10 weeks to each phase. She was minimally improved on the placebo, then became abstinent on the medication and didn't gamble for the duration of the trial. Except for a relapse at week 17, she remained abstinent on open maintenance for an additional seven months. Significant in her personality were compulsive features, including perfectionism and hoarding, and a history of social phobia, all of which respond well to such drugs as clomipramine.

Haller and Hinterhuber (1994) published a double-blind, controlled study (12 weeks each phase) of one gambler treated with carbamazepine. The patient's gambling continued on placebo, with no improvement, but he became abstinent on carbamazepine by week 2 and did not gamble for the duration of the trial. In fact, he remained abstinent on open maintenance (600 mg/day) for 2.5 years. The results are particularly impressive given his prior history of treatment failures. Despite years of behavior therapy, psychoanalysis, and Gamblers Anonymous, his longest previous period of abstinence was three months. Carbamazepine is an anticonvulsant that has been used as a mood stabilizer, particularly in patients with bipolar disorders. There is no mention in the report of emotional instability. We are told only that the patient played roulette to relieve stress and depression. The authors postulated that the efficacy of the medication may have been due to its limbic antikindling effect or its effect on the noradrenergic system.

More recently, Hollander et al. (1998) presented the results of a single-blind placebo lead-in (8 weeks each phase) fluvoxamine study. Of 19 pathological gamblers, 9 dropped out during the placebo phase. Of the 10 who remained, 7 responded with significant improvement, as measured by a marked decrease in cravings and the achievement of abstinence. Two of the three nonresponders also had emotional instability. Since fluvoxamine and the other selective serotonin reuptake inhibitors (SSRIs) can switch depressed patients into a manic phase or bring out an underlying bipolar disorder, there was concern that the medication might exacerbate their emotional instability, particularly in the higher dose (250 mg/day) administered to the nonresponders. The authors recommended that, in future studies in which pathological gamblers are to be given SSRIs, subjects with bipolar disorder should be excluded. Overall, these results suggest that medication may be of some benefit, but more systematic randomized studies are clearly needed. Long-term follow-up (one to two years) is also recommended.

Neurobiological studies (also discussed in Chapter 4) suggest the involvement of serotonin, norepinephrine, and dopamine in pathological gambling. The medications used in the above studies target one or more of these neurotransmitter systems. The norepinephrine system has been associated with arousal and novelty-seeking, dopamine with reward and motivation, and serotonin with impulsivity and compulsivity (Hollander et al., 1998). Another avenue of approach suggested by these studies is the use of medication to treat comorbid conditions. In practice, this is probably the most frequently cited reason for putting gamblers on medication. Comorbid disorders for which medications are commonly prescribed include depression, bipolar disorder, and attention-deficit hyperactivity disorder.

Rosenthal (1997) discussed indications for using medication in the treatment of pathological gamblers. Although some patients experience withdrawal symptoms, including prominent physical symptoms, (Wray and Dickerson, 1981; Meyer, 1989; Rosenthal and Lesieur, 1992), they do not need to be medicated. Also, some gamblers report frequent and intense cravings. Rosenthal (1997) reviewed several approaches to a pharmacotherapy of cravings. One of the most promising involves agents that block the excitement or pleasure of the addictive drug. The best known of these blocking agents is naltrexone, an opioid antagonist used in the treatment of alcoholism. It has also been used in treating those addicted to cocaine and heroin. The effectiveness of the drug in treating pathological gamblers is currently being investigated under controlled conditions by Suck-Won Kim at the University of Minnesota (Kim, 1998).

However, medication is useful only if the patient takes it. It is estimated that, 50 percent of all patients don't take the medications their doctors give them. Greenstein et al. (1981) found that fewer than 10 percent of patients who began naltrexone treatment for opioid dependence were still taking it after two months. For pathological gamblers, compliance is an issue because they are often ambivalent about giving up their gambling or altering long-standing patterns of coping, no matter how ineffective. When they stop gambling, they often feel something has being taken away from them (Taber, 1985).

Addiction-based and Multimodal

This category of treatments, which has a relatively long tradition, includes a broad range of techniques used by inpatient and outpatient programs. The first gambling inpatient program, which started in 1972 at the Brecksville, Ohio, Veterans Administration hospital, was based on a preexisting program for alcoholics. Similarities with substance abuse programs continue and include the use of recovering gamblers as peer counselors, an emphasis on Gamblers Anonymous and other 12-step meetings, and an educational component about addiction, including relapse prevention (Kruedelbach, personal communication to the committee, 1998). This latter component focuses on how to avoid high-risk situations, being able to identify specific gambling triggers, and developing problem-solving skills for dealing with urges or cravings. McCormick (1994) believes that pathological gamblers are deficient in the number of coping skills they have available and in their ability to flexibly choose the skill most appropriate to the stressful, or potentially relapse-triggering, situations they face. In a comparison with nongambling substance abusers, he found that substance abusers with a gambling problem utilize significantly more avoidance and impulsive coping styles.

There are other therapeutic components commonly employed by addiction-based programs. One is autobiography (Adkins et al., 1985). Patients write a history of their gambling problem incorporated into a narrative of the significant events in their life, and then read it to the therapy group. Feedback focuses on the role gambling has played in the person's life, as well as how his or her behavior and perceptions contributed to the development of the problem. The reading of one's autobiography is often a very emotional experience, and many view it both as a rite of passage in the treatment program and as a turning point in their recovery (Adkins et al., 1985).

Joint or family therapy is another therapeutic component of addiction-based treatment. This element is important when dealing with pathological gamblers, because families are often loath to forgive the gambler. Clinical wisdom suggests that it is not until after the individual has stopped gambling that the anger of family members begins to surface. This may be so because gambling can be easy to hide and the financial and interpersonal damage can be swift; those close to the gambler remain distrustful and hold on to their anger to protect themselves. Franklin and Thoms (1989) note that the return of the gambler into the family is often met with resentment and resistance. The spouse and children often are depressed and have problems of their own that are in need of therapy. Alternatively, because the gambling offers intermittent rewards (Heineman, 1994), family members may be angry that the patient has *stopped* gambling.

Another key aspect of the addiction-based approach is after-care planning. This may include identification of a support system, continuing involvement in Gamblers Anonymous, relapse prevention strategies, a budget and plan for financial restitution, a plan for addressing legal issues, ongoing individual or group therapy, family therapy, and medication.

The literature contains several outcome studies of addiction-based treatments. For studies that reported six-month and one-year outcome data, abstinence rates for those contacted were roughly 50 percent (Russo et al., 1984; Taber et al., 1987; Lesieur and Blume, 1991; Stinchfield and Winters, 1996). All studies found that those who abstained from gambling reported greater improvement in interpersonal and intrapersonal functioning than those who returned to some level of gambling; some studies found decreased substance use as well at follow-up (Lesieur and Bloom, 1991; Taber et al., 1987; Stinchfield and Winters, 1996).

Whereas most of the studies involved small samples, a Minnesota study of six state-funded multimodal programs described the outcomes of several hundred clients (Stinchfield and Winters, 1996). This investigation found abstinence rates of 43 percent (at 6 months) and 42 percent (at 12 months), and rates of gambling at less than once a month for 29 percent (at 6 months) and 24 percent (at 12 months) of the contacted subjects. Interestingly, gamblers who started treatment but did not complete it, or who received only an intake evaluation, also reported improvement in virtually all variables related to gambling and psychosocial functioning, even though the extent of change was less dramatic than for those who completed treatment (Rhodes et al., 1997; Stinchfield and Winters, 1996).

Some of the multimodal approaches have been evaluated for long-term effectiveness. Hudac and colleagues (1989) assessed 26 male gamblers four years after they were treated. Of the 26, 8 were abstinent and the others showed less gambling compared with the period prior to treatment. However, the gamblers contacted at the four-year follow-up represented only about one-third of the original treatment sample of 99 pathological gamblers. Schwartz and Linder (1992) found that, after two years following inpatient treatment with a client-centered approach, 13 of 25 assessed clients remained abstinent (33 original subjects were not contacted).

Self-Help

Gambler's Anonymous

Gamblers Anonymous (GA) is believed to be the most commonly used of all approaches to deal with pathological gambling, and it is routinely included in multimodal strategies (Lesieur, 1998). The data suggest that relapse rates tend to be quite high for participants. Stewart and Brown (1988) found that total abstinence was reported by only 8 percent of members surveyed one year after their first attendance and by 7 percent at two years. When those who continued to gamble were compared with those who dropped out of Gamblers Anonymous, Brown (1987) found that dropouts were more likely to perceive that they had less of a gambling problem, found themselves in personality clashes with the members who did attend, and reported that Gamblers Anonymous was too rigid in its abstinence-only policy. Other researchers have examined the role of Gamblers Anonymous in maintaining abstinence. Taber and colleagues (1987) found that 74 percent of abstinent gamblers in their sample attended at least three meetings in the prior month, compared with only 42 percent of those who continued to gamble.

The therapeutic effectiveness of Gamblers Anonymous has also been explored with respect to participation by the gambler's spouse. Johnson and Nora (1992) found that there was a trend for higher abstinence rates for gamblers whose spouses were present at meetings compared with gamblers whose spouses did not attend. Although not statistically significant, the results revealed that 20 out of 44 gamblers whose spouses were present at meetings stopped gambling for at least four years, compared with 13 out of 46 gamblers whose spouses did not participate. In sum, Gamblers Anonymous may be increasing in popularity (Lopez Viets and Miller, 1997), but whether participating in meetings makes a significant and lasting impact is still not known (Brown, 1985; Rosecrance, 1988).

Other Self-Help

Related to the Gamblers Anonymous approach is the use of self-help and psychoeducational literature for pathological gamblers. Dickerson et al. (1990) conducted a preliminary investigation in which he compared use of a self-help manual only with use of the manual plus an interview with an experienced therapist. The manual focused on the definition and underlying causes of problem gambling and how the individual could monitor the problem behaviors and replace them with incompatible but healthier behaviors. The group that received the manual plus interview experienced more rapid improvement during the first three-month follow-up, but progress was not sustained at the six-month follow-up. One interesting aspect of this study was that most clients chose abstinence as their goal rather than a reduction of gambling.

Natural Recovery

Recovery from pathological gambling need not require formal treatment. Understanding how natural recovery occurs is important. First, the factors associated with such natural recovery can be integrated into treatment services. Second, policymakers need to know how many gamblers will recover naturally if they are to estimate the social costs associated with gambling disorders. Natural recovery rates and processes provide the baseline against which social costs and treatment effects and effectiveness can be judged. Thus, estimates of social effects (Prochaska, 1996) and treatment cost-effectiveness cannot be computed until the rates of natural recovery from pathological gambling become calculable. Some economists, for example, compute social cost estimates as if there is no recovery without treatment (Institute of Medicine, 1996). If we assume some rate of natural recovery among pathological gamblers, the social costs of gambling will be lower than estimates that assume no possibility of natural recovery.

Since Winick (1962) first described the process of "maturing out" of narcotics use, the idea of natural recovery has caught the imagination of many clinical investigators. Indeed, natural recovery has become increasingly recognized as a common phenomenon (Institute of Medicine, 1996; McCartney, 1996). Studies about natural recovery have been reported for alcohol problems (e.g., Cunningham et al., 1995; Humphreys et al., 1995; Sobell et al., 1996), smoking (Bernstein, 1970; Diclamente and Prochaska, 1982), cocaine use (Shaffer and Jones, 1989; Toneatto et al., in press), and opiate use (Biernacki, 1990; Klingemann, 1991).

Some investigators have speculated that prevalence studies provide indirect evidence of natural recovery from gambling problems. Volberg (1995) has observed that the difference between higher rates of youth gambling disorders and lower rates of adult gambling disorders suggest the presence of natural recovery, although prospective longitudinal studies would be needed to confirm this conclusion. Wynne's (1994) survey of a Canadian community revealed that 36 percent of respondents who reported a prior gambling problem reported no problems in the past year. In a more direct investigation of natural recovery,

Hodgins and el-Guebaly (1998) used publicity to recruit problem gamblers who had resolved their gambling problems either with or without the help of treatment. Among the subjects in their sample, about half reported that they recovered without treatment. The sole variable that significantly discriminated those who sought treatment from those who did not was the number of DSM-IV pathological gambling symptoms. Those who sought treatment reported about two more symptoms compared with the nonseekers (about eight versus six symptoms). Nevertheless, although research during the past decade has advanced knowledge to some degree about natural recovery from psychoactive substances, natural recovery from gambling has not been examined.

HEALTH CARE SERVICES AND PREVENTION

Although the effectiveness of various treatment approaches is not well substantiated in the literature, it is the committee's view that treatment for most, but perhaps not all, pathological gamblers is warranted. This position is based on three assumptions: First, pathological gambling is a serious disorder associated with several negative consequences. Second, the evidence is that self-help groups alone are not very effective (Brown, 1987). Third, pathological gambling can be a chronically relapsing disorder, often persisting indefinitely even after periods of remission. Yet these assumptions are in need of substantial and rigorous research testing. At this point, we do not know which treatments work best and why they work, and we do not know the extent to which gamblers can recover naturally.

Availability and Access of Treatment Services[2]

Whereas substance abuse has the attention of policymakers, the need to provide treatment for pathological gambling has not been widely recognized. It is difficult to know the extent to which insurance coverage exists for this illness, because consistent re-

---

[2]The committee thanks Roger Svendsen and his team for their investigation of the extent of treatment services.

porting by treatment providers and by jurisdictions on how much they spend treating pathological gamblers is not available. For example, Svendsen (1998), in a survey conducted for the committee, contacted the 20 largest insurance companies in the United States to determine how much they spent on gambling treatment. The companies reportedly would not release the information, arguing that information about reimbursement for any specific disorder would be provided only to participating members or their physicians. Nevertheless, in the same survey, all 34 state affiliates of the National Council on Problem Gambling confirmed their understanding that most health insurers and managed care providers do not reimburse individuals receiving treatment for pathological gambling (Svendsen, 1998). This exclusion from reimbursement occurs despite the fact that pathological gambling has been recognized by the American Psychiatric Association as a mental health disorder since 1980 (American Psychiatric Association, 1980). Such practices not only keep many from seeking treatment, but also require many of those who do seek treatment either to pay out of their own pocket—unlikely for a debt-ridden gambler—or to obtain coverage under the guise of another diagnosis often associated with pathological gambling, such as depression or substance abuse (Letson, 1998).

Current treatment for pathological gambling in the United States, in many ways, may parallel the treatment of substance use disorders (Blume, 1986). Many approaches have been employed in the service of pathological gamblers, although most of the treatment is probably delivered on an outpatient basis. Inpatient care is generally limited to patients with severe acute crises, treatment failures, and severe comorbid disorders, particularly depression (Lesieur, 1998; Blume, 1986). Although there is a growing tendency for treatment programs to focus on pathological gambling, many still operate as specialized tracks within existing substance abuse programs (Lesieur, 1998). Furthermore, despite the growing trend in the United States toward harm reduction strategies and controlled behavior approaches for addiction problems (Marlatt and Tapert, 1993), most gambling treatment programs, like those that treat substance abuse, favor abstinence. Some programs, however, particularly those dealing with problem gamblers in their early stages, do aim at reducing and controlling rather than stopping gambling (Lesieur, 1998).

It is important to consider that treatment for gambling is most likely to be provided by a combination of specialized and non-specialized providers—that is, by a combination of those who treat gambling problems as the focus of their work and those who provide general counseling but occasionally work with gamblers. It may be that nonspecialized providers deliver the majority of addiction treatment services. As an adjunct or alternative to primary treatment, treatment providers often refer gamblers to Gamblers Anonymous and Gam-Anon (Lesieur, 1998; Stinchfield and Winters, 1996). In fact, Gamblers Anonymous appears to be the most readily available form of help for the problem gambler and its out-of-pocket costs are virtually nil. Based on a review of its international services, its Internet web site, and archival records (Svendsen, 1998), Gamblers Anonymous has meetings in all 50 states, with the average number of meetings annually per state being 26 and the median 14, an increase of 36 percent from 1995 to 1998 (see Appendix E).

As already noted, it is the consensus of state affiliates of the National Council on Problem Gambling that the majority of health insurers in the United States do not reimburse those receiving treatment for pathological gambling (Svendsen, 1998). There is nevertheless some funding for gambling treatment, although it is small. Many of the 34 state affiliates, as well as the national organization itself, receive some funding from state or gambling industry organizations (Letson, 1998; Svendsen, 1998). Approximately half of them report public funding specifically to support treatment for problem gambling (Svendsen, 1998); the revenues generated by gambling in the state are used to pay for these services. Amounts for problem gambling treatment services range considerably (from $100,000 to $1.5 million), although most state appropriations are at the low end. Not surprisingly, the affiliate councils see this level of funding as insufficient (Letson, 1998:53). Even in states that spend a good deal on pathological gambling, the amounts are small in comparison to what they take in from legalized gambling revenues. For example, the amount appropriated by the state of New York to its Council on Problem Gambling represents a mere one-tenth of 1 percent of the state's income from legalized gambling (Letson, 1998). For Minnesota, in 1997, it represents about one-half of 1 percent of the state's income from legalized gambling (Svendsen, 1998). Moreover, the majority of state affiliates to the National Council on Problem Gambling probably do not receive this level of funding (Letson, 1998) and, although 47 states have some form of legalized gambling and all 50 states have gambling venues (legal and illegal), only 34 have a council.

    Without a good estimate of the number of pathological gamblers in the United States and the actual number of patients in treatment for this disorder, it is nearly impossible to reliably estimate the gap between the need for and use of treatment services. There are five reasons to expect that a significant gap exists between use of treatment and need for treatment in the area of pathological gambling (Letson, 1998): (1) an unwillingness by many gamblers to seek treatment; (2) a lack of recognition by the public that pathological gambling and problem gambling have significant health consequences; (3) failure of health insurers to recognize lay persons and treatment professionals who are certified by a recognized national or state organization as qualified providers of pathological gambling treatment; (4) lack of funding for treating pathological gambling; and (5) a perception that treatment is or may be ineffective.

Help-Line Services[3]

    A survey designed and conducted for the committee to provide information on problem gambling help lines in the United States reported that gambling help lines now operate in 35 of the 47 states that have some form of legalized gambling (Wallisch, 1998). In addition, the National Council on Problem Gambling, Inc., has a nationwide toll-free number (1-800-522-4700) that some states use as their state number and that other states advertise separately from their own in-state number.

    It is estimated that about 60 to 70 percent of calls to help lines

---

[3]The committee acknowledges Lynn Wallisch for her written report and contribution to this section.

are made by gamblers seeking help for themselves, the rest being made by spouses, family members, friends, therapists, employers, etc., about a problem gambler. Typical services provided by help lines include offering telephone counseling, usually by experienced master's-degree-level counselors (although several help lines lack a professional staff and are concerned about liability issues), information (e.g., about Gamblers Anonymous, Gam-Anon, problem gambling research), referrals to treatment providers, credit and debt counseling referrals, and crisis intervention (some transfer the call directly to a crisis line). Some programs perform other activities, such as gambling education and public awareness, prevention activities, and professional training.

About 60 percent of help lines receive most or all of their funding from the state in which they operate. Funds to operate gambling help lines are also provided by the gambling industry, corporations, and miscellaneous other sources such as memberships, individual contributions, and in-kind donations. Help lines advertise their call-in number in different ways, including running banners on video lottery terminals when not in play (South Dakota); slot machine stickers, posters, and pens (Delaware); billboards (Delaware and Louisiana); bus tails (Delaware); telephone recordings at the Department of Social Services while the caller is on hold (Delaware); targeted mailings to professionals, clergy, and corrections personnel (Minnesota); back of grocery store receipts (Minnesota); the New York Yankees' official billboard outside the stadium (New York); part of collateral materials provided by other agencies (Texas); church newsletters (Texas); postings at Alcoholics Anonymous meeting sites (Texas); listing in *Card Player* magazine (California); and posters conspicuously located inside casinos.

Most help lines cover the entire state, without restriction as to area or population served, and some take calls from nearby states, particularly when a neighboring state does not have its own help line. Because the national number will attempt to find help for any individual in the United States, in theory, no state is entirely without coverage. This diversity of ways of reaching a help line does not mean that all callers will receive equally effective services, however, and confusion can arise. For example, a problem gambler in Rhode Island may call the Rhode Island problem gambling help line and speak with a counselor at Travelers' Aid, or a counselor at the Connecticut Council (because the Connecticut problem gambling help line is advertised as covering Rhode Island), or a counselor with the Texas Council (which picks up Connecticut calls after hours). Depending on how frequently these entities share and update information, they may each have a different set of referrals or use different counseling techniques. This may well be an embarrassment of riches for the caller, but it could also be a potential source of confusion.

Help lines that report data on the number of calls received distinguish between legitimate calls by or about problem gamblers and inappropriate ones that ask for information on how to gamble or for the winning lottery number. These data were provided to the committee either from responses to our mini-survey or were calculated on a weekly basis from data already reported in summary form in help-line reports or datasheets. It is important to keep in mind that a limitation of the data is that some states reported only the number of calls that generated demographic statistics, which may not represent all help-related calls. With these caveats in mind, weekly call volume ranged from about 10 to several hundred. Some states, such as New Jersey, whose 1-800-GAMBLER number is publicized nationally and receives calls from all over the country, and Texas, which contracts to cover calls from a large number of states, reported several hundred calls per week. New England and Maryland reported 100 or more calls per week, and 6 other states (Florida, Minnesota, New York, Iowa, Pennsylvania, and Wisconsin) reported between 50 and 100 calls weekly.

Some help lines have developed information systems about calls and clients. The variability between them is considerable; they ask different questions, do not necessarily ask all questions of all callers, and report data using different summary categories. Some programs make detailed information regularly available, in the form of mailouts, annual reports, or postings to their Internet web site; others report information only as required to do so. Given this heterogeneity of formats and content of data, it is difficult to draw reliable conclusions. However, three systematic investigations of help-line data are worthy of our attention. First, a study by Wallisch and Cox (1997) compared the demographic distribution of callers to the Texas help line with the demographics of problem gamblers in the general population of Texas. The authors found that certain groups of problem gamblers were underrepresented among help-line callers. Notably, gamblers who were younger, female, and Hispanic were less likely to call than would be expected from their numbers in the population of problem gamblers. Given the increasing numbers of statewide prevalence surveys being conducted, extending this type of comparison study between help-line data and prevalence data on the general population would be useful as a way to further inform help-line services about population groups that they underserve. Second, Stinchfield (1998) reported on South Oaks Gambling Screen data from a sample of consecutive callers to the Minnesota help line. The mean score was about 8, which is considerably higher than the standard cutoff score of 5 for defining probable pathological gamblers (Lesieur and Blume, 1987), although it is lower then the mean score obtained from a Minnesota sample of treatment seekers (Stinchfield and Winters, 1996). This finding is interesting, in that it indicates that, at least for the Minnesota sample, help-line callers appear to be a seriously disordered group. Third, Minnesota's Problem Gambling Division commissioned an outcome report of its state help-line callers. A random sample of consecutive callers was called after one month and evaluated on changes in their gambling and their satisfaction with help-line services (Winters et al., 1996). At follow-up, 97 percent of the sample expressed satisfaction with the services received, and 71 percent reported reduction at follow-up in gambling frequency and gambling-related problems compared with baseline measures. While encouraging, the results can only be considered suggestive, primarily because of the absence of a control group in the study. Apparent improvement over time would be expected because the help line was called at a moment of crisis, whereas the follow-up time was chosen by the investigator.

Gambling Counseling Certification and Services[4]

The general purpose of certification of health care providers is to provide a form of recognition based on the contributions that

---

[4]The committee thanks Janet Mann and Marcus Patterson for their written contribution to this section.

they have made to a profession or based on the special expertise that they possess within a practice. Although this form of credentialing does not confer any legal status on those being recognized, it is a means for professional, legislative, and regulatory bodies, private industry, third-party payers, and the public to identify individuals who have demonstrated a particular expertise. Currently, three national organizations have developed a certification process for clinicians who specialize in the treatment of pathological gambling: (1) the American Academy of Health Care Providers in the Addictive Disorders, formed in 1989, offers the Certified Addiction Specialist credential in the areas of alcoholism, drug addiction, eating disorders, compulsive gambling, and sex addiction; (2) the National Council on Problem Gambling, an association formed in 1972 to provide information on problem gambling, began certifying gambling counselors in 1989; and (3) the American Compulsive Gambling Counselor Certification Board, affiliated with the Council on Compulsive Gambling of New Jersey, Inc., and formed in 1989, began offering its credential on a national basis in 1993. In addition, several states have formed certification boards requiring only a minimal level of experience and education for certification. An examination of the various organizations involved with the development of national standards reveals that there is no consistency in experiential and educational levels that these boards recognize.

The current debate surrounding the difference between certification and licensure is an arena that deserves attention. There is a trend toward the licensing of health care professionals who treat alcohol and drug addiction. Unlike certification, licensure confers a legal status on those receiving it. Such a process implies that the treatment of substance abuse is a profession in its own right, not an expertise within another discipline. Many of the associations declare that such a license is too narrow and would unnecessarily restrict or bar other qualified professionals, who may have a background in mental health, marriage, and family counseling, social work or psychology, for example, from practicing addiction counseling. Individuals from any of these disciplines may possess expertise in the treatment of addictive disorders and may therefore wish to acquire a specialty certification in recognition of excellence and proficiency.

Prevention

There are several examples of prevention efforts in the field of pathological gambling, among them teaching gamblers about the odds of the games they play, providing help-line services, and developing public and youth awareness campaigns about the potential risks associated with gambling (American Gaming Association, 1998). However, nothing is known yet about the effectiveness of these efforts.

A clear challenge for developing effective ways to prevent problem gambling is the lack of awareness of the dangers of excessive gambling. In one sense, programs to prevent substance abuse have it easy; the dangers of illicit drug use are relatively easy to identify. With gambling, it's not so easy. Placing a bet does not readily produce immediate adverse effects. Family members may find it harder to detect the effects of excessive gambling by a loved one compared with drug use or smoking. Moreover, advertising for state lotteries and casinos suggest that gambling is a harmless form of recreation. Youth programs receive funding from gambling, such as bingo and raffles, thus further lending support to the notion that gambling is a beneficial activity (Wynne et al., 1996). Many states use advertising and promotional campaigns to foster the acceptance of gambling. They do this by (1) portraying gambling as family entertainment or social recreation, (2) emphasizing community needs for the tax revenues generated, (3) altering the norms surrounding the behavior, so as not to make it deviant, and (4) centering gambling advertisements around successful gamblers (Preston et al., 1998).

Perhaps the most concerted prevention efforts have been directed toward adolescents. Targeting young people makes sense from a public health perspective because gambling often begins early, and thus may act as a gateway to future excessive gambling (Shaffer and Hall, 1994). We found only one youth prevention program that has been empirically evaluated. Gaboury and Ladouceur (1993) describe a three-session program in Quebec organized around an alcohol prevention model. It covered an overview of gambling, discussions of legal issues, how the gambling industry manipulates the chances of winning, beliefs and myths about gambling, and the development of pathological gambling and its consequences. It also covered strategies for controlling gambling. A sample of 289 juniors and seniors from 5 high schools completed the program. Whereas the evaluation showed that the students did learn about gambling and coping skills, what they had learned did not significantly influence their gambling attitudes or behavior six months later. The researchers suggested that future programs should increase involvement of both students and teachers and integrate the prevention program into existing drug and alcoholism prevention programs. Indeed, the reasons attributed to young people's involvement in gambling are similar to those linked to drinking or smoking, including vicarious modeling by parents, perceived pressure from peers, and a susceptibility to illusions of control (Derevensky et al., 1994; Jacobs, 1989; Kearney and Drabman, 1992).

CONCLUSIONS

What is known about the treatment of pathological gambling lags behind even what is known about its prevalence and etiology. A review of the literature indicates that relatively few outcome studies exist, and most of them lack a clear conceptual model and specification of outcome criteria, fail to report compliance and attrition rates, offer little description of actual treatment involved or measures to maintain treatment fidelity by the counselors, and provide inadequate length of follow-up. "At face value, there are few concrete observations that can be said of the effectiveness of treatment approaches for problem (and pathological) gambling beyond the fact that some are effective to some extent over an unknown follow-up period" (Blaszczynski, personal communication to the committee, 1998). This lack of rigorous research is aggravated by the fact that adequate research funding for pathological gambling treatment has not been made available in substantial amounts by the federal government. In contrast, the substance abuse field, which has benefited from treatment research made possible by expansion of research funding by the National Institute on Drug Abuse (NIDA) and the National Institute on Alcohol Abuse and Alcoholism (NIAAA), can point to numerous investigations supporting the effectiveness and cost-effectiveness of drug abuse treatment (Institute of Medicine, 1996:192).

Nevertheless, the committee views professional treatment as an appropriate response in most cases for individuals with a pathological gambling disorder. However, and especially in the absence of research on treatment effectiveness, it is unlikely that recovery from pathological gambling will involve quick and easy treatment. Rather, the treatment process can be characterized by less than complete compliance, a significant probability of relapse after treatment, and a long-term chronic course of symptoms not uncommon to the recovery patterns of alcoholism, drug addiction, and other chronic medical illnesses, such as hypertension and diabetes (McClellan et al., 1998).

The prevailing sentiment among experts in the substance abuse field, backed by two decades of well-funded research, is that for substance abusers, some treatment is better than no treatment (Institute of Medicine, 1996). At this juncture, there appears to be no compelling evidence in the pathological gambling literature to reject the notion that some treatment is better than none. Naturally, as the treatment literature matures for this disorder, a clearer picture of the incremental value of treatment will come into view.

In the near term, it is essential that a comprehensive research agenda on pathological gambling include policy research to identify alternative and optimal funding mechanisms and structures for financing treatment for pathological gambling. It seems wise to model the funding on the system used in substance abuse, in which financing responsibilities are distributed across state and local governments, the federal government (acting on behalf of selected poor, elderly, and chronically disabled individuals), and private insurers acting on behalf of employers and individuals who purchase health insurance. Indeed, private health insurance is now the largest single source of funding for the treatment of alcohol problems (Institute of Medicine, 1990:8). The major concern now being raised in the field of pathological and problem gambling treatment is over rapidly rising health care costs that have virtually blocked access to reimbursable treatment. Clearly, a more detailed understanding of the effectiveness of treatment for pathological gambling, as well as the cost-effectiveness of varying treatments, is required if a truly nondiscriminatory financing policy is to be realized. Research that identifies what keeps pathological gamblers from undertaking treatment and that informs clinical services about how best to locate, attract, and retain patients through treatment is also important.

It is also important to study the effects of managed care contracts and health insurance policies that place severe limits on services for those with a pathological gambling disorder. The extent to which gamblers are shortchanged because of limited access to health care has not been well documented. Furthermore, it is not known to what extent treatment for pathological gambling has been carved out from treatment services for other disorders associated with pathological gambling. It is also not clear if the trend by some states to require separate licensing for pathological gambling counselors will have counterproductive results for clients seeking treatment. Some states offer separate licensing for drug abuse and mental health services and the administration of drug abuse treatment independent of psychiatric, medical, family, and other related services. The results of partitioning these practices may result in less service delivery (McClellan et al., in press) and may defeat the principle of matching patients to the most effective treatments.

As noted by Rosenthal (1992), women constitute one-third of the population of pathological gamblers but are underrepresented in treatment study samples. And there is increasing recognition of the need to set up and evaluate treatment programs designed specifically for women and adolescents. Results from such studies will enable the development of programs targeted at these groups. Other client characteristics that require research attention include outcomes for adolescents (only one study to date has reported outcomes for them), as well as outcomes for members of different ethnic groups. Client characteristics may predict differential responsiveness to various treatment approaches, and this line of investigation could be linked to evaluation of community-based response systems.

In the area of gambling counseling certification and services, the committee sees a need for policy research examining controversial issues and viable options. Such research should describe the extent of certified counseling services, the number of counselors with varying levels of expertise, the demand for services provided, and alternative training and certification structures that are or could be established at colleges, universities, institutes, and health care training programs. Research of this type could lead to opportunities in the treatment community to form consensus and create a blueprint for action that will resolve the confusion and fragmentation currently surrounding the credentialing of gambling treatment professionals.

Future treatment outcome studies need greater methodological rigor. The research literature contains only a handful of controlled outcome studies, and most of them suffer from having small sample sizes, which limits their statistical power to detect reliable effects of group differences. Many studies do not provide information about refusals or dropouts, and, when these data are provided, the results can be discouraging (e.g., Sylvain et al., 1997). Gambling treatment studies should focus particularly on treatments that have manual-guided treatments with careful supervision and documentation of procedures. Poor specification of the therapeutic methods used hinders the replication of successful programs. Not only do therapist's manuals guide interventions, but they also facilitate the clarification of the specific contribution of particular treatment components. Clarifying key outcome measures of gambling treatment research is also a priority, as is measuring such outcomes on the basis of valid instruments.

More research needs to be carried out to identify types of gamblers who may differ in terms of gambling involvement, consequences, and etiology and for whom special treatments may maximize treatment response. The behavior of some pathological and problem gamblers may be biologically based, the direct result of deficits in the brain's neurotransmitter system (Comings, 1998). Patients may also display transient symptoms that minimally meet diagnostic criteria for pathological gambling or emerge as a reaction to emotional, affective, or anxiety-related difficulties (Blaszczynski, 1998). Matching patients to optimal treatment approaches is an ongoing area of research in the substance abuse treatment field. Limited independent research on matching patients to treatment settings suggests that outcomes are improved when patients were matched to settings that address their particular needs (McClellan et al., 1983). Clearly, there is no systematic research on the optimal, most cost-effective configuration of services for different groups of problem gamblers. To even conduct patient matching, three elements are needed: (1) comprehensive assessment tools to identify patient problems and needs, (2) placement criteria to ensure placement in the appropriate setting (e.g., inpatient versus outpatient) and intensity of care, and (3) a means of facilitating movement through a continuum of treatment services (Substance Abuse and Mental Health Services Administration, 1995). Because the gambling treatment field does not contain an adequate knowledge base pertaining to these three elements, matching patients to treatments cannot be adequately studied until the basic research regarding assessment and placement criteria has first been conducted.

Behavioral and cognitive treatment approaches appear to offer promise as effective treatments for pathological gambling. In a recent special issue of the *Journal of Consulting and Clinical Psychology* on empirically supported psychological treatments, cognitive-based treatments were cited as perhaps the treatment most widely studied and most highly regarded by proponents of clinical trial methodologies (DeRubeis and Crits-Christoph, 1998:38). It has also been observed that cognitive treatments are an emerging approach for the treatment of addictions (Crits-Christoph et al., 1998; DeRubeis and Crits-Christoph, 1998). Nevertheless, this is not to say that eclectic approaches to treating pathological gamblers should be ignored. As Blaszczynski and Silove (1995) and Lesieur (1998) cogently argue, there is growing recognition that multiple treatment components should be considered given the client's specific configuration of problems. Thus, clients with dysphoria should be evaluated for antidepressant medication; marital counseling may be indicated in the presence of extreme family estrangement; and substance abuse counseling may be necessary for those whose addictive behavior also includes alcohol or other drug abuse.

There is a particular need for studies of the role of Gamblers Anonymous in recovery and treatment outcomes. If there is a high dropout rate from Gamblers Anonymous, as the literature suggests, then it is important to investigate its causes and strategies for reducing it. Another important understudied research area is the role of therapist characteristics in the treatment of problem gambling behaviors. In addition, the effect of treatment settings is unclear. Although favorable outcomes have been reported from both inpatient and outpatient programs, their differential effects are still unknown. More research on treating spouses of pathological gamblers is also called for (Lesieur, 1998). It is typical for spouses to be directed to Gam-Anon programs to help deal with their partner's gambling. Given the view that a spouse may be involved in the gambling addiction, it has been argued that the treatment of husband and wife together is a necessary component to the rehabilitation process for married couples (Heineman, 1987; Steinberg, 1993).

Pharmacotherapy research needs to be expanded to determine if this approach has an important role in the treatment of pathological gamblers. We still do not know if medications provide therapeutic effect by ameliorating the pathological gambler's cravings, ruminations, or negative feelings.

Research persuasively demonstrates that one of the most reliable predictors of treatment outcome for substance abuse addiction is the patient's readiness to change, regardless of treatment strategy (Prochaska et al., 1992). Consequently, the pathological gambling treatment field should direct research attention to studying the patients' overall readiness to change and the specific stage of change as predictors of treatment outcome.

REFERENCES

Adkins, B.J., J.I. Taber, and A.M. Russo
    1985   The spoken autobiography: A powerful tool in group psychotherapy. *Social Work* 30:435-439.
American Gaming Association
    1998   *Responsible Gaming Resource Guide, Second Edition*. Washington, DC: American Gaming Association.
American Psychiatric Association
    1980   *DSM-III: Diagnostic and Statistical Manual of Mental Disorders*, 3rd ed. Washington, DC: American Psychiatric Association.
Arribas, M.P., and J.J. Martinez
    1991   Tratamiento individual de jugadores patologicos: Descripcion de casos. *Analisis y Modificacion de Conducta* 17:255-269.
Bannister, G., Jr.
    1977   Cognitive and behavior therapy in a case of compulsive gambling. *Cognitive Therapy and Research* 1:223-227.

Barker, J.C., and M. Miller
 1966   Aversion therapy for compulsive gambling. *Lancet* 1:491-492.
Bergler, E.
 1936   On the psychology of the gambler. *American Imago* 22:409-441.
 1943   The gambler: A misunderstood neurotic. *Journal of Criminal Psycho-pathology* 4:379-393. (Reported in *Selected Papers of Edmund Bergler, M.D. 1933-1961*. New York: Grune and Stratton, 1969.)
 1958   *The Psychology of Gambling*. New York: International Universities Press.
Bernstein, D.
 1970   The modification of smoking behavior: An evaluation review. In *Learning Mechanisms in Smoking*, W. Hunt, ed. Chicago: Aldine.
Biernacki, P.
 1990   *Pathways from Heroin Addiction: Recovery Without Treatment*. Philadelphia: Temple University Press.
Blackman, S., R.V. Simone, D.R. Thoms, and S. Blackman
 1989   The Gamblers Treatment Clinic of St. Vincent's North Richmond Community Mental Heath Center: Characteristics of the clients and outcome of treatment. *International Journal of the Addictions* 24(1):29-37.
Blaszczynski, A.
 1998   Views on the Treatment of Pathological Gambling. Comments to the National Research Council, Committee on the Social and Economic Impact of Pathological Gambling. University of New South Wales, Australia.
Blaszczynski, A., N. McConaghy, and A. Frankova
 1991   Control versus abstinence in the treatment of pathological gambling: A two to nine year follow-up. *British Journal of Addiction* 86:299-306.
Blaszczynski, A., and D. Silove
 1995   Cognitive and behavioral therapies for pathological gambling. *Journal of Gambling Studies* 11:195-220.
Blume, S.
 1986   Treatment for the addictions: Alcoholism, drug dependence and compulsive gambling in a psychiatric setting. *Journal of Substance Abuse Treatment* 3(2):131-133.
Boyd, W.H., and D.W. Bolen
 1970   The compulsive gambler and spouse in group psychotherapy. *International Journal of Group Psychotherapy* 20:77-90.
Brown, R.
 1985   The effectiveness of Gamblers Anonymous. Pp. 259-284 in *The Gambling Studies: Proceedings of the Sixth National Conference on Gambling and Risk Taking*, W.R. Eadington, ed. Reno: Bureau of Business & Economic Research, University of Nevada.
 1986   Dropouts and continuers in Gamblers Anonymous: IV. Evaluation and summary. *Journal of Gambling Behavior* 3:202-210.
 1987   Pathological gambling and related patterns of crime: Comparisons with alcohol and other drug addictions. *Journal of Gambling Behavior* 3:98-114.

Brownell, K.D., G.A. Marlatt, E. Lichenstein, and G.T. Wilson
  1986   Understanding and preventing relapse. *American Psychologist* 41:765-782.
Bujold, A., R. Ladouceur, C. Sylvain, and J.M. Boisvert
  1994   Treatment of pathological gamblers: An experimental study. *Journal of Behavior Therapy and Experimental Psychiatry* 25:275-282.
Ciarrocchi, J., and R. Richardson
  1989   Profile of compulsive gamblers in treatment: Update and comparisons. Seventh International Conference on Gambling and Risk Taking, 1987, Reno, NV. *Journal of Gambling Behavior* 5:53-65.
Comess, L.
  1960   The Analysis of the Gambler. Ph.D. dissertation, Southern California Psychoanalytic Institute.
Comings, D.E.
  1998   The molecular genetics of pathological gambling. *CNS Spectrums* 3:20-37.
Cotler, S.B.
  1971   The use of different behavioral techniques in treating a case of compulsive gambling. *Behavior Therapy* 2:579-584.
Crits-Christoph, P., L. Siqueland, J. Chittams, J.P. Barber, A.T. Beck, A. Frank, B. Liese, L. Luborsky, D. Mark, D. Mercer, L.S. Onken, L.M. Najavits, M.E. Thase, and G. Woody
  1998   Training in cognitive, supportive-expressive, and drug counseling therapies for cocaine dependence. *Journal of Consulting and Clinical Psychology* 66:484-492.
Cunningham, J.A., L.C. Sobell, M.B. Sobell, and G. Kapur
  1995   Resolution from alcohol problems with and without treatment: Reasons for change. *Journal of Substance Abuse* 7(3):365-372.
DeCaria, C.M., E. Hollander, R. Grossman, C.M. Wong, S.A. Mosovich, and S. Cherkasky
  1996   Diagnosis, neurobiology, and treatment of pathological gambling. *Journal of Clinical Psychiatry* 57:80-84.
Derevensky, J., R. Gupta, and G. Della Cioppa
  1994   A Developmental Perspective on Gambling Behavior in Children and Adolescents. Paper presented at the Ninth International Conference on Gambling and Risk Taking, Las Vegas, NV, June. McGill University, Montreal, Canada.
DeRubeis R.J., and P. Crits-Christoph
  1998   Empirically supported individual and group psychological treatments for adult mental disorders. *Journal of Consulting and Clinical Psychology* 66:37-52.
Dickerson, M.
  1989   Gambling: A dependence without a drug. *International Review of Psychiatry* 1(1-2):157-171.
Dickerson, M.G., J. Hinchy, and S.L. England
  1990   Minimal treatments and problem gamblers: A preliminary investigation. *Journal of Gambling Studies* 6:87-102.

Dickerson, M.G., and D. Weeks
    1979   Controlled gambling as a therapeutic technique for compulsive gamblers. *Journal of Behavior Therapy and Experimental Psychiatry* 10:139-141.

Diclamente, C.C., and J.O. Prochaska
    1982   Self-change and therapy change of smoking behavior: A comparison of processes of change in cessation and maintenance. *Addictive Behaviors* 7(2):133-142.

Echeburura, E., C. Baez, and J. Fernandez-Montalvo
    1994   Effectividad diferencial de diversas modalidades terapeuticas en el tratamiento psicologico del juego patologico: Un estudio experimental. *Analisis y Modificacion de Conducta* 20:617-643.

Franklin, J., and D.R. Thoms
    1989   Clinical observations of family members of compulsive gamblers. Pp. 135-146 in *Compulsive Gambling: Theory, Research and Practice*, H.J. Shaffer, S.A. Stein et al., eds. Lexington, MA: Lexington Books.

Freedman, A.M., H.I. Kaplan, B.J. Sadock
    1975   *Comprehensive Textbook of Psychiatry, II.* Baltimore: Williams and Wilkins.

Freud, S.
    1928   Dostoevsky and parricide. Pp. 175-196 in *Standard Edition of the Complete Psychological Works of Sigmund Freud*, J. Strachey, trans., ed. London: Hogarth, 1961, Vol XXI.

Gaboury, A., and R. Ladouceur
    1989   Erroneous perceptions and gambling. *Journal of Social Behavior and Personality* 4:411-420.
    1993   Evaluation of a prevention program for pathological gambling among adolescents. *Journal of Primary Prevention* 14(1):21-28.

Galdston, J.
    1960   The gambler and his love. *American Journal of Psychiatry* 117:553-555.

Goorney, A.B.
    1968   Treatment of a compulsive horse race gambler by aversion therapy. *British Journal of Psychiatry* 114:328-333.

Greenberg, D., and I. Marks
    1982   Behavioral psychotherapy of uncommon referrals. *British Journal of Psychiatry* 141:148-153.

Greenberg, D., and H. Rankin
    1982   Compulsive gamblers in treatment. *British Journal of Psychiatry* 140:364-366.

Greenson, R.R.
    1947   On gambling. *American Imago* 4:61-77.

Greenstein, R.A., C.P. O'Brien, A.T. McLellan, G.E. Woody, J. Grabowski, M. Long, G. Coyle-Perkins, and A. Vittor
    1981   Naltrexone: A short-term treatment for opiate dependence. *American Journal of Drug and Alcohol Abuse* 8(3):291-300.

Haller, R., and H. Hinterhuber
    1994   Treatment of pathological gambling with carbamazepine. *Pharmacopsychiatry* 27:19.

Hand, I.
1998   Pathological gambling: A negative state model and its implications for behavioral treatments. *CNS Spectrums* 3:58-71.
Harkavy, E.
1954   The psychoanalysis of a gambler. *International Journal of Psychoanalysis* 35:285.
Harris, H.I.
1964   Gambling addiction in an adolescent male. *Psychoanalytic Quarterly* 33:513-525.
Heineman, M.
1987   A comparison: The treatment of wives of alcoholics with the treatment of wives of pathological gamblers. *Journal of Gambling Behavior* 3:27-40.
1994   Compulsive gambling: Structured family intervention. *Journal of Gambling Studies* 10(1):67-76.
Hodgins, D.C., and N. el-Guebaly
1998   Recovery from Gambling Problems: A Comparison of Resolved and Active Gamblers. Unpublished manuscript. University of Calgary and Foothills Medical Centre, Calgary Alberta.
Hollander, E., T. Begaz, and M. DeCaria
1998   Pharmacologic approaches in the treatment of pathological gambling. *CNS Spectrums* 3:72-82.
Hollander, E., M. Frenkel, C. Decaria, S. Trungold, and D.J. Stein
1992   Treatment of pathological gambling with clomipramine. *American Journal of Psychiatry* 149:710-711.
Hudak, C.J., R. Varghese, and R.M. Politzer
1989   Family, marital, and occupational satisfaction for recovering pathological gamblers. *Journal of Gambling Behavior* 5:201-210.
Humphreys, K., R.H. Moos, and J.W. Finney
1995   Two pathways out of drinking problems without professional treatment. *Addictive Behaviors* 20:427-441.
Institute of Medicine
1990   *Broadening the Base of Treatment for Alcohol Problems.* Washington, DC: National Academy Press.
1996   *Pathways of Addiction: Opportunities in Drug Abuse Research.* Washington, DC: National Academy Press.
Jacobs, D.F.
1989   A general theory of addictions: Rationale for and evidence supporting a new approach for understanding and treating addictive behaviors. Pp. 249-292 in *Compulsive Gambling: Theory, Research, and Practice*, H.J. Shaffer, S.A. Stein, and T.N. Cummings, eds. Lexington, MA: D.C. Heath and Company.
Johnson, E.E., and R.M. Nora
1992   Does spousal participation in Gamblers Anonymous benefit compulsive gamblers? *Psychological Reports* 71:914.
Kaufman, E.
1994   *Psychotherapy of Addicted Persons.* New York: Guilford Press.

Kearney, C.A., and R.S. Drabman
  1992   Risk-taking/gambling-like behavior in preschool children. *Journal of Gambling Studies* 8(3):287-297.
Khantzian, E.J.
  1981   Some treatment implications of the ego and self disturbances in alcoholism. Pp. 163-188 in *Dynamic Approaches to the Understanding and Treatment of Alcoholism*, M.H. Bean, E.J. Khantzian, J.E. Mack, G.E. Vaillant, and N.E. Zinberg, eds. New York: Free Press.
Khantzian, E.J., K.S. Halliday, and W.E. McQuliffe
  1990   *Addiction and the Vulnerable Self: Modified Dynamic Group Therapy for Substance Abusers*. New York: Guilford Press.
Kim, S.W.
  1998   Opioid antagonists in the treatment of impulse-control disorders. *Journal of Clinical Psychiatry* 59(4):159-162.
Klingemann, H.K.H.
  1991   The motivation for change from problem alcohol and heroin use. *British Journal of Addiction* 86:727-744.
Knapp, T.J., and B.C. Lech
  1987   Pathological gambling: A review with recommendations. *Advances in Behavior and Research Therapy* 9:21-49.
Koller, K.M.
  1972   Treatment of poker-machine addicts by aversion therapy. *The Medical Journal of Australia* 1:742-745.
Kraft, T.
  1970   A short note on forty patients treated by systematic desensitization. *Behavior Research and Therapy* 8:219-220.
Krystal, H., and H.A. Raskin
  1970   *Drug Dependence: Aspects of Ego Function*. Detroit: Wayne State University Press.
Ladouceur, R., J.M. Boisvert, and J. Dumont
  1994   Cognitive-behavioral treatment for adolescent pathological gamblers. *Behavior Modification* 18:230-242.
Laufer, M.
  1966   Object loss and mourning during adolescence. In *The Psychoanalytic Study of the child, Vol. 21*. New York: International Universities Press.
Lesieur, H.R.
  1988   Altering the DSM-III criteria for pathological gambling. *Journal of Gambling Behavior* 4(1):38-47.
  1998   Costs and treatment of pathological gambling. *Annals of the American Academy* 556:153-171.
Lesieur, H.R., and S.B. Blume
  1987   The South Oaks gambling screen (SOGS): A new instrument for the identification of pathological gamblers. *American Journal of Psychiatry* 144(9):1184-1188.
  1991   Evaluation of patients treated for pathological gambling in a combined alcohol, substance abuse, and pathological gambling treatment unit

using the Addiction Severity Index. *British Journal of Addiction* 86:1017-1028.

Lesieur, H.R., S.B. Blume, and R. Zoppa
1986 Alcoholism, drug abuse and gambling. *Alcoholism: Clinical and Experimental Research* 10:33-38.

Letson, L.M.
1998 Problem and pathological gambling: A consumer perspective. *CNS Spectrums* 3:48-57.

Linden, M.D., H.G. Pope, Jr., and J.M. Jonas
1986 Pathological gambling and major affective disorder: Preliminary findings. *Journal of Clinical Psychiatry* 47:201-203.

Lindner, R.M.
1950 The psychodynamics of gambling. *Annals of the American Academy of the Political and Social Sciences* 26:93-107.

Lopez Viets, V.C., and W.R. Miller
1997 Treatment approaches for pathological gamblers. *Clinical Psychology Review* 17:689-702.

Lorenz, V.C., and R.A. Yaffee
1988 Pathological gambling: Psychosomatic, emotional, and marital difficulties as reported by the spouse. *Journal of Gambling Behavior* 4:13-26.

Marlatt, G.A., and J.R. Gordon, eds.
1985 *Relapse Prevention: Maintenance Strategies in the Treatment of Addictive Behaviors.* New York: Guilford Press.

Marlatt, G.A., and S.F. Tapert
1993 Harm reduction: Reducing the risks of addictive behaviors. In *Addictive Behaviors Across the Life Span: Prevention, Treatment and Policy Issues,* J.S. Bauer, G.A. Marlatt, and R.J. McMahon, eds. Newbury Park, CA: Sage Publications.

McCartney, J.
1996 A community study of natural change across the addictions. *Addiction Research* 4:65-83.

McClellan, A.T., G.R. Grissom, D. Zanis, M. Randall, P. Brill, and C.P. O'Brien
in press Improved outcomes from problem-service "matching" in substance abuse patients: A controlled study in a four-program, EAP network. *Archives of General Psychiatry.*

McClellan, A.T., G. Woody, L. Luborsky, C. O'Brien, and K. Druley
1983 Increased effectiveness of substance abuse treatment: A prospective study of patient treatment matching. *Journal of Nervous and Mental Diseases* 171:597-605.

McClellan, T., C. O'Brien, N. Hoffmann, and H. Kleber
1998 Is Drug Dependence a Treatable, Medical Illness? Paper presented to the Physician Leadership on National Drug Policy, Washington, DC. March.

McConaghy, N.
1991 A pathological or compulsive gambler? *Journal of Gambling Studies* 7:55-64.

McConaghy, N., M.S. Armstrong, A. Blaszczynski, and C. Allock
  1983   Controlled comparison of aversive therapy and imaginal desensitization in compulsive gambling. *British Journal of Psychiatry* 142:366-372.
  1988   Behavior completion versus stimulus control in compulsive gambling: Implications for behavioral assessment. *Behavior Modification* 12:371-384.
McConaghy, N., A. Blaszczynski, and A. Frankova
  1991   Comparison of imaginal desensitization with other behavioral treatments of pathological gambling. *British Journal of Psychiatry* 159:390-393.
McCormick, R.A.
  1994   The importance of coping skill enhancement in the treatment of the pathological gambler. *Journal of Gambling Studies* 10:77-86.
Meyer, G.
  1989   *Glucksspieler in Selbsthilfegruppen: Erste Ergebnisse Einer Empirischen Untersuchung.* Hamberg: Neuland.
Moore, T.
  1998   Evaluating a Large Systems Treatment Intervention: An Update of the Oregon State-Wide Evaluation Study. Presentation to the 12th National Conference of Problem Gambling, June 19, Las Vegas, NV.
Moskowitz, J.A.
  1980   Lithium and Lady Luck: Use of lithium carbonate in compulsive gambling. *New York State Journal of Medicine* 80:785-788.
Murray, J.B.
  1993   Review of research on pathological gambling. *Psychological Reports* 72:791-810.
Niederland, W.G.
  1967   A contribution to the psychology of gambling. *Psychoanalytic Forum* 2:175-185.
Preston, F.W., B.J. Bernhard, R.E. Hunter, and S.L. Bybee
  1998   Gambling as stigmatized behavior: Regional relabeling and the law. *Annals of the American Academy of Political and Social Science* 556:186-196.
Prochaska, J.O.
  1996   A Transtheoretical Approach to Addictive Treatment: Considering Stages of Change to Optimize Treatment Outcomes. Paper presented at the Drugs and Addictions Treatment Briefing, Harvard University, May 6.
Prochaska, J.O., C.C. DiClemente, and J.C. Norcross
  1992   In search of how people change: Applications to addictive behaviors. *American Psychologist* 47:1102-1114.
Rabow, J., L. Comess, N. Donovan, and C. Hollos
  1984   Compulsive gambling: Psychodynamic and sociological perspectives. *Israel Journal of Psychiatry and Related Sciences* 21:189-207.
Rankin, H.
  1982   Case histories and shorter communications. *Behavior Research and Therapy* 20:185-187.

Reider, N.
1960 Percept as a screen: Economic and structural aspects. *Journal of the American Psychoanalytic Association* 8:82-99.
Rhodes, W., J.J. Norman, S. Langenbahn, P. Harmon, and D. Deal
1997 *Evaluation of the Minnesota State-Funded Compulsive Gambling Treatment Programs.* Cambridge, MA: Abt Associates Inc.
Rosecrance, J.
1988 Active gamblers as peer counselors. *International Journal of the Addictions* 23: 751-766.
Rosenthal, R.J.
1986 The pathological gambler's system of self-deception. *Journal of Gambling Behavior* 2:108-120.
1987 The psychodynamics of pathological gambling: A review of the literature. In *The Handbook of Pathological Gambling*, T. Galski, ed. Springfield, IL: Charles C. Thomas.
1992 Pathological gambling. *Psychiatric Annals* 22:72-78.
1997 The Role of Medication in the Treatment of Pathological Gambling. Paper presented at the Tenth International Conference on Gambling and Risk-Taking, Montreal, Canada, June 2. Department of Psychiatry, University of California, Los Angeles.
Rosenthal, R.J., and H.R. Lesieur
1992 Self-reported withdrawal symptoms and pathological gambling. *American Journal of the Addictions* 1:150-154.
Rosenthal, R.J., and L.J. Rugle
1994 A psychodynamic approach to the treatment of pathological gambling: Part I. Achieving abstinence. *Journal of Gambling Studies* 10:21-42.
Russo, A.M., J.I. Taber, R.A. McCormick, and L.F. Ramirez
1984 An outcome study of an inpatient treatment program for pathological gamblers. *Hospital and Community Psychiatry* 35:823-827.
Salzmann, M.M.
1982 Treatment of compulsive gambling. *British Journal of Psychiatry* 141:318-319.
Schore, A.N.
1994 *Affect Regulation and the Origin of the Self: The Neurobiology of Emotional Development.* Hillsdale, NJ: Lawrence Erlbaum.
Schwarz, J., and A. Lindner
1992 Inpatient treatment of male pathological gamblers in Germany. *Journal of Gambling Studies* 8:93-109.
Seager, C.P.
1970 Treatment of compulsive gamblers by electrical aversion. *British Journal of Psychiatry* 117:545-553.
Seager, C.P., M.R. Pokorny, and D. Black
1966 Aversion therapy for compulsive gambling. *Lancet* 1:546.

Shaffer, H.J.
  1995   Denial, ambivalence and countertransference hate. In *Alcoholism: Dynamics and Treatment*, J.D. Levin and R. Weiss, eds. Northdale: Jason Aronson.
  1997   Psychology of stage change. Pp. 100-106 in *Substance Abuse: A Comprehensive Textbook, 3rd Edition*, J.H. Lowinson, P. Ruiz, R.B. Millman, and J.G. Langrod, eds. Baltimore: Williams and Wilkins.

Shaffer, H.J., and M.N. Hall
  1994   *The Emergence of Youthful Gambling and Drug Use: The Prevalence of Underage Lottery Use and the Impact of Gambling*. Boston: Harvard Medical School, Division on Addictions.

Shaffer, H.J., and S.B. Jones
  1989   *Quitting Cocaine: The Struggle Against Impulse*. Lexington, MA: Lexington Books.

Sharpe, L., and N. Tarrier
  1993   Towards a cognitive-behavioral theory of problem gambling. *British Journal of Psychiatry* 162:407-412.

Simmel, E.
  1920   Psychoanalysis of the gambler. *International Journal of Psychoanalysis* 1:352-353.

Sobell, L.C., J.A. Cunningham, and M.B. Sobell
  1996   Recovery from alcohol problems with and without treatment: Prevalence in two population surveys. *American Journal of Public Health* 86:966-972.

Steinberg, M.A.
  1993   Couples treatment issues for recovering male compulsive gamblers and their partners. *Journal of Gambling Studies* 9(2):153-167.

Stewart, R.M., and R. Brown.
  1988   An outcome study of Gamblers Anonymous. *British Journal of Psychiatry* 152:284-288.

Stinchfield, R.D.
  1998   Reliability, Validity and Classification Accuracy of the SOGS. Paper presented at the Twelfth National Conference on Problem Gambling, June 18-20, Las Vegas, NV. University of Minnesota Medical School.

Stinchfield, R.D., and K.C. Winters
  1996   *Treatment Effectiveness of Six State-Supported Compulsive Gambling Treatment Programs in Minnesota*. Minneapolis: Department of Psychiatry, University of Minnesota.

Substance Abuse and Mental Health Services Administration
  1995   Overview of the FY94 National Drug and Alcoholism Treatment Unit Survey (NDATUS): Data from 1993 and 1980-1993. Advance Report Number 9A, August 1995. Rockville, MD: Substance Abuse and Mental Health Services Administration.

Svendsen, R.
  1998   *Health Care Service Issues for the Treatment of Pathological Gamblers: Survey Results*. Anoka: Minnesota Institute on Public Health.

Sylvain, C., and R. Ladouceur
  1992   Correction cognitive et habitudes de jeu chez les jouers de poker video. *Revue Canadienne des Sciences du Comportement* 24:479-489.
Sylvain, C., R. Ladouceur, and J.M. Boisvert
  1997   Cognitive and behavioral treatment of pathological gambling: A controlled study. *Journal of Consulting and Clinical Psychology* 65:727-732.
Taber, J.I.
  1985   Pathological gambling: The initial screening interview. *Journal of Gambling Behavior* 1(1):230-234.
Taber, J.I., R.A. McCormick, A.M. Russo, B.J. Adkins, and L.F. Ramirez
  1987   Follow-up of pathological gamblers after treatment. *American Journal of Psychiatry* 144:757-761.
Toneatto, T., L.C. Sobell, M.B. Sobell, and E. Rubel
in press Natural recovery from cocaine dependence. *Psychology of Addictive Behaviors*.
Ulman, R.B., and H. Paul
  1998   *Narcissus and Wonderland: The Self-Psychology of Addiction and Its Treatment.* New York: Analytic Press.
U.S. Bureau of the Census
  1997   Estimates for recorded music and video games include persons 12 and older. Pp. 565-566 in *Statistical Abstract of the United States 1997.* Washington, DC: U.S. Department of Commerce.
Volberg, R.A.
  1994   The prevalence and demographics of pathological gamblers: Implications for public health. *American Journal of Public Health* 84:237-241.
  1995   *Wagering and Problem Wagering in Louisiana.* Report to the Louisiana Economic Development and Gaming Corporation. Roaring Spring, PA: Gemini Research.
Volberg, R.A., and H.J. Steadman
  1988   Refining prevalence estimates of pathological gambling. *American Journal of Psychiatry* 145(4):502-505.
Von Hattingberg, H.
  1914   Analerotik, angstlust and eigensinn. *Internationale Zeitschrift fur Psychoanalyse* 2:244-258.
Walker, M.B.
  1992   *The Psychology of Gambling.* Oxford: Pergamon Press.
  1993   Treatment strategies for problem gambling: A review of effectiveness. Pp. 533-566 in *Gambling Behavior and Problem Gambling,* W.R. Eadington and J. Cornelius, eds. Reno, NV: Institute for the Study of Gambling and Commerical Gaming.
Wallisch, L.S.
  1998   *Problem Gambling Helplines Nationwide.* Austin: Texas Commission on Alcohol and Drug Abuse.

Wallisch, L., and S. Cox
  1997 Gambling in Texas Before and After the Lottery: Information from the Texas Gambling Surveys of Adults and Adolescents and the Gambling Telephone Hotline. Paper presented to the 10th International Conference on Gambling and Risk-Taking, Montreal, Canada, June 3. Texas Commission on Alcohol and Drug Abuse, Austin.
Weissman, P.
  1963 The effects of preoedipal paternal attitudes on development and character. *International Journal of Psychoanalysis* 44:121-131.
Winick, C.
  1962 Maturing out of narcotic addiction. *United Nations Bulletin on Narcotics* 14:1-7.
Winters, K.C., P.L. Bengston, and R.D. Stinchfield
  1996 *Findings from a Follow-up Study of Callers to the Minnesota Problem Gambling Hotline.* Minneapolis: Department of Psychiatry, University of Minnesota.
Wong, N.
  1989 Theories of personality and psychopathology: Classical psychoanalysis. Pp. 356-403 in *Comprehensive Textbook of Psychiatry, 5th Edition*, H.I. Kaplan and B. Sadock, eds. Baltimore: Williams and Wilkins.
Wray, I., and M.G. Dickerson
  1981 Cessation of high frequency gambling and "withdrawal" symptoms. *British Journal of Addiction* 76:401-405.
Wurmser, L.
  1974 Psychoanalytic considerations of the etiology of compulsive drug use. *Journal of the American Psychoanalytic Association* 22:820-843.
  1978 *The Hidden Dimension: Psychodynamics of Compulsive Drug Use.* New York: Jason Aronson.
Wynne, H.J.
  1994 Female Problem Gamblers in Alberta. Report prepared for the Alberta Alcohol and Drug Abuse Commission, Edmonton, Canada.
Wynne, H., G. Smith, and D. Jacobs
  1996 Adolescent Gambling and Problem Gambling in Alberta. Edmonton: Alberta Alcohol and Drug Abuse Commission.
Yaffee, R., V. Lorenz, and R. Politzer
  1993 Models explaining gambling severity among patients undergoing treatment in Maryland: 1983-1989. Pp.657-677 in *Gambling Behavior and Problem Gambling*, W.R. Eadington and J.A. Cornelius, eds. Reno: University of Nevada.

7

Organization and Technology of Gambling

Most research on the causes of pathological gambling examines gamblers themselves—their family back grounds, personality traits, experiences with gambling, attitudes about risk, motivations to gamble, and genetic attributes. Such research can lead to a better understanding of individual risk factors in pathological gambling and to better ways to predict and treat gambling problems. Another perspective examines changes in the social and technological environment surrounding gambling. From this perspective, we can ask whether changes in the organization of the gambling enterprise and technologies of gambling lead to more or fewer pathological or problem gamblers, or to new disorders associated with gambling. These are critical questions for developing sensible policies.

Most of the research on these questions is only indirectly related to pathological gambling. At the level of games and betting, there is considerable experimental research on the effects of game structure and game presentation on people's propensity to take risks or to make "nonrational" gambles (e.g., Cole and Hastie, 1978; Mikesell and Zorn, 1987; Ladouceur and Gaboury, 1988). Papers have been authored about how, at the level of society, legalization has potentially affected the prevalence of gambling and pathological gambling (Rose, 1995, 1998). There also has been discussion, but not much empirical research, on how changes in the gambling industry have changed the social context of gambling (e.g., Clotfelter and Cook, 1989). More recently, researchers and policymakers are debating whether the spread of computer-based (video or machine) gambling is changing the prevalence or nature of pathological gambling (Fisher, 1994; Fisher and Griffiths, 1995). Research has not established whether distinctive types of gambling organization and technology cause systematic changes in pathological gambling, but some of the research suggests such links may exist (Griffiths, 1993, 1995, 1998).

HISTORY

Much of what we know about the effects of earlier changes in the gambling industry and gambling technologies—such as the introduction of slot machines and the legalization of casinos in Nevada—comes from historical, biographical, and ethnographic narratives (e.g., Chavetz and Simon, 1967; Skolnick, 1978; Thompson, 1986; Fabian, 1990). This work suggests a close relationship between the social context and technology of gambling, gambling behavior, and social outcomes. For example, according to Barrett (personal communication to the committee, 1998), the most significant early technological development in horse racing was the invention at the turn of the century of a wagering system and calculating machine called the Pari Mutuel System. (The system survives today as "pari-mutuels.") The system allowed some bettors to improve their outcomes by predicting races more skillfully and/or by betting more wisely than most bettors, who underestimate the utility of betting on favorites compared with long shots (Griffiths, 1994; Metzger, 1985; Ladouceur et al., 1998). The system also gave rise to distinctive social roles (bookmaker, professional racetrack gambler, punter) and distinctive supporting technologies (e.g., the racing form).

Different domains of gambling have evolved distinctive cultures, norms, technologies, and social groups who have dominated gambling markets in their respective domains. For example, bingo has its callers and parlors and mainly women patrons. In general, "female" gambling domains are those in which gambling is likely to be less skill-based or to involve less social assertiveness than "male" domains (Kiesler et al., 1985). Kallick and colleagues (1979) noted that, in the United States, Jewish men were overrepresented at the racetracks and were also likely to have gambling problems. This demographic pattern, which is not as discernible in current studies, perhaps was related to the proximity of racetracks to Jewish communities. In any event, there developed among these men a subculture of the track and racing lore. Close social networks were formed among those who bet at the track or in offtrack venues; they would trade tips and loans. Rosecrance (1986) and Zurcher (1970) have also provided accounts of the role of social groups in gambling. It is possible that the subculture of some gambling domains buffers the effects of pathological and problem gambling. For example, friends who gamble together may exert mutual social pressure to limit their gambling expenditures. Such social processes surrounding the technology of gambling have obvious implications for the advent of home gambling and machine games that may also encourage solo gambling.

NATURE AND STRUCTURE OF GAMES

A large body of research suggests that today's gambling technologies and venues take advantage of people's normal responses to reward contingencies and to people's cognitive biases, perceptions of risk, and tendency to compartmentalize mental accounts of their expenditures (e.g., Fischhoff et al., 1981; Wagenaar, 1988; Varey et al., 1990; Kahneman and Tversky, 1979; Tversky and Kahneman, 1992). Some authors argue that gambling represents the purchase of an intangible leisure good, like purchasing a ticket to the movies (Vogel, 1994). However, because gamblers no doubt expect, or hope for, something tangible (money), gambling might be less similar to viewing a movie than to shopping for a luxury watch or car. The value of the activity draws in part from the social desirability of obtaining a rare tangible good and in part from the drama or pleasure of the activity itself. Risk may be part of the pleasure. Gambling is influenced both by the actual risks and rewards of games and by how people imagine these risks and rewards.

Reward Contingencies

Most of the early experimental literature related to gambling focused on the tangible rewards in gambling and were derived from studies of learning through reinforcement and conditioning. Animal and human studies showed that behavior that is rewarded intermittently and randomly is likely to be repeated in the same situation and will be highly resistant to extinction (i.e., the behavior ceases only after many unrewarded trials). Thus, variable and multiple rewards in a gambling situation evoke more gambles and higher bets than single, consistent rewards do (Knapp, 1976). Because most commercial games comprise intermittent rewards of varying magnitude, early learning research suggested that what it called compulsive gambling is a learned or conditioned behavior; however, since few gamblers become compulsive, intermittent and variable reward alone cannot explain problem or pathological gambling.

One possibility is that additional aspects of gambling reward experiences are likely to result in habitual or problem gambling. For instance, people are likely to continue gambling when they are ahead and can gamble "with the house's money" (Thaler and Johnson, 1990). As mentioned in Chapter 2, it has also been shown that near-wins (e.g., the slot machine shows two apples and one pear) are particularly motivating (Skinner, 1953) (see also Kahneman and Tversky, 1979, for cognitive explanations of this effect). With some exceptions (e.g., Ladouceur et al., 1995), this research has been conducted in hypothetical gambling situations or involved small amounts of money (e.g., Wagenaar, 1988). A few studies report that pathological gamblers say they experienced a jackpot or winning streak early on (e.g., Moran, 1970), which is consistent with the laboratory research, although these studies lack baseline data. Perhaps every gambler remembers his or her first big win.

Cognitive Distortions

Research on the cognitive processes involved in judgment and choice has been fruitful in helping to elucidate gambling choices and preferences and, by extension, the kinds of technologies that may encourage habitual or excessive gambling (Wagenaar, 1988). For example, several specific cognitive distortions have been noted as possible contributors to pathological and problem gambling, including: (1) the misunderstanding of the concepts of chance and randomness, (2) attitudinal and belief inertia, and (3) improper resetting of mental accounts. Each of these, discussed below, may contribute to biases in people's assessment of chance processes. Not surprisingly, many popular and profitable gambling products feature games that capitalize on biased judgments; many of these products are attractive to people even in the presence of very unlikely rewards. For example, many gamblers seem to think that multiple gambles give them "more ways to win" even when the multiple gambles are actually disadvantageous to them (Cohen and Chesnick, 1970). And many gamblers also believe independent, random events are somehow connected (Ladoucer and Dube, 1997).

People generally have a strong need to impose order or meaning on random processes, and researchers have investigated whether people can generate random sequences of binary events (such as flipping a coin). Results show that they are often poor at both recognizing and creating such sequences (Wagenaar, 1988), may impose too many alternations on a sequence, or may equate randomness with a balance of event frequencies (Wagenaar, 1972). These tendencies contribute to the gambler's fallacy, which dictates that past losing events are less likely to occur in the future (Cook and Clotfelter, 1993). For example, after several heads have appeared sequentially in the tossing of a coin, it is hard for many to resist the temptation to believe that the next toss will not be heads once again, even though the odds are still 50 percent heads versus 50 percent tails.

In addition to trying to identify predictable patterns in random sequences, people also try to control random outcomes. Langer (1975) refers to this effect as the illusion of control. Gamblers have a variety of methods for exerting their control in gambling situations. For example, Henslin (1967) noted that some gamblers believe they can influence the outcomes of a die roll by tossing it softly for a low number and hard when a high number is desired. Keren and Wagenaar (1985) found that blackjack players would often switch to new tables after a streak of losses in order to change their luck. Other blackjack players would try to *interfere* with the shuffled order of cards by drawing an extra card that they would normally never draw. In this way, they believed they could break an unlucky predetermined pattern and put themselves on a winning streak.

The attempt to impose order on random sequences also relates to overestimating the importance of minimal skill involved in some types of gambling. This was described by Gilovich et al. (1985) who claim that the "hot hand," apparent in basketball when a player's performance is perceived to be significantly better than expected, may be no more than a long sequence of randomly generated events. That is, players occasionally may perform better than expected simply due to chance, and to believe otherwise may be a cognitive distortion. However, playing basketball involves skill. So, although a successful string of free throws may be the result of chance, it is also possible that a player's shooting on a particular day may have been much more skillful than normal and due to little if any chance at all. As previously indicated, some forms of gambling (e.g., cards and track betting) involve both chance and limited skill. Cognitive distortions can occur when gamblers over- or underestimate the chance and the skill involved.

Other forms of gambling, such as slot machines, involve no skill at all but can nonetheless affect illusions of control. Griffiths (1994) asked those who gambled frequently and infrequently, "Is there any skill involved in playing the slot machine?" Those who gambled infrequently tended to say, "mostly chance," whereas frequent gamblers often said, "equal chance and skill." When asked, "How skillful do you think you are compared with the average person?" frequent gamblers thought they were often above average in skill, whereas infrequent gamblers said they were either below average or totally unskilled.

Gamblers favor lotteries featuring complex games; they fail to multiply probabilities and believe they are more likely to win these games than they really are (Cole and Hastie, 1978). These perceptions may explain some of the attractions of slots, lotteries, and multiple-game video machines. Gamblers also favor long shots (Griffith, 1994; Metzger, 1985), a bias that causes them to win less than they might otherwise in sports betting. Experience does not necessarily increase accuracy. With experience, many gamblers lose their fear of taking risks, place larger bets, and bet more on long shots (Ladouceur and Mayrand, 1986).

Gamblers' reduced fear with experience may be associated with their tendency to create stories about events and anthropomorphize gambling objects. Gamblers imbue artifacts such as dice, roulette wheels, and slot machines with character, calling out bets as though these random (or uncontrollable) generators have a memory or can be influenced (Langer, 1975). More generally, gamblers desire, and think they can have, more influence than they actually do on random events (Langer, 1975). They choose lucky numbers, get strong hunches about future random events, value numbers they choose more than numbers they don't, think they can influence a dealer's shuffle, and bet more on their own hands than on others' hands (Phillips and Amrhein, 1989; Chau and Phillips, 1995; Lacey and Pate, 1960). They develop retrospective stories about systematic turns of luck, resulting in the gambler's fallacy about past losses (Rule and Fischer, 1970) and a belief in winning streaks (Myers and Fort, 1963; Cohen et al., 1969). They also remember wins and explain away losses (Gilovich, 1983) and become more comfortable with risk and what they are "learning" as they make repeated gambles (Rachlin, 1989). The illusion of luck turning or of control increasing with experience encourages betting (Lupfer and Jones, 1971). Rachlin (1990) suggests that gamblers frame their games in strings, ending each string after a win. He claims people are especially attracted to large prizes because any win would more than eliminate losses.

Pathological gambling often involves chasing losses (Lesieur and Custer, 1984). This behavior is addressed by Rachlin (1990), who argues that people who persist in gambling despite heavy losses do not adequately update their mental accounts. Normally, people keep track of their spending, winnings, and cash amounts mentally. Rachlin (1990) describes how gamblers may not reset their mental accounts often enough to recognize the full extent of their losses; that heavy gamblers temporarily discount losses more in long, negative strings than in short, positive strings. Negative strings can be evaluated positively in the mind of the gambler if losses are discounted. Furthermore, gamblers postpone their resetting as they continue to gamble, which can make negative strings falsely appear even more positive. This model of chasing losses can describe at least some of the cognitive distortion in pathological gambling.

Moreover, peoples' attitudes, beliefs, and opinions are remarkably resistant to change, even when confronted with overwhelming evidence to the contrary (Klayman and Ha, 1987). This state of attitudinal and belief inertia is exacerbated by biased memories of past events. Some theorists have argued that people show evidence of a hindsight bias (Fischhoff, 1975). After an outcome has occurred, people may claim that they "knew it all along" (Wagenaar, 1988)—which may illustrate another form of omnipotence or an illusion of control. In addition, gamblers may have better recall for absolute wins than for relative net winnings—because they gamble frequently, they may win frequently, and some of their wins may be quite large. Nonetheless, those who gamble also lose frequently, and given the fact that the odds are against them, losses usually surpass wins by a considerable margin. Yet it is the wins, especially the big wins, that tend to be remembered, and loses tend to be discounted or forgotten.

An important question is whether electronic slots, video poker, and video lottery machines, all of which are spreading rapidly and involve chance-based betting, are more or less harmful than more traditional games, such as racetrack betting and playing poker and blackjack. There are arguments on both sides of this question, and empirical research has not settled the matter. In part the question depends on who gambles. Games that are part skill-based might attract particular groups, such as men (Chantal et al., 1995; Oster and Knapp, 1998), educated people, or people who desire control (Langer, 1975; Chantal et al., 1995); such groups may be more or less prone to pathological gambling. On one hand, problem gambling could result from skill-based betting per se, if people's belief in their gambling skills encouraged them to hold misplaced illusions of control or respond overly to short-term streaks (Phillips and Amrhein, 1989). On the other hand, skill-based gambling might be less likely to lead to pathological gambling than wagering in purely chance games. If wagering involves skill, then negative feedback (losses) could cause further study or rational adjustments in strategy. Game speed may be important. Skill-based betting may be experienced as slow or unexciting compared with most chance betting situations (Barrett and Russell, 1998). Although the absence of time pressure tends to encourage betting in the laboratory (Phillips and Amrhein, 1989), gambling without time pressures in real-world settings could be experienced as relaxing and might encourage gamblers to bet limited amounts to extend their play time.

Game Structure

The characteristics of game technologies, such as the number of gambles offered per time period, the physical and informational environment of games, game rules, speed of play, probabilistic structure, cost per play, and jackpot size, appear to affect gambling preferences and habits. For instance, repetitive and multiple interactive games can be created in which the gambler's illusions of increasing skill and premonitions of impending luck are encouraged through reward contingencies. These technology attributes, of course, are more easily manipulated by those who develop and offer games than are attributes of gamblers themselves. New computer-based video machines, in particular, can be programmed to emit the most empirically profitable stimuli and reward contingencies. Often today's machines and games are tested with customers in real gambling settings; those that pay off best are retained and those that customers tire of are discarded (McKay, personal communication to the committee, 1998). Hence these products adapt to the marketplace, evolving to present more enticing gambling situations.

State lottery commissions have increasingly changed the structure of lotteries to take advantage of cognitive biases and responses to reward. A powerful phenomenon is people's attraction to bets featuring large rewards with small probabilities of winning as opposed to bets with smaller rewards and bigger probabilities of winning (Herrnstein, 1990). In the 1990s, numerous front-page stories documented public zeal over multimillion-dollar jackpots with infinitesimal chances of winning. Cook and Clotfelter (1993) provided a thorough account, both theoretical and empirical, of the effect of odds and jackpots on lotto play. They note that the size of the market may influence lotto ticket sales and determine whether a long-odds game is feasible to implement in states like Delaware with relatively small populations. Lyons and Ghezzi's (1995) time series analysis of Oregon's and Arizona's lotteries is one of the few quasi-experimental studies showing how these preferences interact with changes in technology. The authors showed that Oregon's lottery was modified five times and Arizona's four times from 1985 to 1991. Each modification resulted in lower odds of winning and/or a bigger jackpot. On one hand, reducing the odds was unrelated in either state to changes in betting, suggesting that people like low stakes and do not discriminate different odds or changes in the odds when the odds are small anyway (see also Waerneryd, 1996; Huber et al., 1997). On the other hand, increasing the jackpot was strongly related to increased betting. Betting also increased when lotteries were drawn twice weekly instead of weekly, which could be explained either by increased opportunity to play or by reduced risk aversion with more familiarity (Rachlin, 1989). Sales trends suggested that ever-larger jackpots were required to sustain previous levels of play.

Lyons and Ghezzi's (1995) time series study strongly suggests that gambling can be manipulated by lottery organizations through adjustments of lottery structure and rewards. However their study did not examine all aspects of the game environment. For instance, Orgeon has added instant scratch-off numbers games, keno, video poker, sports betting, and the multistate Lotto American game. Both states border Nevada and California, which offer competing products. The behavior of the Oregon and Arizona lottery commissions suggests strongly that lottery organizations model one another in devising competitive market strategies; hence changes in the environment of gambling arise from interstate as well as intrastate competition. Advances in telecommunications and the spread of Internet-supported gambling suggest that gambling is becoming a global business, responsive to competitive pressures across the world.

"Stimulus" Context of Games

A dimension of games that has not received much research attention is the physical and informational environment in which games are presented. This environment includes such factors as informational variations in advertising and instructions, visual differences in the architecture of casinos, and what interface designers call the "form factor" of games (e.g., whether the slot machine has an arm or buttons, takes coins or reads plastic cards, and so forth). Advertising and other information affect what people know about gambling and how they think about it. For instance, lottery organizations publicize winners of big jackpots and use slogans that emphasize the pleasures of playing and winning (see Michael, 1993). Casinos design their architecture to make customers feel as though they are visiting a fantastic, but legitimate world (along the lines of Disneyland); rooms, lighting, sound, and the array of game areas are meant to create feelings of welcome, excitement, comfort, and luxury (Skea, 1995; Kranes, 1995).

Research on working memory and the consequences of cognitive load suggest that gambling situations with many distractions cause changes in how people make decisions and judgments. Generally, this research shows that multiple conflicting stimuli, multiple calls on attention, and noisy environments cause increases in cognitive load (effort of processing information and using working memory), which in turn cause people to process information using guesses and stereotypes and to respond more automatically to stimuli (Gopher and Donchin, 1986). Casinos, racetracks, and increasingly lines at multistate lottery venues feature crowds and crowd suspense and a celebratory atmosphere. Casinos have large rooms, lines of noisy machines, the sound of coins spilling into trays, flashing neon lights, multimedia presentations, loud announcements over the sound system, and the smells of food, perfume, and alcohol (Skea, 1995; Hirsch, 1995). This barrage of distracting stimuli is likely to induce high levels of cognitive load, which in turn could reduce introspection, increase the use of guessing in gambles, and more generally encourage thoughtless gambling.

LEGALIZATION AND SOCIAL INFLUENCE

Legalization is assumed to dramatically change the organization and technology of gambling as new businesses enter the market. In the past few decades, researchers have examined the effects of changes in the legal status of gambling. In particular, the entry of legal gambling enterprises into a locale creates many new opportunities for the public to gamble easily and without stigma. Researchers interested in legalization have emphasized how legalization may have increased people's access to gambling by giving them closer proximity to gambling establishments and making gambling products and services more available.

It is not known whether increased access changes fundamental gambling patterns or switches gamblers from one venue to another. Hybels (1979) argued that related types of gambling (e.g., wagering related to horse racing) may be complementary, that is, when a new kind of gambling is introduced in a particular gambling domain, people gamble more. Lesieur and Sheley (1987) noted that illegal and legal gambling can cooccur; they describe "line sellers," who sell (illegal) tickets on the basis of the display board at legal bingo games. There is conflicting evidence on whether new games displace other gambling or augment total gambling. Kaplan (1990) argues that the decline in racetrack attendance preceded the establishment of state lotteries and that racetrack attendance doesn't differ much between lottery and nonlottery states. However, Coate and Ross (1974) and McDonald (1976) reported that the opening of offtrack betting venues in New York City hurt racetrack attendance. Thalheimer and Ali (1992) found that opening a telephone betting service reduced racetrack attendance and betting overall. This evidence points to a tentative conclusion that, once people have had access to many gambling options, their gambling expenditures level off and are relatively fixed.

Legalization has been linked to pathological gambling. Volberg (1994) reported that the percentage of pathological gamblers as a percentage of the total population was less than 0.5 percent of the population in states where gambling had been legal for less than 10 years, whereas it was 1.5 percent in states where gambling had been legal for more than 20 years. Two prevalence studies reviewed by the committee show increases in the number of pathological gambling before and after legalized gambling (Cox et al., 1997; Emerson and Laundergan, 1996). However, some studies have failed to show that legalization results in increased pathological or problem gambling (Jacobs, personal communication to the committee, 1998). Hraba and colleagues (1990) found that participation in a state lottery was associated with a greater involvement in general gambling, which is in turn connected with problem gambling, but Winters and colleagues (1995) found that the Minnesota lottery switched adolescents from illegal to legal gambling and did not increase overall involvement in gambling in the state. The before-and-after study by Wallisch (1996) in Texas did not show consistent increases in the number of pathological gamblers.

Even when more pathological gamblers are concentrated in locations with more opportunities to gamble, the mechanisms behind this phenomenon are little understood. For example, legal gambling could increase the number of people who gamble at least a few times; if pathological gambling is some constant proportion of people who experiment with gambling, then the numbers of pathological gamblers will also increase. Another possibility is that legalization encourages people to gamble more frequently and to spend more money on gambling. This increased gambling activity could place more people at risk for developing gambling problems by increasing their comfort with games, their familiarity with gambling as entertainment, and their likelihood of socializing with other gamblers.

The spread of professional, legal gambling services (e.g., gambling offered by casino companies and government lottery agencies) over the past few decades has probably contributed to increases in public acceptance of gambling as recreation. It has been proposed that more middle-class parents consider gambling safe, family-oriented, and fun, and fewer worry about whether their teenagers gamble than they did in the past (Kearney et al., 1996). These attitude changes could encourage more adolescents to experiment with adult forms of gambling.

Because legalization typically increases the advertising of gambling and the openness of people's gambling behavior, the public is increasingly exposed to gambling behavior. Research on social influence shows that people's behavior typically conforms to that of others in the situation, particularly when the behavior is public and unambiguous (Cialdini, 1993). Adults, as well as children and teenagers, are influenced by their peers (Harris and

Liebert, 1991). This conformity behavior occurs even in the presence of contradicting general values and prior learning. For example, children who are honest at home and have honest parents may cheat in school if their friends do. A reasonable hypothesis derived from this research is that, if people are exposed to settings in which people gamble, then behavioral norms (what most people in the situation actually do) will influence their gambling attitudes and behavior.

Exposure to gambling in others has been shown to be correlated with gambling or gambling problems. As discussed in earlier chapters, those who gamble as adults (especially illegally) report that they were exposed to gambling as children (Kallick et al., 1979; Downes et al., 1976). In the study by Kallick et al., people who made illegal bets reported three times the amount of childhood exposure to gambling than those who did not gamble. College students who played the lottery were more likely than those who did not to report that they had friends and parents who gambled. However, biases in retrospective memory seriously compromise these survey results. That is, even if everyone has the same exposure, people who gamble would be much more likely to think about others' gambling, to create cognitive associations with gambling, and to remember their parents' and friends' gambling activities. Pathological gamblers may be more likely to remember their parents as having gambled heavily than others would, even if there were no real differences between the two sets of parents. In effect, unless retrospective surveys are very carefully designed and conducted, they cannot determine whether social influence through exposure plays a causal role in pathological gambling.

Another aspect of the social context of gambling that may influence people's propensity to develop problems with gambling is their practice of gambling in the company of friends or family. For instance, men who frequent the racetrack or who play poker together in the same group may develop (or reinforce) friendships around this activity. Many Americans used to invite one another to their homes for informal card games, sometimes limiting themselves to penny wagers. Elderly people and married women gambled with friends and family in bingo parlors or church basements; in some English communities, the bingo game was women's single opportunity to socialize outside the house (Dixey, 1987). Many large casinos today are attractive to elderly people because they can attend with friends or family. Racetracks, casinos, and card rooms often feature restaurants and other spaces where people can meet. In England and Europe, there are exclusive gambling clubs where people can socialize with others in their social circle.

Two opposing hypotheses seem reasonable. On one hand, it is possible that gambling with friends or family (compared with gambling alone or in the presence of strangers) is unlikely to result in excessive gambling, at least in the short run. Pleasurable social interaction increases positive feelings. Although positive feelings increase people's perceived probability of winning, they also reduce betting (Nygren et al., 1996), perhaps by increasing gamblers' happiness or reducing their boredom or loneliness. As well, social pressures from family and friends who are present may reduce gamblers' alcohol consumption or limit their expenditures. On the other hand, if friends and family gamble excessively, other members of these friendship and family groups could be led to do the same. Those who grow up in families in which family members gamble frequently, and those who have friends with gambling problems, could learn to use gambling as a response to stress, or perhaps to underestimate their gambling problems. In one study, problem gamblers were more likely than other gamblers to engage in team lottery play (Hraba and Lee, 1995).

EFFECTS OF CHANGING TECHNOLOGY

Americans seem to love technology and the products and services made possible by technology. In 1995, people over 18 spent about 3,400 hours watching TV and videos, listening to the radio and recorded music, playing home video games, and reading printed books, newspapers, and magazines (Bureau of the Census, 1997). Interaction with a home computer is fast approaching the popularity of these older technologies and activities. The first home computers were introduced as a hobbyist kit in 1975. Today, about 40 percent of all U.S. households own a personal computer; roughly a third of these homes have access to the Internet. Computer technologies in homes, offices, and public places combine and increase the functionality of older technologies, providing new ways to use information and to communicate with others. None of the major changes in the organization of computing and in computing technology was foreseen even halfway in the century—the rise of high-technology industries, the shifts in office employment from clerical to technical labor, the popularity of electronic mail, the adoption of home computers, and the phenomenal spread of the Internet (from 150 sites in 1993 to 2.45 million in 1997).

The organization and technology of gambling has changed no less dramatically and no less surprisingly in the past few decades. Some indicators of this change can be gleaned from analyses of gambling revenues and consumer spending. For example, in an analysis of the demand for commercial gambling, Christiansen (1998, Table 2:41) listed sources of revenue from gambling in 1982 and 1996. In 1996 but not in 1982, revenues from the following types of gambling were sufficiently well measured (or noticeable) to be listed: intertrack wagering (horses), intertrack wagering (greyhounds), offtrack betting (greyhounds), video lotteries, cruise ship casinos, deepwater cruise ships, cruises-to-nowhere, other commercial casino gambling, noncasino devices, and Indian reservation Class II (e.g., bingo) and Class III (casino) gambling. During this period, consumer expenditures on gambling increased at an annual rate of 11.4 percent, comparable to the growth of cable TV, home computers, and the Internet. At the same time, a redistribution of revenue sources occurred across types of gambling. People spent less at the racetrack and on traditional table games and bingo, and more on casinos, lotteries, card rooms, and sports betting.

Changes in the marketing of gambling may alter the demographics of gambling and pathological gambling. Gambling enterprises have traditionally attracted new or repeat customers through a variety of mechanisms, such as easy credit, low prices of entry (nickel slots; $1 lottery tickets), or "comps" and "freebies" (free games, food, or drinks; reduced hotel costs; shows and other entertainment for nongambling family members). As gambling has become more acceptable as a business investment (Eadington, 1982), popular marketing techniques have been applied to increase gambling sales and profits. Increasingly, businesses target particular market segments. For example, whereas racetracks traditionally attracted men and people who could or would take time off from work, casinos may offer baby-sitting facilities for parents and weekend package getaways for working people to reduce their effort and concerns about budget and time. Casinos also evaluate how to use floor space in relation to their market (Dandurand, 1990). For example, they may identify a market niche, such as elderly women who gamble $2 slots, and design safe places for these women to put their purses. Lotteries may attract gamblers who are female, minority, low income, or elderly because they are practically effort-free and do not require risky social behaviors or large investments (Lorenz, 1990).

During the period when legalization and the open marketing of gambling opened large new markets to gambling, technical advances in computing and telecommunications made possible the creation of new automated gambling devices and services, better casino security and policing against cheating, development of remote gambling services, consolidated operations across states and venues, and better collection and use of market data from such information sources as credit ratings, Internet hits, and membership (club card) records. The rapidly growing high-technology gambling industry suggests that future advances in multimedia, digitization, satellites, and the like will lead to many future technological changes in gambling.

Technological change is evident even in the traditional horse racing industry. A decade ago, competition with other forms of legal gambling threatened the owners of horses, training facilities, and racetracks with slimmer profits as new forms of gambling gave customers new entertainment options. New technology in the form of satellite wagering facilities or "betting parlors," simulcast races, and video poker machines that could run 48 hours a day may have saved some racetracks. Racetracks today offer new wagering options on chance-based games made possible by computers (e.g., picking the exact order of finishing or wagering that an even-numbered horse will win). New games such as picking the winner of six races can offer large payoffs with low probabilities of a win, approaches that increase profits and attract customers. Changes in computers and telecommunications are changing the way racing games are being distributed.

Wagering on horse races is now available to many people without leaving their homes. The Internet offers hundreds of web sites where people can bet on a variety of sports, including racing. A new effort by Television Video Games/On Demand Services joins television technology with racetrack products (Barrett, personal communication to the committee, 1998). It is not clear what effect these new gambling opportunities will have; for example, complexity in games can actually reduce risk-taking (Johnson and Bruce, 1997).

In evaluating the impact of technological change on pathological gambling, we cannot make predictions based on technical features alone (Shaffer, 1996). For instance, the telephone, TV, and the Internet are all technologies that have the potential to reduce the importance of physical distance as a constraint on gambling. They reduce the financial and behavior costs of getting information about gambling and increase people's gambling options. However, people could use both the telephone and the Internet, instead, to augment their traditional face-to-face communication for social contact. They could expand their number of friends and acquaintances and reduce the difficulty of coordinating interaction with them. Alternatively, because these technologies disproportionately reduce the costs of communication with geographically distant friends and acquaintances, they may lead to shifts in people's portfolios to more distant contacts. In addition, the Internet, through such things as interactive games and distribution lists, fosters communication among strangers. As a result, people who use these technologies heavily may have a smaller proportion of their total social contacts with family and close friends. Gambling via cable or satellite television and the Internet provides asocial entertainment and information that could compete with social contact as a way for people to spend their time.

Game Machines

Several writers have argued that playing computer-based game machines is more likely to lead to pathological gambling than other forms of gambling (e.g., Fisher and Griffiths, 1995; Fabian, 1995). Morgan and colleagues (1996) reported that video lottery gambling is the predominant type of gambling behavior engaged in by gamblers seeking treatment. Fisher and Griffiths (1995) argue that England's legal "fruit machines" (slots) are especially risky for adolescents. They claim that game machines, better than other technologies, can be designed and programmed to encourage frequent gambling. Gupta and Derevensky (1996) asked heavy and light video-game-playing children (ages 9-14) in Canada to complete a questionnaire and to play a computer blackjack game. The high-frequency video game players were more likely to report being regular gamblers. Heavy-playing boys also bet more on the blackjack tasks. The authors speculate that experience with video games, in which practice can improve performance, leads teenagers to have the illusion that gambling machine games are somehow solvable. Griffiths (1990) found that troubled teenagers (problem gamblers, those who had been charged with crimes) were likely to hang out in video arcades and to play fruit machines frequently. However, this study and others on the correlates of children's machine gambling are only suggestive of a causal link between playing game machines and pathological gambling, and reasonable alternative explanations exist. For example, background and personal factors leading British adolescents to get into trouble could also lead them to hang out in arcades, play slots, and also to have illusions of skill in their gambling and other areas of their lives.

If new game machines such as video poker machines can be tailored to their users, they might be able to deliver more effective reward contingencies. Such an effect could increase the probability of problem gambling. Kilby (1987) discussed an older rating system for casino players whereby records were kept of frequent patrons' conversions of currency to chips. Those who cashed in more money might be given more "comps" such as free food, drinks, or games. Today, plastic club cards used with game machines are a far more sophisticated version of the old system; they can record exactly how much a gambler is wagering on which types of games. In theory, these cards can track gambler preferences, wagers, and outcomes; future rewards and games can be "personalized" to those patterns (Popkin and Hetter, 1994). The cards also can be used to tally frequent gambler credits, encouraging loyalty to the casino or other venue.

Telecommunications technology also could be used in tailoring gambling to customer preferences and responses. Current gambling sites on the Internet require customers to provide their name, postal address, email address, social security number, and credit card information. Some sites require customers also to provide the name of the customer's mother's maiden name or other specific identifying information. Typically software has to be downloaded to the customer's machine as well; the customer's machine has a unique address that allows records to be kept over time about the use of that machine. Software can record gamblers' identity when they start a gambling session and passively log the time they spend gambling, the game they play, the time they spend logged into the Internet, the address that identifies the web pages they connect to, and in some cases the electronic mail addresses they exchange email with. Although current Internet gambling sites are fairly traditional in their design and have problems with slow response time and errors, the technology provides opportunity for much more sophisticated, adaptive applications in the future.

Home Gambling

Many scholars, technologists, and social critics debate how computer technologies, and the Internet in particular, are transforming economic and social life (e.g., Anderson and Van Der Heijden, 1998). It has been posited that home gambling and the Internet may attract adolescent gamblers, or cause people to get addicted to gambling and cut themselves off from normal social constraints on gambling, as they hunker alone over their terminals playing games in electronic casinos or betting with anonymous strangers through chat rooms. However, it could also be argued that gambling problems at home, whether via the Internet or some other telecommunications technology, will be rare. It has been claimed that the Internet actually offers people more and better entertainment and social opportunities by freeing them from the constraints of geography or isolation brought on by stigma, illness, or schedule (e.g., Rheingold, 1993).

There are at least two reasons why computer-based gambling at home should be studied further, using methodologies that can distinguish the effects of gambling at home from other factors.

One reason is that gambling at home may increase people's susceptibility to pathological gambling through the ease and frequency with which they can gamble. Another reason is that gambling at home may contribute to other personal problems. In particular, gambling at home is likely to increase passive leisure activity and solo gambling, and it may displace time spent on active, social interaction (including social gambling excursions with others and table games at home).

Computer-based gambling at home may have effects similar to those of watching television. Empirical work suggests that television-watching reduces social interaction (Jackson-Beeck and Robinson, 1981; Neuman, 1991; Maccoby, 1951). At the individual level, social disengagement is associated with poor quality of life and diminished physical and psychological health. Time studies show that social interactions are among the most pleasant experiences people have (Robinson and Godbey, 1997). People who have close ties with local friends, neighbors, and family have available to them social support that seems to buffer them from life stresses (Cohen and Wills, 1985). One study also shows that the social support that people get from distant acquaintances, friends, and family is less effective in buffering daily stress than the support they get from their local friends and neighbors (Wellman and Wortley, 1990b). Compared with people who have little social contact in their lives, people with more social contact are physically healthier, mentally healthier, and happier (e.g., Cohen and Wills, 1985).

Gambling at home also may encourage passive, sedentary activity, as watching television does. Recent epidemiological research has linked television-watching with reduced physical activity and diminished physical and mental health (Anderson and Van Der Heijden, 1998). Gambling by adolescents is correlated with watching television and other passive leisure-time activities (Junger and Wiegersma, 1995).

CONCLUSIONS

Computers and telecommunications are changing the gambling industry, individuals' opportunities to gamble, and the social context of gambling. The effects of these technologies, especially of home gambling and the Internet, are highly uncertain. Putnam (1995) and Condry (1993) have pointed to the television as a technology that has caused Americans to withdraw from personal and civic relationships, to the detriment of the television watchers themselves and the community as a whole. However, even for the case of television, which has been around for years, we have only a weak causal chain, suggesting that television viewing reduces social involvement or activity which in turn reduces physical and psychological health. The chain for the case of gambling machines and home gambling is even weaker. Studies of the prevalence of pathological or problem gambling for different types of gambling do not generally control for extraneous factors, including survey questions, locale, and year in which the survey was done. Computer-based video machine gambling is new enough that it is not well represented even in the modest number of surveys that address the issue. Hence the impact of technology remains an important but open question. We do not know whether problem gamblers are more attracted to video or machine gambling than gamblers without problems, and we do not understand the mechanisms that account for the associations reported in the literature.

Research is needed that allows us to better understand the link between use of gambling technologies and subsequent changes in gambling disorders. By conducting natural experiments and prospective studies, preferably with national samples, it would be possible to estimate the extent to which conclusions from correlational cross-sectional studies are valid or widespread and to determine some of their limiting conditions. By differentiating social and asocial types of gambling, and by employing careful measures such as time diaries and assessments of the size and type of social circles that gamblers maintain, researchers would be able to test several of the plausible mechanisms by which use of technology may change vulnerability to pathological gambling.

Research on the organization and technology of gambling should be evaluated in the context of the sparse research on social and technological change more generally. Little empirical research exists even about the social effects of such important technologies as the television and the telephone. Laboratory studies on technology in gambling have tended to focus on the structure of gambles rather than gambling habits and social outcomes. These studies have led to important theories about the nature of betting, but their implications for technology and gambling problems have not been tested. Few if any gambling organizations would be willing to run public experiments on these issues, and even if they did, the link to pathological gambling would be difficult to trace. Field research on the organization and technology of gambling is rare, although there is a body of literature on the effects of legalization, most of which relies on cross-sectional surveys and self-reports of gambling behaviors. Since legalization is likely to change reporting along with the technology, markets, attitudes, and constraints of gambling, it is hard to draw conclusions about how a particular aspect of legalization is affecting people.

One way to study the effects of new technology or organization in natural settings is through natural experiments; natural experiments elicit data to which time series analyses can be applied (see Lyons and Ghezzi, 1995). Another approach would be to conduct prospective, longitudinal studies of individuals. This approach has long been used in studies of health and disease (e.g., the Framingham heart study). However, it is possible that little is to be gained from a dedicated longitudinal prospective study of pathological gambling, since only a tiny percentage of the sample is likely to develop a gambling problem. Still, it would seem feasible and worthwhile to add measures of gambling and related leisure activities and outcomes (e.g., debts) to other prospective longitudinal studies in health or mental health. Doing so would not only add valuable information about gambling over time, but would also provide important information about baseline date and comorbidity.

Even prospective studies can pose threats to valid causal claims. First, statistical controls may not adequately equate groups (e.g., gamblers and nongamblers) on other factors. Preexisting factors (ranging from cohort characteristics to biological stress) could cause people to be predisposed to gambling and as well to be attracted to a particular type of game or gambling setting. Second, unmeasured variables that change over time may induce both gambling of certain types and changes in outcomes such as problem gambling. Measuring gambling in relationship to how people spend their time and money more generally might be useful in understanding other factors that may be related to both normal, social gambling and problem gambling. Detailed studies using time and expenditure measures; measures of social network size, social activities, and stress; psychological measures of social support and physical and mental health could contribute to understanding of the relationships between problem gambling, how people use technology, time, and money, social interaction, and the size of social networks.

REFERENCES

Anderson A., and H. Van Der Heijden
    1998   Media, culture, and the environment. *Environmental Politics* 7(4):188-189.

Barrett, L.F., and J.A. Russell
    1998   Independence and bipolarity in the structure of current affect. *Journal of Personality and Social Psychology* 74(4):967-984.

Bureau of the Census
    1997   Estimates for recorded music and video games include persons 12 and older. Pp. 565-566 in *Statistical Abstract of the United States*. Washington, DC: U.S. Department of Commerce.

Chantal, Y., R.J. Vallerand, and E.F. Vallieres
    1995   Motivation and gambling involvement. *Journal of Social Psychology* 135(6):755-763.

Chau, A.W., and J.G. Phillips
    1995   Effects of perceived control upon wagering and attributions in computer blackjack. *Journal of General Psychology* 122.

Chavetz, H., and C. Simon
    1967   *Play the Devil: A History of Gambling in the United States*. New York: C.N. Potter.

Cialdini, R.B.
    1993   *Influence: Science and Practice, 3rd ed.* New York: Harper Collins College Publishers.

Clotfelter, C.T., and P.J. Cook
    1989   *Selling Hope: State Lotteries in America.* Cambridge, MA: Harvard University Press.

Coate, D., and G. Ross
    1974   The effect of off-track betting in New York City on revenues to the city and state governments. *National Tax Journal* 27:63-69.

Cohen, J., L.E. Boyle, and A.P.W. Shubsachs
    1969   Rouge et noir: Influence of previous play on choice of binary event outcome and size of stake in a gambling situation. *Acta Psychologica* 31:340-352.

Cohen, J., and E.I. Chesnick
  1970   The doctrine of psychological chances. *British Journal of Psychology* 61(3):323-334.
Cohen, S., and T.A. Wills
  1985   Stress, social support, and the buffering hypothesis. *Psychological Bulletin* 98(2):310-357.
Cole, W.R., and R. Hastie
  1978   The effects of lottery game structure and format on subjective probability and attractiveness of gambles. *Personality and Social Psychology Bulletin* 4(4):608-611.
Condry, J.
  1993   Thief of time, unfaithful servant: Television and the American child. *Daedalus* 122(1):249-278.
Cook, C.T., and P.J. Clotfelter
  1993   The peculiar scale economies of lotto. *American Economic Review* 83(3):633-634.
Cox, S., H.R. Lesieur, R.J. Rosenthal, and R.A. Volberg
  1997   *Problem and Pathological Gambling in America: The National Picture.* Columbia, MD: National Council on Problem Gambling.
Dandurand, L.
  1990   Market niche analysis in the casino gaming industry. *Journal of Gambling Studies* 6:73-85.
Dixey, R.
  1987   It's a great feeling when you win: Women and bingo. *Leisure Studies* 6(2):199-214.
Downes, D.M., B. Davies, and M.E. David
  1976   *Gambling, Work and Leisure: A Study Across Three Areas.* London: Routledge and Kegan.
Eadington, W.R.
  1982   *Studies in the Business of Gambling.* Reno: Bureau of Business and Economic Research, University of Nevada.
Emerson, M.O., and J.C. Laundergan
  1996   Gambling and problem gambling among adult Minnesotans: Changes 1990 to 1994. *Journal of Gambling Studies* 12(3):291-304.
Fabian, A.
  1990   *Card Sharps, Dream Books, and Bucket Shops: Gambling in 19th-Century America.* Ithaca, NY: Cornell University Press.
Fabian, T.
  1995   Pathological gambling: A comparison of gambling at German-style slot machines and "classical" gambling. *Journal of Gambling Studies* 11(3):249-263.
Fischhoff, B.
  1975   Hindsight = foresight: The effect of outcome knowledge on judgment under uncertainty. *Journal of Experimental Psychology, Human Perception & Performance* 1:288-299.

Fischhoff, B., S. Lichtenstein, P. Slovic, S.L. Derby, and R. Keeney
  1981   *Acceptable Risk.* New York: Cambridge University Press.
Fisher, S.E.
  1994   Identifying video game addiction in children and adolescents. *Addictive Behaviors* 19(5):545-553.
Fisher, S.E., and M. Griffiths
  1995   Current trends in slot machine gambling: Research and policy issues. Special Issue: Slot Machine Gambling. *Journal of Gambling Studies* 11(3):239-247.
Gilovich, T.
  1983   Biased evaluation and persistence in gambling. *Journal of Personality and Social Psychology* 44:1110-1126.
Gilovich, T., R. Vallone, and A. Tversky
  1985   The hot hand in basketball: On the misperception of random sequences. *Cognitive Psychology* 17:295-314.
Gopher, D., and E. Donchin
  1986   Workload—An examination of the concept. Pp. 41-48 in *Handbook of Perception and Human Performance*, K.R. Boff, L. Kaufman, and J.P. Thomas, eds. New York: John Wiley.
Griffith, R.M.
  1949   Odds adjustment by American horse-race bettors. *American Journal of Psychology* 62:290-294.
Griffiths, M.D.
  1990   The acquisition, development, and maintenance of fruit machine gambling in adolescents. *Journal of Gambling Studies* 6(3):193-204.
  1993   Fruit machine gambling: The importance of structural characteristics. *Journal of Gambling Studies* 9:133-152.
  1994   The role of cognitive bias and skill in fruit machine gambling. *British Journal of Psychology* 85:351-369.
  1995   Technological addictions. *Clinical Psychology Forum* 76:14-19.
  1998   Gambling Technologies: Lessons from Scholarly Literature and Prospects for Pathological Gambling. Presentation to the National Research Council Committee on the Social and Economic Impact of Pathological Gambling, September 2. Nottingham Trent University, Nottingham, Australia.
Gupta, R., and J.L. Derevensky
  1996   The relationship between gambling and video-game playing behavior in children and adolescents. *Journal of Gambling Studies* 12(4):375-394.
Harris, J.R., and R.M. Liebert
  1991   *The Child: A Contemporary View of Development, 3rd ed.* Englewood Cliffs, NJ: Prentice-Hall, Inc.
Henslin, J.M.
  1967   Craps and magic. *American Journal of Sociology* 73:316-330.
Herrnstein, R.
  1990   Behavior, reinforcement and utility. *American Psychologist* (45):356.

Hirsch, A.R.
1995 Effects of ambient odors on slot-machine usage in a Las Vegas casino. *Psychology and Marketing* 12(7):585-594.

Hraba, J., and G. Lee
1995 Problem gambling and policy advice: The mutability and relative effects of structural, associational and attitudinal variables. *Journal of Gambling Studies* 11(2):105-121.

Hraba J., W. Mok, and D. Huff
1990 Lottery play and problem gambling. *Journal of Gambling Studies* 6:355-377.

Huber, O., R. Wider, and O.W. Huber
1997 Active information search and complete information presentation in naturalistic risky decision tasks. *Acta Psychologica* 95(1):15-29.

Hybels, J.H.
1979 The impact of legalization on illegal gambling participation. *Journal of Social Issues* 35(3):27-35.

Jackson-Beeck, M., and J.P. Robinson
1981 Television nonviewers: An endangered species? *Journal of Consumer Research* 7(4):356-359.

Johnson, J.E.V., and A.C. Bruce
1997 A profit model for estimating the effect of complexity on risk taking. *Psychological Reports* 80(3 Pt 1):763-772.

Junger, M., and A. Wiegersma
1995 The relations between accidents, deviance and leisure time. *Criminal Behaviour and Mental Health* 5(3):144-174.

Kahneman, D., and A. Tversky
1979 Prospect theory: An analysis of decision under risk. *Econometrica* 47:263-291.

Kallick, M., D. Suits, T. Dielman, and J. Hybels
1979 *A Survey of American Gambling Attitudes and Behavior.* Research report series, Survey Research Center, Institute for Social Research. Ann Arbor: University of Michigan Press.

Kaplan, H.
1984 The social and economic impact of state lotteries. *Annals of the American Academy of Political and Social Science* 474(July):81.

Kaplan, H.R.
1990 The effects of state lotteries on the parimutuel industry. *Journal of Gambling Studies* 6:331-344.

Katz, J.E., and P. Aspden
1997 A nation of strangers? *Communications of the ACM* 40(12):81-86.

Kearney, C.A., T. Roblek, J. Thurman, and P.D. Turnbough
1996 Casino gambling in private school and adjudicated youngsters: A survey of practices and related variables. *Journal of Gambling Studies* 12(3):319-327.

Keren, G., and C. Lewis
    1994   The two fallacies of gamblers: Type I and type II. *Organizational Behavior and Human Decision Processes* 60(1):75-89.
Keren, G., and W.A. Wagenaar
    1985   On the psychology of playing blackjack: Normative and descriptive considerations with implications for theory. *Journal of Experimental Psychology General* 114(2):133-158.
Kiesler, S., L. Sproull, and J. Eccles
    1985   Poolhalls, chips, and war games: Women in the culture of computing. *Psychology of Women Quarterly* 9:451-462.
Kilby, J.
    1987   Casinos and Good Players: The Ideal Rating System. Paper presented to the Seventh Conference on Gambling and Risk Taking, August 23, Reno, NV.
Klayman, J., and Y. Ha
    1987   Confirmation, disconfirmation, and information in hypothesis testing. *Psychological Review* 94:211-228.
Knapp, T.J.
    1976   A functional analysis of gambling behavior. In *Gambling and Society*. Springfield, IL: Thomas.
Kranes, D.
    1995   Play grounds. Special Issue: Gambling: Philosophy and policy. *Journal of Gambling Studies* 11(1):91-102.
Lacey, O.L., and J.L. Pate
    1960   An empirical study of game theory. *Psychological Reports* 7:527-530.
Ladouceur, R., and D. Dube
    1997   Monetary incentive and erroneous perceptions in American roulette. *Psychology: A Journal of Human Behavior* 34(3-4):27-32.
Ladouceur, R., D. Dube, I. Giroux, N. Legendre, et al.
    1995   Cognitive biases in gambling: American roulette and 6/49 lottery. *Journal of Social Behavior and Personality* 10(2):473-479.
Ladouceur, R., and A. Gaboury
    1988   Effects of limited and unlimited stakes on gambling behavior. *Journal of Gambling Behavior* 4:119-126.
Ladouceur, R., I. Giroux, and C. Jacques
    1998   Winning on the horses: How much strategy and knowledge are needed? *Journal of Psychology* 132(2):133-142.
Ladouceur, R., and M. Mayrand
    1986   Psychological characteristics of monetary risk-taking by gamblers and non-gamblers in roulette. *International Journal of Psychology* 21(4-5):433-443.
Langer, E.J.
    1975   The illusion of control. *Journal of Personality and Social Psychology* 32:311-328.
Lesieur, H.R., and R.L. Custer
    1984   Pathological gambling: Roots, phases, and treatment. *Annals of the American Academy of Political and Social Science* 474:146-156.

Lesieur, H.R., and J.F. Sheley
1987   Illegal appended enterprises: Selling the lines. *Social Problems* 34:249-260.
Lorenz, V.C.
1990   State lotteries and compulsive gambling. *Journal of Gambling Studies* 6(4):383-396.
Lupfer, M., and M. Jones
1971   Risk taking as a function of skill and chance orientations. *Psychological Reports* 28:27-33.
Lyons, C.A., and P.M. Ghezzi
1995   Wagering on a large scale: Relationships between public gambling and game manipulations in two state lotteries. *Journal of Applied Behavior Analysis* 28(2):127-137.
Maccoby, E.E.
1951   Television: Its impact on school children. *Public Opinion Quarterly* 15:421-444.
McDonald, J.
1976   How horseplayers got involved in the urban crisis. In *An Economic Analysis of Crime*, L.J. Kaplan and D. Kessler, eds. Springfield, IL: Thomas.
Metzger, M.A.
1985   Biases in betting: An application of laboratory findings. *Psychological Reports* 56(3):883-888.
Michael, J.
1993   *Pot of Gold. A Novel.* New York: Poseidon Press.
Mikesell, J.L., and C.K. Zorn
1987   State lottery sales: Separating the influence of markets and game structure. *Growth and Change* 18:10-19.
Moran, E.
1970   Varieties of pathological gambling. *British Journal of Psychiatry* 116:593-597.
Morgan, T., L. Kofoed, J. Buchkoski, and R.D. Carr
1996   Video lottery gambling: Effects on pathological gamblers seeking treatment in South Dakota. *Journal of Gambling Studies* 12(4):451-460.
Myers, J.L., and J.G. Fort
1963   A sequential analysis of gambling behavior. *Journal of General Psychology* 69:299-309.
Neuman, S.B.
1991   *Literacy in the Television Age: The Myth of the TV Effect.* Norwood, NJ: Ablex Publishing Corporation.
Nygren, T.E., A.M. Isen, P.J. Taylor, and J. Dulin
1996   The influence of positive affect on the decision rule in risk situations: Focus on outcome (and especially avoidance of loss) rather than probability. *Organizational Behavior and Human Decision Processes* 66(1):59-72.

Oster, S.L., and T.J. Knapp
   1998   Sports betting by college students: Who bets and how often? *College Student Journal* 32(2):289-292.
Phillips, J.G., and P.C. Amrhein
   1989   Factors influencing wagers in simulated blackjack. *Journal of Gambling Behavior* 5(2):99-111.
Popkin, J., and K. Hetter
   1994   America's gambling craze. *US News and World Report* March 14:42-43,46,48-56.
Putnam, R.
   1995   Tuning in, tuning out: The strange disappearance of social capital in America. *Public Speeches* 28(December):664-683.
Rachlin, H.
   1989   *Judgment, Decision, and Choice.* New York: W.H. Freeman.
   1990   Why do people gamble and keep gambling despite heavy losses? *Psychological Science* 1(5):294-297.
Rheingold, H.
   1993   *The Virtual Community: Homesteading on the Electronic Frontier.* Reading, MA: Addison-Wesley Publishing Company.
Robinson, J.P., and G. Godbey
   1997   *Time for Life: The Surprising Ways Americans Use Their Time.* University Park: Pennsylvania State University Press.
Rose, I.N.
   1995   Gambling and the law: Endless fields of dreams. *Journal of Gambling Studies* 11:15-33.
   1998   Technology and the Future of Gambling. Unpublished manuscript. Whittier Law School, Costa Mesa, CA.
Rosecrance, J.
   1986   Adapting to failure: The case of horse race gamblers. *Journal of Gambling Behavior* 2(2):81-94.
Rule, B.G., and D.G. Fischer
   1970   Impulsivity, subjective probability, cardiac response, and risk-taking: Correlates and factors. *Personality* 1:251-260.
Shaffer, H.J.
   1996   Understanding the means and objects of addiction: Technology, the Internet, and gambling. *Journal of Gambling Studies* 12(4):461-469.
Skea, W.H.
   1995   "Postmodern" Las Vegas and its effects on gambling. *Journal of Gambling Studies* 11(2):231-235.
Skinner, B.F.
   1953   *Science and Human Behavior.* New York: Macmillan.
Skolnick, J.
   1978   *House of Cards: Legalization and Control of Casino Gambling.* Boston: Little Brown.

Thaler, R.H., and E.J. Johnson
  1990   Gambling with the house money and trying to break even: The effects of prior outcomes on risky choice. *Management Science* 36:643-660.
Thalheimer, R., and M.M. Ali
  1992   Demand for parimutuel horse race wagering with special reference to telephone betting. *Applied Economics* 24(1):137-142.
Thompson, D.
  1986   *Nevada: A History of Change.* Reno, NV: Danberg Foundation.
Tversky, A., and D. Kahneman
  1992   Advances in prospect theory: Cumulative representation of uncertainty. *Journal of Risk and Uncertainty* 5.
Varey, C., B. Mellers, and M. Birnbaum
  1990   Judgments of proportions. *Journal of Experimental Psychology* 16:613-625.
Vogel, H.L.
  1994   *Entertainment Industry Economics: A Guide for Financial Analysis,* Third Edition. Cambridge, England: Press Syndicate of the University of Cambridge.
Volberg, R.A.
  1994   The prevalence and demographics of pathological gamblers: Implications for public health. *American Journal of Public Health* 84:237-241.
Waerneryd, K.E.
  1996   Risk attitudes and risky behavior. *Journal of Economic Psychology* 17(6):749-770.
Wagenaar, W.
  1972   Generation of random sequences by human subjects: A critical survey of the literature. *Psychological Bulletin* 77:65-72.
  1988   Paradoxes of gambling behavior. *American Journal of Psychology* 103:290-297.
Wallisch, L.S.
  1996   *Gambling in Texas: 1995 Surveys of Adult and Adolescent Gambling Behavior.* Austin: Texas Commission on Alcohol and Drug Abuse.
Wellman, B., and S. Wortley
  1990a Brothers' keepers: Situating kinship relations in broader networks of social support. *Sociological Perspectives* 32(3):273-306.
  1990b Different strokes from different folks: Community ties and social support. *American Journal of Sociology* 96(3):558-588.
Winters, K.C., R.D. Stinchfield, and L.G. Kim
  1995   Monitoring adolescent and gambling in Minnesota. *Journal of Gambling Studies* 11:165-183.
Zurcher, L.A.
  1970   The "friendly" poker game: A study of an ephemeral role. *Social Forces* 49(2):173-185.

Appendixes

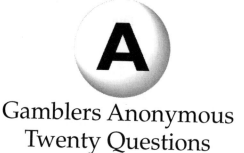

Gamblers Anonymous
Twenty Questions

1. Did you ever lose time from work or school due to gambling?
2. Has gambling ever made your home life unhappy?
3. Did gambling affect your reputation?
4. Have you ever felt remorse after gambling?
5. Did you ever gamble to get money with which to pay debts or otherwise solve financial difficulties?
6. Did gambling cause a decrease in your ambition or efficiency?
7. After losing did you feel you must return as soon as possible and win back your losses?
8. After a win did you have a strong urge to return and win more?
9. Did you often gamble until your last dollar was gone?
10. Did you ever borrow to finance your gambling?
11. Have you ever sold anything to finance gambling?
12. Were you reluctant to use "gambling money" for normal expenditures?
13. Did gambling make you careless of the welfare of yourself and your family?
14. Did you ever gamble longer than you had planned?
15. Have you ever gambled to escape worry or trouble?

16. Have you ever committed, or considered committing, an illegal act to finance gambling?
17. Did gambling cause you to have difficulty in sleeping?
18. Do arguments, disappointments or frustrations create within you an urge to gamble?
19. Did you ever have an urge to celebrate any good fortune by a few hours of gambling?
20. Have you ever considered self destruction as a result of your gambling?

Source: Gamblers Anonymous.

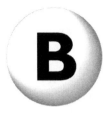

Diagnostic and Statistical Manual of Mental Disorders Criteria for Pathological Gambling

CRITERIA FROM THE 1980 DSM-III

Disorders of Impulse Control Not Elsewhere Classified: Pathological Gambling

The essential features are a chronic and progressive failure to resist impulses to gamble and gambling behavior that compromises, disrupts, or damages personal, family, or vocational pursuits. The gambling preoccupation, urge, and activity increase during periods of stress. Problems that arise as a result of the gambling lead to an intensification of the gambling behavior. Characteristic problems include loss of work due to absences in order to gamble, defaulting on debts and other financial responsibilities, disrupted family relationships, borrowing money from illegal sources, forgery, fraud, embezzlement, and income tax evasion.

Commonly these individuals have the attitude that money causes and is also the solution to all their problems. As the gambling increases, the individual is usually forced to lie in order to obtain money and to continue gambling, but hides the extent of the gambling. There is no serious attempt to budget or save money. When borrowing resources are strained, antisocial behavior in order to obtain money for more gambling is likely. Any criminal behavior—e.g., forgery, embezzlement, or fraud—is typically nonviolent. There is a conscious intent to return or repay the money.

Associated features. These individuals most often are overconfident, somewhat abrasive, very energetic, and "big spenders"; but there are times when they show obvious signs of personal stress, anxiety, and depression.

Age at onset and course. The disorder usually begins in adolescence and waxes and wanes, tending to be chronic.

Impairment. The disorder is extremely incapacitating and results in failure to maintain financial solvency or provide basic support for oneself or one's family. The individual may become alienated from family and acquaintances and may lose what he or she has accomplished or attained in life.

Complications. Suicide attempts, association with fringe and illegal groups, and arrest for nonviolent crimes that may lead to imprisonment are among the possible complications.

Predisposing factors. These may include: loss of parent by death, separation, divorce, or desertion before the child is 15 years of age; inappropriate parental discipline (absence, inconsistency, or harshness); exposure to gambling activities as an adolescent; a high family value on material and financial symbols; and lack of family emphasis on saving, planning, and budgeting.

Prevalence. No information.

Sex ratio. The disorder is apparently more common among males than females.

Familial pattern. Pathological Gambling and Alcoholism are more common in the fathers of males and in the mothers of females with the disorder than in the general population.

Differential diagnosis. In **social gambling**, gambling with friends is engaged in mainly on special occasions and with predetermined acceptable losses.

During a **manic or hypomanic episode** loss of judgment and excessive gambling may follow the onset of the mood disturbance. When manic-like mood changes occur in Pathological Gambling they typically follow winning.

Problems with gambling are often associated with **Antisocial Personality Disorder** and in Pathological Gambling antisocial behavior is frequent. However, in Pathological Gambling any antisocial behavior that occurs is out of desperation to obtain money to gamble when money is no longer available and legal resources have been exhausted. Criminal behavior is rare when the individual has money. Also, unlike the individual with Antisocial Personality Disorder, the individual with Pathological Gambling usually has a good work history until it is disrupted because of the gambling.

Diagnostic Criteria for Pathological Gambling

A. The individual is chronically and progressively unable to resist impulses to gamble.

B. Gambling compromises, disrupts, or damages family, personal, and vocational pursuits, as indicated by at least three of the following:

    1. arrest for forgery, fraud, embezzlement, or income tax evasion due to attempts to obtain money for gambling

    2. default on debts or other financial responsibilities

    3. disrupted family or spouse relationship due to gambling

    4. borrowing of money from illegal sources (loan sharks)

    5. inability to account for loss of money or to produce evidence of winning money, if this is claimed

    6. loss of work due to absenteeism in order to pursue gambling activity

    7. necessity for another person to provide money to relieve a desperate financial situation

C. The gambling is not due to Antisocial Personality Disorder.

CRITERIA FROM THE 1987 DSM-III-R

Impulse Control Disorders Not Elsewhere Classified: Pathological Gambling

The essential features of this disorder are a chronic and progressive failure to resist impulses to gamble, and gambling behavior that compromises, disrupts, or damages personal, family, or vocational pursuits. The gambling preoccupation, urge, and activity increase during periods of stress. Problems that arise as a result of the gambling lead to an intensification of the gambling behavior. Characteristic problems include extensive indebtedness and consequent default on debts and other financial responsibilities, disrupted family relationships, inattention to work, and financially motivated illegal activities to pay for gambling.

Associated features. Generally, people with Pathological Gambling have the attitude that money causes and is also the solution to all their problems. As the gambling increases, the person is usually forced to lie in order to obtain money and to continue gambling. There is no serious attempt to budget or save money. When borrowing resources are strained, antisocial behavior in order to obtain money is likely.

People with this disorder are often overconfident, very energetic, easily bored, and "big spenders"; but there are times when they show obvious signs of personal stress, anxiety, and depression.

Age at onset and course. The disorder usually begins in adolescence in males, and later in life in females. It waxes and wanes, but tends to be chronic.

Impairment. The disorder is extremely incapacitating and results in failure to maintain financial solvency or provide basic support for oneself or one's family. The person may become alienated from family and acquaintances.

Complications. Psychoactive Substance Abuse and Dependence, suicide attempts, association with fringe or illegal groups (more common in males), civil actions, and arrest for typically nonviolent crimes involving only property are among the possible complications.

Predisposing factors. Among the predisposing factors are inappropriate parental discipline (absence, inconsistency, or harshness); exposure to gambling activities as an adolescent; and a high family value placed on material and financial symbols and a lack of family emphasis on saving, planning, and budgeting. Females with this disorder more likely than others to have a husband with Alcohol Dependence or who is absent from the home.

Prevalence. Recent estimates place prevalence at 2%-3% of the adult population.

Sex ratio. The disorder is more common among males than females.

Familial pattern. Pathological Gambling and Alcohol Dependence are more common among the parents of people with Pathological Gambling than in the general population.

Differential diagnosis. In **social gambling,** gambling is with friends, and acceptable losses are predetermined.

During a **manic** or **hypomanic episode,** loss of judgment and excessive gambling may follow the onset of the mood disturbance. When manic-like mood changes occur in Pathological Gambling, they are generally related to winning streaks, and they are usually followed by depressive episodes because of subsequent gambling losses. Periods of depression tend to increase as the disorder progresses.

Problems with gambling are often associated with **Antisocial Personality Disorder**, and in Pathological Gambling antisocial behavior is frequent. In cases in which both disorders are present, both should be diagnosed.

Diagnostic Criteria for 312.31 Pathological Gambling

Maladaptive gambling behavior, as indicated by at least four of the following:

(1)   frequent preoccupation with gambling or with obtaining money to gamble

(2)   frequent gambling of larger amounts of money or over a longer period of time than intended

(3)   a need to increase the size or frequency of bets to achieve the desired excitement

(4)   restlessness or irritability if unable to gamble

(5)   repeated loss of money by gambling and returning another day to win back losses ("chasing")

(6)   repeated efforts to reduce or stop gambling

(7)   frequent gambling when expected to meet social or occupational obligations

(8)   sacrifice of some important social, occupational, or recreational activity in order to gamble

(9)   continuation of gambling despite inability to pay mounting debts, or despite other significant social, occupational, or legal problems that the person knows to be exacerbated by gambling

CRITERIA FROM THE 1994 DSM-IV

Impulse-Control Disorders Not Elsewhere Classified: Pathological Gambling

Diagnostic Features

The essential feature of Pathological Gambling is persistent and recurrent maladaptive gambling behavior (Criterion A) that disrupts personal, family, or vocational pursuits. The diagnosis is not made if the gambling behavior is better accounted for by a Manic Episode (Criterion B).

The individual may be preoccupied with gambling (e.g., reliving past gambling experiences, planning the next gambling venture, or thinking of ways to get money with which to gamble) (Criterion A1). Most individuals with Pathological Gambling say that they are seeking "action" (an aroused, euphoric state) even more than money. Increasingly larger bets, or greater risks, may be needed to continue to produce the desired level of excitement (Criterion A2). Individuals with Pathological Gambling often continue to gamble despite repeated efforts to control, cut back, or stop the behavior (Criterion A3). There may be restlessness or irritability when attempting to cut down or stop gambling (Criterion A4). The individual may gamble as a way of escaping from problems or to relieve a dysphoric mood (e.g., feelings of helplessness, guilt, anxiety, depression) (Criterion A5). A pattern of "chasing" one's losses may develop, with an urgent need to keep gambling (often with larger bets or the taking of greater risks) to undo a loss or series of losses. The individual may abandon his or her gambling strategy and try to win back losses all at once. Although all gamblers may chase for short periods, it is the long-term chase that is more characteristic of individuals with Pathological Gambling (Criterion A6). The individual may lie to family members, therapists, or others to conceal the extent of involvement with gambling (Criterion A7). When the individual's borrowing resources are strained, the person may resort to antisocial behavior (e.g., forgery, fraud, theft, or embezzlement) to obtain money (Criterion A8). The individual may have jeopardized or lost a significant relationship, job, or educational or career opportunity because of gambling (Criterion A9). The individual may also engage in "bailout" behavior, turning to family or others for help with a desperate financial situation that was caused by gambling (Criterion A10).

Associated Features and Disorders

Distortions in thinking (e.g., denial, superstitions, overconfidence, or a sense of power and control) may be present in individuals with Pathological Gambling. Many individuals with Pathological Gambling believe that money is both the cause of and solution to all their problems. Individuals with Pathological Gambling are frequently highly competitive, energetic, restless, and easily bored. They may be overly concerned with the approval of others and may be generous to the point of extravagance. When not gambling, they may be workaholics or "binge" workers who wait until they are up against deadlines before really working hard. They may be prone to developing general medical conditions that are associated with stress (e.g., hypertension, peptic ulcer disease, migraine). Increased rates of Mood Disorders, Attention-Deficit/Hyperactivity Disorder, Substance Abuse or Dependence, and Antisocial, Narcissistic, and Borderline Personality Disorders have been reported in individuals with Pathological Gambling. Of individuals in treatment for Pathological Gambling, 20% are reported to have attempted suicide.

Specific Culture and Gender Features

There are cultural variations in the prevalence and type of gambling activities (e.g., pai go, cockfights, horse racing, the stock market). Approximately one-third of individuals with Pathological Gambling are females. Females with the disorder are more apt to be depressed and to gamble as an escape. Females are underrepresented in treatment programs for gambling and represent only 2%-4% of the population of Gamblers Anonymous. This may be a function of the greater stigma attached to female gamblers.

Prevalence

The limited data available suggest that the prevalence of Pathological Gambling may be as high as 1%-3% of the adult population.

Course

Pathological Gambling typically begins in early adolescence in males and later in life in females. Although a few individuals are "hooked" with their very first bet, for most the course is more insidious. There may be years of social gambling followed by an abrupt onset that may be precipitated by greater exposure to gambling or by a stressor. The gambling pattern may be regular or episodic, and the course of the disorder is typically chronic. There is generally a progression in the frequency of gambling, the amount wagered, and the preoccupation with gambling and obtaining money with which to gamble. The urge to gamble and gambling activity generally increase during periods of stress or depression.

Familial Pattern

Pathological Gambling and Alcohol Dependence are both more common among the parents of individuals with Pathological Gambling than among the general population.

Differential Diagnosis

Pathological Gambling must be distinguished from social gambling and professional gambling. **Social gambling** typically occurs with friends or colleagues and lasts for a limited period of time, with predetermined acceptable losses. In **professional gambling,** risks are limited and discipline is central. Some individuals can experience problems associated with their gambling (e.g., short-term chasing behavior and loss of control) that do not meet the full criteria for Pathological Gambling.

Loss of judgment and excessive gambling may occur during a **Manic Episode**. An additional diagnosis of Pathological Gambling should only be given if the gambling behavior is not better accounted for by the Manic Episode (e.g., a history of maladaptive gambling behavior at times other than during a Manic Episode). Alternatively, an individual with Pathological Gambling may exhibit behavior during a gambling binge that resembles a Manic Episode. However, once the individual is away from the gambling, these manic-like features dissipate. Problems with gambling may occur in individuals with **Antisocial Personality Disorder;** if criteria are met for both disorders, both can be diagnosed.

Diagnostic Criteria for 312.31 Pathological Gambling

A.   Persistent and recurrent maladaptive gambling behavior as indicated by five (or more) of the following:

(1) is preoccupied with gambling (e.g., preoccupied with reliving past gambling experiences, handicapping or planning the next venture, or thinking of ways to get money with which to gamble)

(2) needs to gamble with increasing amounts of money in order to achieve the desired excitement

(3) has repeated unsuccessful efforts to control, cut back, or stop gambling

(4) is restless or irritable when attempting to cut down or stop gambling

(5) gambles as a way of escaping from problems or of relieving a dysphoric mood (e.g., feelings of helplessness, guilt, anxiety, depression)

(6) after losing money gambling, often returns another day to get even ("chasing" one's losses)

(7) lies to family members, therapist, or others to conceal the extent of involvement with gambling

(8) has committed illegal acts such as forgery, fraud, theft, or embezzlement to finance gambling

(9) has jeopardized or lost a significant relationship, job, or educational or career opportunity because of gambling

(10) relies on others to provide money to relieve a desperate financial situation caused by gambling

B. The gambling behavior is not better accounted for by a Manic Episode.

Source: American Psychiatric Association (1980): *Diagnostic and Statistical Manual of Mental Disorders,* Third Edition. Washington, DC: American Psychiatric Association.

American Psychiatric Association (1987): *Diagnostic and Statistical Manual of Mental Disorders,* Third Edition Revised. Washington, DC: American Psychiatric Association.

American Psychiatric Association (1994): *Diagnostic and Statistical Manual of Mental Disorders,* Fourth Edition. Washington, DC: American Psychiatric Association.

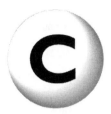

Legal-Age Gambling Opportunities and Restrictions

I. Nelson Rose

State	Lottery	Pari-Mutuel Betting	Casinos and Slot Machines	Charity Bingo & Pull-tabs
Alabama		18/19		19
Alaska			18	19/21
Arizona	18	18	18	18
Arkansas		18		
California	18	18	18/21	18
Colorado	18	18	21	18
Connecticut	18	18	18/21	18
Delaware	18	18	21	18
District of Columbia	18		18	18
Florida	18	18		18
Georgia	18			None
Hawaii				
Idaho	18	18		None/18
Illinois	18	17	18/21	18
Indiana	18	18	21	18
Iowa	18	18	21	None
Kansas	18	18		18
Kentucky	18	18		18
Louisiana	21	18	21	18?
Maine	18	18		16
Maryland	18	18	18	16-18
Massachusetts	18	18		18

State	Lottery	Pari-Mutuel Betting	Casinos and Slot Machines	Charity Bingo & Pull-tabs
Michigan	18	18	18?	18
Minnesota	18	18	18	18
Mississippi			21	18
Missouri	18	18	21	18
Montana	18	18	18	16
Nebraska	18/19	18		18
Nevada	21?	21	21	21?
New Hampshire	18	21		18
New Jersey	18	18	21	18
New Mexico	18	18/21	18	None?
New York	18	18	18	None
North Carolina			?	None?
North Dakota		18/21	21	18/21
Ohio	18	18		18/60
Oklahoma		18		?
Oregon	18	18	18/21	18
Pennsylvania	18	18	18	None
Puerto Rico	18	18	18	18
Rhode Island	18	18	18	18
South Carolina			21	?
South Dakota	18/21	18	21	?
Tennessee				
Texas	18	21		18
Utah				
Vermont	18	18		18
Virgin Islands	18			?
Virginia	18	18		18
Washington	18	18	18?	18
West Virginia	18	18	18?	18
Wisconsin	18	18	21/18*	None
Wyoming		18		?

NOTE: A question mark without a number means that form of gambling is legal in that state, but the minimum age requirements, if any, are not known. A number with a question mark means there is a state limit, but it is unclear whether it applies. This is usually the case with Indian gaming, for which tribes are often free to set their own limits.

* Four of 15 tribes have not yet agreed to raise the minimum age to 21.

STATE BY STATE ANALYSIS

ALABAMA—Alabama Code §15-8-150 makes it a crime to bet with a minor.

Pari-mutuel betting: The minimum age for betting horse and greyhound racetracks is 18 in some counties, 19 in others: Birmingham and Macon—19, Greene and Mobile—18. Association of Racing Commissioners International, Inc., *Pari-Mutuel Racing: 1996* at 59; Alabama Code §11-65-44.

Bingo: Non-profit organizations can run bingo games for charitable or educational purposes. The state has separate statutes for various counties and at least one city—all set the minimum playing age as well as the minimum age for conducting or assisting bingo at 19.

ALASKA—Alaska has been considering allowing casino gambling on cruise ships between ports in the state, during the course of an international voyage.

Slot machines: Alaska Statutes §43.35.040 sets the minimum age at 18 and forbids the location of coin-operated amusement and gaming devices within a radius of 100 yards of a school building.

Bingo and pull-tabs: State statutes set the minimum age for bingo at 19, but the age for pull-tabs was raised from 19 to 21 on June 26, 1993. Alaska Statutes §§05.15.180 and 05.15.187.

ARIZONA

Lottery: It is a misdemeanor to sell a lottery ticket to anyone under 18, but it is not unlawful to give the minor a lottery ticket as a gift. Arizona Revised Statutes §5-515.

Pari-mutuel betting: Arizona puts the legal wagering age at 18, according to the Association of Racing Commissioners International, Inc.'s *Parimutuel Racing: 1996* at 59. The state's statutes

---

By I. Nelson Rose, J.D. Harvard 1979, Professor of Law at Whittier Law School. The author would like to thank his research assistants, Ranjit Indran, James B. Lewis, Kimberly Phillips, and Michael Shelton-Frates for their help with this project.

set the minimum age at the age of majority: Arizona Revised Statutes §5-112 states, "A permittee shall not knowingly permit a minor to be a patron of the pari-mutuel system of wagering." This also would allow an operator to raise the defense that it did not know a child was underage.

Casinos: Charities can operate casino nights. The state has entered into compacts with many tribes, authorizing the operation of slot machines and non-banked (revolving deal) card games. The minimum ages for Indian casinos in Arizona is 18.

ARKANSAS

Pari-mutuel betting: Arkansas's horse racing statute expressly prohibits "any person under eighteen (18) years of age to be a patron of the pari-mutuel or certificate system of wagering conducted or supervised by it." But it is unclear if such persons are prohibited from attending horse races. The dog racing counterpart, prohibits employing a minor or allowing "any minor to be a patron at the racetrack." This language seems closer to prohibiting the presence of children. Arkansas Statutes §§23-110-405 and 23-111-308.

CALIFORNIA

Lottery: California has a complete set of restrictions, typical of the state lotteries that have addressed youth gambling:

> (a) No tickets or shares in Lottery Games shall be sold to persons under the age of 18 years. Any person who knowingly sells a ticket or share in a Lottery Game to a person under the age of 18 years is guilty of a misdemeanor. Any person under the age of 18 years who buys a ticket or share in a Lottery is guilty of a misdemeanor. In the case of Lottery tickets or shares sold by Lottery Game Retailers or their employees, these persons shall establish safeguards to assure that the sales are not made to persons under the age of 18 years. In the case of the dispensing of tickets or shares by vending machines or other devices, the Commission shall establish safeguards to help assure that the vending machines or devices are not operated by persons under the age of 18 years.

(b) All tickets or shares in Lottery Games shall include, and any devices which dispense tickets or shares in Lottery Games shall have posted in a conspicuous place thereupon, a notice which declares that state law prohibits the selling of a Lottery ticket or share to, and the payment of any prize to, a person under the age of 18 years.

California Government Code §8880.52.

"No prize shall be paid to any person under the age of 18 years." Id. §8880.32.

Pari-mutuel betting: The age limit of 18 for horse races was established by regulations of the Racing Control Board, not by the legislature in a statute.

Casinos: California law allows cities and counties the local option of licensing gaming clubs, limited to non-banked table games. There are more than 300 gaming clubs operating throughout the state—age limits appear to be usually 21. The only state limit is a restriction limiting operators and owners to be at least 18. California Business & Professions Code §19809. Indian tribes are operating slot machines without compacts, in technical violation of the controlling federal law, the Indian Gaming Regulatory Act. All non-compacted Indian gaming, even when legal, is regulated by the tribe, which can change the age limits whenever it wishes. The Cabazon Band of Mission Indians, for example, announced in September, 1995 that it was raising the minimum age from 18 to 21 for its casino near Palm Springs and that it was firing all casino workers under 21.

Bingo: Minors (currently age 18) are not allowed to participate in bingo games. California Penal Code §326.5.

COLORADO

Lottery: Colorado Revised Statutes §24-35-214 makes it illegal to sell a lottery ticket to anyone under 18 or for any person under 18 to purchase a ticket. However it permits the receipt of a lottery ticket given as a gift to a person under 18. The difference can be significant: "Any prize won by a person under 18 years of age who purchased a winning ticket in violation of section 24-35-

214(1)(c) shall be forfeited. If a person otherwise entitled to a prize or a winning ticket is under 18 years of age, the director may direct payment of the prize by delivery to an adult member of the minor's family or a guardian of the minor of a check or draft payable to the order of such minor."

Pari-mutuel betting: It is illegal to purchase or to sell a pari-mutuel ticket to any person under the age of 18. Colorado Revised Statutes §12-60-601.

Casinos: Privately owned casinos are limited to three little mountain towns, with $5 maximum bets. Colorado also has signed compacts with two Indian tribes; age limits are 21.

Bingo and pull-tabs: State law prohibits anyone under 18 from playing bingo or buying pull-tabs. However, it also allows anyone 14 or older to "assist in the conduct of bingo or pull tabs." Colorado Revised Statutes §12-9-107.

CONNECTICUT—Connecticut's off-track betting operation, owned and operated by a private company, Autotote, is taking telephone wagers from around the nation.

Lottery: Games limited to players over 18.

Pari-mutuel betting: Connecticut allows betting on jai-alai, as well as on racing. Connecticut not only bars anyone under 18 from betting, but General Statutes §12-576 prohibits "the presence of any minor under the age of 18 being present in any room, office, building or establishment when off-track betting takes place."

Casinos: Charity "Las Vegas Nights" are limited to those over 18. Connecticut General Statutes §186a. The state prohibits anyone under 16 from even being present in a room where gambling is taking place. Connecticut has signed compacts with two Indian tribes. The Mashantucket Pequot Tribe apparently felt that 18 was too young, and put its age limit at 21. The tribe's casino, Foxwoods, may be the most profitable casino in the world, with blackjack, craps, etc. and 4,000 slot machines.

Bingo and pull-tabs: In its "Sealed tickets" statute Connecticut prohibits the sale to any person less than 18 years of age. Connecticut General Statutes §7-169h.

DELAWARE

Lottery: Delaware has the strongest restriction of any state lottery, having locked its 18-year-old age limit into the state constitution. Delaware Constitution Article 2, §17. However state statutes, while prohibiting the sale of lottery tickets to persons under 18, expressly allow the purchase of a ticket for the purpose of making a gift by a person 18 years of age or older to a person less than that age. Delaware Code Title 29, §4810.

Pari-mutuel betting and slot machines: While racetracks appear to put the limit at age 18, the state recently amended its laws to allow video lottery machines in racetracks, with an age limit of 21. Delaware Code Title 29, §4810.

Bingo: A person has to be 18 or over to participate in any charitable gambling, the prize for which is money; yet, anyone over 16 may participate in Bingo and other charitable games. This must limit 16-year-olds and 17-year-olds to games where prizes are merchandise. Delaware Code Title 28, §1139.

DISTRICT OF COLUMBIA

Lottery: Limited to players over 18.

Casinos and Bingo: Charities in the District of Columbia can run "Monte Carlo Night Parties" as well as bingo. The minimum age to participate as well to be present is 18, but minors under 18 may to be present if accompanied by an adult. D.C. Code §2-2534.

FLORIDA

Lottery: Limited to players over 18.

Pari-mutuel betting: Florida has not only dog and horse tracks, but also jai-alai. State statutes prohibit wagering by a person under the age of 18 but permit admittance if the minor is accompanied by a parent or legal guardian. Florida Statutes §550.0425.

Bingo: State law prevents anyone under 18 from being allowed to play any bingo game or be involved in the conduct of a bingo game in any way. Florida Statutes §849.0931.

GEORGIA—The state legislature has enacted a unique law creating civil liability along with the more common criminal punishments. "A parent shall have a right of action against any person who shall play and bet at any game of chance with his minor child for money or any other thing of value without the parent's permission." Georgia Code §51-1-18.

Lottery: State statutes not only prohibit anyone under 18 from buying lottery tickets but also requires conspicuous labels, prohibiting minors from using any electronic or mechanical devices related to the lottery. Georgia Code §50-27-10.

Bingo: State law allows a person under 18 to play Bingo if accompanied by an adult. Georgia Code §16-12-58.

HAWAII—Hawaii, Utah and Tennessee are the only states with no commercial gambling. Hawaii, like many other states, does allow "social gambling"—minimum age is 18. Hawaii Revised Statutes §712-1231.

IDAHO—The Coeur d'Alene tribe has set up a telephone and Internet lottery, the "US Lottery."

Lottery: Idaho Code §67-7413 prohibits the knowing sale of tickets to anyone under 18.

Pari-mutuel betting: Minors are prohibited from using the pari-mutuel system. Idaho Code §54-2512.

Bingo: A person under 18 may not play bingo for a cash prize or in games where the prize exceeds $25.00 worth of merchandise. Idaho Code §67-7703. Therefore, children under 18 may play bingo for money for smaller prizes.

ILLINOIS—Illinois is unique in defining a minor (at least under the horse racing statutes) as "any individual under the age of 17 years." Illinois Revised Statutes chapter 230, §5/3.08. The state also makes a distinction between casino gambling run by charities—age 18—and casino gambling run for profit on riverboats—age 21.

Lottery: It is unlawful to sell a ticket to anyone under the age of 18, but adults may buy tickets as gifts to minors. "If the person entitled to a prize or any winning ticket is under the age of 18 years, and such prize is less than $2500, the Director may direct payment of the prize by delivery to an adult member of the minor's family or a guardian of the minor of a check or draft payable to the order of such minor. If the person entitled to a prize or any winning ticket is under the age of 18 years, and such prize is $2500 or more, the Director may direct payment to the guardian of such minor. . . ." Illinois Revised Statutes chapter 20, §§1605/15 and 1605/18.

Pari-mutuel betting: Minors (defined as age 17) are forbidden from being admitted as a patron during a racing program unless accompanied by a parent or guardian. Exceptions are made for employees, licensees, owners, trainers, jockeys, or drivers. Illinois Revised Statutes chapter 230, §5/26.

Casinos: The state has both riverboat and charity casinos. The state riverboat statute prohibits any person under 21 betting or even being permitted on an area of a riverboat where gambling is being conducted. An exception is made for employees, but workers must be at least 21 to perform any function involved in gambling. Illinois Revised Statutes chapter 230, §10/11.

Illinois charitable casinos do a multi-million dollar business. The "Charitable Games Act" allows the following games: roulette, blackjack, poker, pull-tabs, craps, bang, beat the dealer, big six, gin rummy, five card stud poker, chuck-a-luck, keno, hold-em poker and merchandise wheel with a $10.00 maximum bet. Unlike for-profit riverboat casinos, charity casinos are open to anyone over 18. Illinois Revised Statutes chapter 230, § 30/8.

Bingo and pull-tabs: Minimum age for bingo and pull-tabs is 18. Illinois Revised Statutes chapter 230, §§20/4 and 25/2. In fact, persons under 18 may not be in the area where bingo is being played, unless accompanied by a parent or guardian.

INDIANA

Lottery: Minimum age 18, but prizes may not be paid to anyone under 18, unless the ticket was received as a gift. Indiana Code §§4-30-9-3, 4-30-11-3, 4-30-12-1, 4-30-13-1.

Pari-mutuel betting: Minimum age to work at a racetrack is 16, but the racing commission can license children even younger, who are working for their parent or legal guardian. Indiana Code §4-31-6-5.

Casinos: Indiana has riverboat gambling, even though, at this writing, none of the casinos are in operation. The minimum age for an occupational license is 18; however, anyone under 21 is prohibited from being in the area of a riverboat where gambling is being conducted. Indiana Code §§4-33-8-3, 4-33-9-12.

Bingo and pull-tabs: Players must be over 18. Indiana Code §4-32-9-34; Indiana Administrative Code title 45, regulation 18-3-2 (Department of State Revenue).

IOWA

Lottery: Iowa law prohibits the sale of a lottery ticket to a person under the age of 18, but allows adult to buy tickets for them as gifts. Iowa Code §§99E.16.

Pari-mutuel betting: Iowa Code §99D.11, in a simple sentence, prohibits a person under 18 from making a pari-mutuel wager. No one may knowingly permit a person under the age of 18 to make a pari-mutuel wager. Id. at §99D.24.

Casinos: Iowa raised the minimum gambling age on its riverboat casinos from 18 to 21 in 1989. It against the law for a licensee to knowingly allow a minor to participate in the gambling, or even to be in the area of the excursion boat where gambling is being conducted. Iowa Code §§99B.6 and 99F.9.

Bingo: Iowa makes some specific exemptions to its general prohibition on gambling by anyone under 21. There are no age limits at all for games of chance at carnivals, so long as only non-cash merchandise worth no more than $25 is given as prizes. Bingo similarly has no age limit; cash prizes may be given and are usually limited to $100; however, the bingo game may offer a jackpot of up to $800.

KANSAS—The general law of Kansas defines a minor as "a person under 21 years of age"; yet, the lower age of 18 is used for both legal and illegal gambling. Kansas Statutes §§41-2601(l) and (m).

Lottery: Kansas goes further than most states in keeping the presence of children out of the state lottery. Besides the usual restriction that licensees must be at least 18, the state legislature has prohibited the Kansas lottery from "recruiting for employment or as a volunteer any person under 18 years of age for the purpose of appearing, being heard or being quoted in any advertising or promotion of any lottery in any electronic or print media." Kansas Statutes §§74-8708, 74-8718, 74-8722.

Pari-mutuel betting: The legislature put the same ban on the Kansas racing commission, prohibiting the use of children in commercials. It is a crime to sell a pari-mutuel ticket to a person knowing such person to be under 18 years of age. Those under 18 are also specifically barred from buying the ticket. Kansas Statutes §§74-8810 and 74-8839.

Casinos: The state is in the middle of a protracted fight over Indian casinos. Although the legislature created a joint committee on gaming compacts, no mention was made of minimum age limits. Kansas Statutes §46-2303.

Bingo and pull-tabs: Minimum age limit of 18 to participate in the management, operation or conduct of any game of bingo. Kansas Statutes §79-4706. Although "conduct" is not the best word, this statute probably covers playing the game as well.

KENTUCKY

Lottery: It is a violation to knowingly sell a lottery ticket to someone under 18, and a misdemeanor to do it a second time. This would not prohibit adults from buying lottery tickets for minors. Kentucky Revised Statutes §154A.990.

Pari-mutuel betting: Although Kentucky statutes do not expressly cover pari-mutuel betting, Kentucky places an age restriction of 18 on all activities (except drinking); therefore, it is legal for anyone 18 or older to bet at race tracks. Kentucky Revised Statutes §2.015. The state's racing commissioners also report the minimum age as being 18. Association of Racing Commissioners International, Inc., *Pari-Mutuel Racing: 1996* at 59.

Bingo: Kentucky has a "Charitable Gaming" Act, which controls bingo games. The age limit is 18. A charitable organization may permit persons under 18 to play bingo if they are accompanied by a parent or legal guardian and if only non-cash prizes are awarded. Kentucky Revised Statutes §238.545.

LOUISIANA—The latest state to raise the minimum age for some forms of gambling. Casino gaming was always limited to players over 21, but state Senator Dardenne's SB33 in 1998 amended La.R.S. §§ 27:319, 47:9025(B)(2) and 47:9070, raising the age from 18 to 21 for State Lottery and privately-owned video poker machines. A 19-year-old and the owner of a bar with video poker machines filed suit in January 1999, claiming the new law violates the state constitutional provision against age discrimination. AP Newswire J5840 (Jan. 7, 1999). The amendment provides that winnings of underage video pokers players are paid to the state. A video poker licensee, or its agent or employee, who allows persons under 21 but at least 15 to play, reasonably believing the minor is over 21, is fined $1,000 for the first violation, $1,000 for the second violation in a year, and loses its license for a third violation. A licensee who knowingly lets a minor over 15 play, or even inadvertently lets a child under 15 play, will have its license revoked. The minor is fined up to $100. The State Lottery is treated more leniently: Knowingly selling a ticket to a minor leads to a fine of $100 to $500; the minor is fined up to $100; but adults may purchase lottery tickets for children as gifts. Louisiana has everything except sports betting: Riverboat casinos, two Indian casinos, America's first urban land-based casino in New Orleans, video poker machines everywhere with large numbers at truckstops and racetracks, electronic bingo machines, pari-mutuel betting, and a state lottery.

Lottery: See paragraph above. The law provides that no ticket shall knowingly be sold to any person under the age of 21, but does not prohibit the purchase of a ticket by a person over 21 for the purpose of making a gift to a minor. Louisiana Revised Statutes 47:9025 and 47:9070.

Pari-mutuel betting: The state legislature told the state racing commission to adopt rules and regulations to exclude and eject "persons . . . who are not of age." Louisiana Revised Statutes 4:193. Another state statute holds that any minor age six or above may, with the permission of the racing association, be allowed to attend any race meeting if accompanied by a parent, grandparent, or legal guardian but in no case shall any minor in attendance be allowed to engage in wagering. An applicant for licensure as a jockey, apprentice jockey, exercise person, groom, or hot walker must be at least 16. Louisiana Revised Statutes 4:150 and 4:157.

Casinos and slot machines: Anyone under 21 is not permitted to play any table game or slot machine, loiter in the designated gaming area of a riverboat, or be employed as a gaming employee. Non-riverboat gaming devices are similarly limited to players over 21. The legal burden is placed both on the minor and on the gambling operator. Louisiana Revised Statutes 4:525, 4:544 and 4:660.

Bingo and pull-tabs: Louisiana Revised Statutes 33:4861.11 prohibits any licensee from allowing any person under 18 to assist in "the holding, operation, or conduct of any game of chance," including electronic bingo machines. This statutory language is vague but probably covers players.

MAINE

Lottery: Maine has one of the weakest regulatory schemes for its state lottery. Tickets may not be sold to anyone under 18, but may not be bought by adults as gifts for minors. The minor who buys illegally is subject to no punishment. In addition, there is no penalty for unintentionally selling to a minor. The only punishment comes in when a lottery agent knowingly sells to a minor, but this is punished as a civil, not criminal, violation with a maximum fine of only $200. Maine Revised Statutes Title 8, §§374 and 380.

Pari-mutuel betting: Off-track betting facilities are open to children under age 16 when accompanied by a parent, legal guardian or custodian. A person under the age of 18 is not only prohibited from participating in a pari-mutuel pool, but may not come within 15 feet of a betting window or other place for accepting wagers. Maine Revised Statutes title 8, §§275-D and 278.

Bingo and pull-tabs: No one under the age of 16 years is permitted to take part in the conduct of, or participate in, the game of "Beano" or "Bingo," nor shall such minor be admitted to the playing area unless accompanied by parent, guardian or other responsible person. Maine Revised Statutes title 17, §319.

MARYLAND—Maryland's gambling laws contain a number of unique quirks.

Lottery: The state follows the other states in requiring that no ticket be sold to a person the seller knows is under 18, while allowing adults to buy tickets for minors as gifts. Lottery sellers must be at least 21. Maryland State Government Code §§9-112 and 9-124.

Pari-mutuel betting: The state's racing commissioners report the minimum age as being 18. Association of Racing Commissioners International, Inc., *Pari-Mutuel Racing: 1996* at 59.

Casinos and slot machines: Charities in some parts of Maryland can operate casinos, including slot machines.

Bingo: Maryland's bingo laws are unique in two aspects: the state legislature has passed specific statutes for individual counties, rather than a single law covering the entire state; and some statutes explicitly allow 16-year-olds to play bingo. Maryland Criminal Law Code Art. 27, "Gaming."

MASSACHUSETTS

Lottery: The state follows the other states in requiring that no ticket be sold to a person the seller knows is under 18, while allowing adults to buy tickets for minors as gifts. Lottery sellers must be at least 21. Massachusetts General Laws chapter 10, §§24 and 29.

Pari-mutuel betting: Massachusetts does not even allow minors (age 18) to attend its horse and dog races, let alone make bets. But the penalties are very small. First time violators are fined no more than $100.00. Even permitting a minor to make bets subjects a track to a fine of no more than $100.00. Massachusetts General Laws chapter 128A, §§9 and 10.

Bingo and pull-tabs: In Massachusetts, Bingo is called "Beano." State law requires "that no person under 18 years of age shall be permitted in that portion of any building or premises of the licensee during such time as such game is being played." Massachusetts General Laws chapter 10, §38.

Casinos: The governor of Massachusetts has agreed to allow an Indian tribe to own a casino, with a minimum gambling age of 21.

MICHIGAN

Lottery: It is a misdemeanor to knowingly sell, or offer to sell, a lottery ticket to anyone under 18. Although tickets may not be sold to minors, an adult may buy one as a gift for someone under 18. State law also requires a person to be at least 18 in order to acquire a lottery resale license. Michigan Compiled Laws §§432.11 and 432.29.

Pari-mutuel betting: "A holder of a race meeting license shall not knowingly permit a person less than 18 years of age to be a patron of the pari-mutuel wagering conducted or supervised by the holder." Michigan Compiled Laws §431.72.

Casinos and slot machines: Charities are allowed to run "Millionaire parties," i.e., casinos. Michigan has signed compacts with many tribes, now operating high-stakes casinos throughout the state. The legislature has voted a minimum age of 18 for all charity casinos. Michigan Compiled Laws §432.110a. Indian casinos appear to be abiding by this age limit.

Bingo and pull-tabs: Charity game ticket may not be sold to anyone under 18. However, like lottery tickets, charity pull-tabs may be bought for minors as gifts by adults. Michigan Compiled Laws §432.107a.

MINNESOTA—Minnesota is the only state that, at least on paper, came close to having a comprehensive plan for dealing with the minimum age for gambling, and it failed. After the compacts were signed, the state legislature passed a statute mandating that Indian casinos be restricted to adults over 21, and added that the minimum age for all other forms of legal gambling in the state would also be raised from 18 to 21 if more than half the tribes agreed to that limit. The tribes took this as a trick to get them to re-open compact negotiations and rejected the move to 21.

Lottery: Minnesota is unusual in setting up a complex system for dealing with underage lottery players, including prohibiting minors from receiving prizes. This would seem to preclude gifts by adults.

Minnesota Statutes §349A.12. Prohibited acts:

Subdivision 1. Purchase by minors. A person under the age of 18 years may not buy or redeem for a prize a ticket in the state lottery.

Subdivision 2. Sale to minors. A lottery retailer may not sell and a lottery retailer or other person may not furnish or redeem for a prize a ticket in the state lottery to any person under the age of 18 years.

It is an affirmative defense, meaning the burden is on the lottery retailer, to prove by a preponderance of the evidence that he reasonably and in good faith relied upon the minor's showing a false identification.

Pari-mutuel betting: The age restrictions are identical to the state lottery. Minnesota Statutes §§240.13 and 240.25.

Casinos: More legal full-scale Indian casinos than Atlantic City, with minimum age limits presently at 18.

Bingo and pull-tabs: No one under 18 may buy a pull-tab, tipboard ticket, paddlewheel ticket, or raffle ticket, or a chance to participate in a bingo game other than a bingo game exempt or excluded from licensing; violation is a misdemeanor. A licensed organization or employee who allows a person under age 18 to participate in lawful gambling is guilty of a misdemeanor.

Michigan Statutes §349.2127.

MISSISSIPPI—Mississippi is one of the toughest states on both minors and casinos who violate the law: The underage gambler may not keep the winnings and the casino may not say it thought the minor was over 21.

Casinos: Mississippi has true riverboat casinos and dockside casinos that are technically over water but cannot move.

Mississippi Code §75-76-155. Age requirement for patrons and gaming employees; penalties for violations; belief as to person's age no excuse.

(1) A person under the age of twenty-one (21) years shall not:

(a) Play, be allowed to play, place Wagers, or collect winnings, whether personally or through an agent, from any gaming authorized under this chapter.

(b) Be employed as a gaming employee.

(2) Any licensee, employee, dealer or other person who violates or permits the violation of any of the provisions of this section, and any person under twenty-one (21) years of age who violates any of the provisions of this section shall, upon conviction, be punished by a fine of not more than One Thousand Dollars ($1,000.00) or imprisoned in the

county jail not more than six (6) months, or by both such fine and imprisonment.

(3) In any prosecution or other proceeding for the violation of any of the provisions of this section, it is no excuse for the licensee, employee, dealer or other person to plead that he believed the person to be twenty-one (21) years old or over.

Bingo and pull-tabs: Charity bingo operators are given the unusual option of excluding anyone under 18. The state charitable bingo law provides that no licensee shall allow anyone under 18 to play a bingo game unless accompanied by his or her parent or legal guardian, except that a licensee may prohibit all persons under 18 from entering the licensed premises by posting a written notice to that effect. Mississippi Code §97-33-67. The state allows video pull-tab and video bingo machines.

MISSOURI

Lottery: Tickets may not be sold to anyone under 18; however gifts by adults to minors are permitted. No one under 21 may be licensed as a lottery game retailer. Missouri Revised Statutes §§313.260 and 313.280.

Pari-mutuel betting: A strangely worded statute prohibits minors from "knowingly making or attempting to make any wager on any horse race." I do not know how a minor could accidentally make a bet. Racetrack licensees may not knowingly permit anyone under 18, unless accompanied by a parent or guardian, into any pari-mutuel wagering area. Licensees are also prohibited from knowingly permitting any individual under 18 to place a wager. Missouri Revised Statutes §313.670.

Casinos: Missouri has two unusual provisions: The state legislature explicitly gave cities the option to completely exclude minors from riverboat casinos; and a minor's parent or conservator may sue to recover any money lost gambling. The other provisions of the Excursion Gambling Boat Statute are typical: "A person under twenty-one years of age shall not make a wager on an excursion gambling boat and shall not be allowed in the area of the excursion boat where gambling is being conducted; provided that employees of the licensed operator of the excursion gambling boat who have attained eighteen years of age shall be permitted in the area in which gambling is being conducted when performing employment-related duties, except that no one under twenty-one years of age may be employed as a dealer or accept a wager on an excursion gambling boat." It is a misdemeanor to permit a person under 21 to make a wager. Missouri Revised Statutes §§434.060 and 313.817.

Bingo and pull-tabs: Children as young as 16 may play or participate in the conducting of bingo, and even those under 16 may attend, when accompanied by a parent or guardian. Missouri Revised Statutes §313.040.

MONTANA—The state has legalized video poker and keno machines. Montana also has card clubs and allows calcutta betting on sports events. Indian tribes are operating casinos.

Lottery: Tickets may not be sold to or by anyone under 18. Montana Code §§23-7-110, 23-7-301.

Pari-mutuel betting: Montana Code §23-4-301 prohibits the licensee permitting a minor to use the pari-mutuel system.

Casinos: A person under 18 may not "purposely or knowingly" participate in a gambling activity. The law also disallows an operator from purposely or knowingly allowing a person under 18 years of age to participate in a gambling activity. The Video Gaming Machine Control Law requires operators to place gaming devices in such a way as to prevent access by persons under 18. Montana Code §§23-5-158 and 23-5-603.

Charity bingo and pull-tabs: A "bingo caller" is defined as a person 18 years of age or older. Montana Code §23-5-112.

NEBRASKA—Nebraska has the unusual arrangement of having no state lottery, but allowing cities and counties to run lotteries. It then makes a strange age distinction:

Lottery: Villages, cities and counties can operate lotteries in Nebraska—minimum age to buy a ticket: 19. However, charity lotteries and raffles—minimum age to buy a ticket: 18. Compare Nebraska Revised Statutes §§9-646, 9-810, and 9-814 with §9-345, 9-430, 9-426. It is a minor misdemeanor for anyone under 19 to knowingly buy a governmental lottery ticket, and a more serious misdemeanor to knowingly sell one. While most states either allow adults to buy lottery tickets as gifts, or are silent on the issue, Nebraska explicitly prohibits anyone from buying a ticket for the benefit of a person under 19.

Pari-mutuel betting: Knowingly aiding or abetting any minor to make a pari-mutuel wager is a misdemeanor. Nebraska Revised Statutes §2-1207.

Bingo and pull-tabs: Age 18 minimum; lotteries are allowed to sell "pickle cards," i.e. pull-tabs. The state also allows keno, which has become a big business.

NEVADA

Lottery: The Nevada Constitution still prohibits all lotteries, except charity raffles. The enabling statute does not mention a minimum age for buying a raffle ticket. The age limit of 21 for casinos probably applies.

Pari-mutuel betting: Almost complete prohibition for everyone under 21. Notice the statutory prohibition on "loitering," allowing casinos to have minors pass through. Also note the minor is not allowed to collect; nothing is said to prevent casinos from keeping children's money, win or lose.

A person under the age of 21 years shall not:

(a) Play, be allowed to play, place wagers at, or collect winnings from, whether personally or through an agent, any gambling game, slot machine, race book, sports pool or pari-mutuel operator.

(b) Loiter, or be permitted to loiter, in or about any room or premises wherein any licensed game, race book, sports pool or pari-mutuel wagering is operated or conducted.

(c) Be employed as a gaming employee except in a counting room. Any licensee, employee, dealer or other person who violates or permits the violation of any of the provisions of this section and any person, under 21 years of age, who violates any of the provisions of this section is guilty of a misdemeanor.

Nevada Revised Statutes §463.350.

Casinos: See Pari-mutuel betting, above. There are many additional specific restrictions, all set at age 21. Nevada Revised Statutes §129.130 prohibits gaming or employment in gaming of a person under 21. Section 205.460 makes it unlawful to allow a person under 21 to enter a gambling establishment or engage in gambling in a gambling establishment. Section 609.210 specifies that every person who employs, or causes to be employed, exhibits or has in his custody for exhibition or employment, any minor, and every parent, relative, guardian, employer, or other person having the care, custody, or control of any minor, who in any way procures or consents to the employment of the minor, in any area of a casino where there is gaming or where the sale of alcoholic beverages is the primary commercial activity unless the minor is in the casino area to provide entertainment pursuant to an employment contract, is guilty of a misdemeanor.

NEW HAMPSHIRE

Lottery: Tickets may not be sold to anyone under 18; however, gifts by adults are allowed. New Hampshire Revised Statutes §287-F:8

Pari-mutuel betting: Limited to bettor over 21. New Hampshire Revised Statutes §284:33.

Bingo and pull-tabs: State law prohibits anyone under 18 to be admitted to or play bingo games. New Hampshire Revised Statutes §§287-E:7, 287-E:10 and 287-E:12.

NEW JERSEY—Mostly as historic accidents, New Jersey has chosen a different standard for each type of gambling permitted by law. Pari-mutuel: minors. Bingo: 18 with no exceptions. State lottery: 18, but tickets may be received by children as gifts. Casinos: drinking age.

Lottery: Tickets may not be sold to anyone under 18; gifts by adults are allowed. Minimum age for lottery agents is 21. New Jersey Revised Statutes §§5:9-15 and 5:9-7.

Pari-mutuel betting: Strict restrictions on minors, which is currently 18. New Jersey Statutes §5:5-65.

Casinos: Atlantic City casinos must exclude anyone not old enough to drink alcoholic beverages, currently 21. New Jersey Statutes §5:12-119. As explained in the text, the state allows a casino to claim it did not know the minor was under 21 only when the casino is charged with a criminal offense; strict liability is imposed for all non-criminal procedures, including administrative fines.

Bingo: Prohibited to anyone under 18. New Jersey Statutes §5:8-32.

NEW MEXICO—Tribes opened casinos without compacts. The Governor then signed compacts, but the State Supreme Court and federal courts ruled he did not have the power to authorize forms of gambling not permitted under New Mexico state law. The Legislature approved a compromise: compacts for tribes, with a heavy state tax, and slot machines for race tracks and fraternal organizations. The tribes reluctantly agreed to the compacts, but are challenging the tax aspect, which does appear to violate the federal Indian Gaming Regulatory Act. The state is unique in allowing betting on bicycle races.

Lottery: Tickets may not be sold to anyone under 18, but gifts by adults are permitted. Lottery retailers must be at least 18. New Mexico Statutes §§6-24-14, 6-24-15, and 6-24-32.

Pari-mutuel betting: Betting on bicycle races is limited to age 21. The horse racing statutes do not give a minimum age for placing a bet. The state's racing commissioners report the minimum age as being 18. Association of Racing Commissioners International, Inc., *Pari-Mutuel Racing: 1996* at 59.

Casinos: Compacts require Indian casinos to limit players to a minimum gambling age of 21.

Bingo and pull-tabs: New Mexico gambling statutes do not specify a minimum age for players.

NEW YORK—New York has signed a compact with the Oneida tribe, resulting in an Indian casino without slot machines; Turning Stone is probably the most profitable table-games-only casino in the world. New York off-track betting operations are taking telephone wagers from around the nation. The state also allows charities to run casino nights; minimum age is 18. New York General Municipal Law §195-a.

Lottery: Tickets may not be sold to anyone under 18; however, adults may buy tickets for the purpose of making a gift to a minor.

The New York courts upheld the right of the underage recipient to collect if his ticket wins. New York Tax Law §1610, *Pando v. Fernandez* 485 N.Y.S.2d 162, 127 Misc.2d 224 (1984), affirming that the minor's age is no bar but reversing on other grounds, 499 N.Y.S.2d 950, 118 A.D.2d 474 (1986).

Pari-mutuel betting: Tracks and off-track betting operations are required to prevent betting by anyone who is actually and apparently under 18 years of age. This gives racing operators the excuse that the minor looked over 18. New York Racing and Pari-mutuel Law §104.

Bingo and pull-tabs: New York General Municipal Law §486 allows anyone under 18 to participate in bingo games, if accompanied by an adult.

Casinos: New York has signed a compact with the Oneida tribe creating Turning Stone, the largest casino in the world without slot machines. The state also allows charities to run casino nights.

NORTH CAROLINA—North Carolina has signed a compact to allow the Cherokee Tribe to operate video gaming at its bingo hall.

Bingo: State Bingo statutes do not specify a minimum age for players.

NORTH DAKOTA

Lottery: North Dakota is the only state where voters refused to authorize a state lottery, in part because the state already has so many other forms of gambling, including charity casinos.

Pari-mutuel betting: North Dakota allows a primitive form of pari-mutuel betting, called Calcutta Pool, on all sporting events other than high school contests—age limit 18. North Dakota Century Code §53-06.1-07.3. North Dakota is apparently the only state to put a higher limit—minimum age 21—on pari-mutuel wagering at OTBs than at the track. The state's racing commissioners report the minimum age as being 18. Association of Racing Commissioners International, Inc., *Pari-Mutuel Racing: 1996* at 59.

Casinos: North Dakota Century Code §53-06.1-07.1 prevents any person under 21 from directly or indirectly playing games of pull-tabs, punchboards, twenty-one, calcuttas, sports pools, paddlewheels, or poker. Low limit blackjack, for charity, is common throughout the state. Tribes operate full-scale casinos under compacts.

Bingo and pull-tabs: Although pull-tabs are restricted to players over 21, bingo is limited to players over 18, unless accompanied by an adult. North Dakota Century Code §53-06.1-07.1.

OHIO

Lottery: Ohio Revised Code §3770.08 prohibits the sale of a lottery ticket or chance to a person under 18 years of age.

Pari-mutuel betting: "Minors," currently age 18, are barred from participating. Regulation 3731.2.

Bingo: A wonderful minimum age: Participants and operators in Bingo games conducted by multipurpose senior centers must be at least 60 years old. Employees at other bingo halls must be over 18. Ohio Revised Code §§173.121 and 2915.09.

OKLAHOMA

Pari-mutuel betting: Oklahoma Statutes title 3A §208.4 prevents any organization licensee from knowingly permitting any minor to be a patron of the pari-mutuel system of wagering conducted by the organization licensee.

OREGON—The state lottery operates video poker machines and takes bets on sports events. Tribes in the state are operating full-scale casinos pursuant to compacts.

Lottery: The state has a strict scheme for dealing with minors. Lottery tickets may not be sold to anyone under 18. If someone under 18 wins the lottery, they may not be paid the prize. This effectively eliminates adults buying tickets as gifts. Oregon Revised Statutes §§461.250, 461.300, and 461.600.

Pari-mutuel betting: If a track has a reasonable doubt that a patron is over 18, it must require the bettor to make a written statement of age and furnish evidence of his true age and identity. The state statutes prevent any person under 18 from entering a race course, except when accompanied by a person 18 years of age or older who is the person's parent, guardian, or spouse; or when in the performance of a duty incident to employment. It further prohibits any person under 12 from entering after 6 p.m.

This statute also prohibits any person under 18 from loitering in the wagering area of a race course. Oregon Revised Statutes §§462.190 and 462.195.

Casinos: Video poker is limited to age 21 and older, because the devices are limited to establishments with liquor licenses. However, the first Indian/State casino compact put the minimum age at 18 for video poker machines; all later compacts put the age at 21. Compacts were also signed putting the minimum age at 18 for bingo and blackjack. So, the present situation allows one Indian casino to let 18-year-olds gamble at all of its games; the other Indian casinos must restrict machine gambling to age 21, but may allow 18-year-olds to play every other game. The compacts for blackjack are only temporary, and the state will insist that the age for that game be raised to 21. Besides the Indian casinos, the state has cardrooms for poker and blackjack under a vaguely worded statute allowing "contests of chance." Oregon Revised Statutes §163.575 makes it a crime of endangering the welfare of a minor if the person knowingly induces, causes, or permits a person under 18 to participate in gambling.

PENNSYLVANIA

Lottery: Lottery tickets may not be sold to anyone under 18, but adults may give tickets as gifts to minors. Lottery agents must be over 21. Pennsylvania Consolidated Statutes title 72 §§3761-6, 3761-10.

Pari-mutuel betting: Pennsylvania Consolidated Statutes title 4 §325.228 states, "No licensed corporation shall permit any person who is actually and apparently under 18 years of age to wager at a race meeting conducted by it. No licensed corporation shall permit any person who is under 18 years of age to attend a horse race meeting conducted by it unless the person is accompanied by a parent or guardian."

Casinos: Charities can operate casinos under Pennsylvania's "Small Games of Chance Act," minimum age limit is 18. Pennsylvania Consolidated Statutes title 10 §320.

Bingo: Persons under 18 are not permitted to play bingo unless accompanied by an adult. Pennsylvania Consolidated Statutes title 10 §305.

PUERTO RICO—Puerto Rico allows betting on cockfights, bolitas, and various other forms of gambling, including full-scale casinos with an unusual twist: the slot machines are owned and operated by the Commonwealth government itself.

Lottery: Sales prohibited to persons under 18. Puerto Rico Laws title 15 §§809 and 814.

Pari-mutuel betting: No age limit is mentioned in the statute. The state's racing commissioners report the minimum age as being 18. Association of Racing Commissioners International, Inc., *Pari-Mutuel Racing: 1996* at 59.

Casinos: "No gambling room shall be permitted to advertise or otherwise offer their facilities to the public of Puerto Rico; or to admit persons under 18 years of age." Puerto Rico Laws title 15 §77. Despite the obvious infringement on free speech, this statute was declared constitutional by the United States Supreme Court in *Posadas de Puerto Rico Assoc. v. Tourism Co.*, 478 U.S. 328, 92 L.Ed.2d 266, 106 S.Ct. 2968 (1986).

Bingo: Puerto Rico Laws title 15 §71 equates bingo to other gambling games such as roulette, dice, and cards, thus bingo would be governed under §77's 18-year-old age limit.

RHODE ISLAND—The Rhode Island state lottery operates video lottery terminals at racetracks.

Lottery: "No person under the age of eighteen (18) years may play a video lottery game authorized by this chapter, nor shall any licensed video lottery retailer knowingly permit a minor to play a video lottery machine or knowingly pay a minor with respect to a video lottery credit slip. Violation of this section shall be punishable by a fine of five hundred dollars ($500)." Lottery tickets may not be sold to anyone under 18, but adults may give tickets as gifts to minors. Lottery agents must be over 21. General Laws of Rhode Island §42-61.2-5, 11-19-32, and 42-61-9.

Pari-mutuel: Licensees may not admit anyone under 18 into a building where pari-mutuel betting or simulcast is taking place, nor knowingly permit any minor to be a patron of the pari-mutuel system or any other betting system. General Laws of Rhode Island §§41-4-2 and 41-11-4.

Bingo and pull-tabs: Anyone under 18 is not permitted to play. General Laws of Rhode Island §11-19-32.

SOUTH CAROLINA—South Carolina accidentally legalized video gaming devices, with off-beat restrictions, through a series of strange statutes and court decisions. In 1988, Terry Blackmon, a grocery store owner, was indicted for paying players for the free replays they won on his store's video poker machines. The State Supreme Court ruled that a poorly worded anti-slot machine statute actually legalized the devices. The legislature had exempted "coin-operated nonpayout machines with a free play feature." The Court declared that video gaming devices were legal, so long as the machine itself did not dispense money. However, the Court later ruled that an even more ancient statute allowed losers to sue and get their money back. In June 1993 the state legislature enacted a new law in an attempt to clarify that at least some of these "video game machines" are legal, so long as they are approved by local voters, and pay no more than $125 per day. But the State Supreme Court continues to render conflicting decisions and lawsuits against video poker are pending. In the most recent case, the Court ruled three-to-two that not all video games are created equal. Under the majority's reading of South Carolina laws, video poker machines are legal, but video slot machines are illegal and can be ordered destroyed. *State v. Four Video Slot Machines*, S.C., 453 S.E.2d 896 (1995); *State v. Blackmon*, 304 S.C. 270, 403 S.E.2d 660 (1991); *Berkebile v. Outen*, 311 S.C. 50, 426 S.E.2d 760 (1993); Code of Laws of South Carolina §§32-1-10, 12-21-2791, and 61-9-410. No one under 21 may play or collect winnings.

SOUTH DAKOTA—South Dakota was one of the first states to allow its state lottery to set up video lottery terminals, slot machines without coin drops. The state also allows full-scale, low-stake casinos in Deadwood and on Indian land.

Lottery: Lottery tickets may not be sold to anyone under 18. However, to play a video lottery terminal a gambler must be at least 21. South Dakota Codified Laws §§42-7A-13, 42-7A-32, 42-7A-44, and 42-7A-48.

Pari-mutuel betting: South Dakota Codified Laws §42-7-76 prohibits a racetrack licensee from permitting any individual under the age of 18 to place a bet on a race.

Casinos: Participation in casino games is limited to gamblers

21 and older. South Dakota Codified Laws §§42-7B-35, 42-7B-4, and 42-7B-25.

TENNESSEE

Pari-mutuel betting: Tennessee had legalized horse racing, but the statute contained a sunset clause, causing it to expire by its own terms before a track could be licensed or built. The age limit was clearly stated: Code §4-36-310 stated in its entirety, "No person under eighteen (18) years of age shall be permitted to wager at any race meeting."

TEXAS

Lottery: Lottery tickets may not be sold to anyone under 18, but adults may give tickets as gifts to minors. Texas Government Code §466.253.

Pari-mutuel betting: Minimum age for betting is defined as the minimum age for buying alcoholic drinks.

Bingo and pull-tabs: Texas Civil Code Art. 179d prohibits any person from knowingly permitting any individual under 18, unless accompanied by a parent or guardian over 18, to be admitted to a bingo parlor.

UTAH—Utah, Hawaii, and Tennessee are the only states prohibiting all forms of commercial gambling. Utah, unlike Hawaii, does not even allow social bets.

VERMONT

Lottery: Vermont limits its state lottery to persons who have "attained the age of majority," currently 18. However, minors may receive lottery tickets as gifts. Vermont Statutes title 13 §2143, title 31 §§654 and 661.

Pari-mutuel betting: Vermont Statutes title 31 §613 prohibits a minor from participating in any pari-mutuel pools or even to be admitted to any pari-mutuel enclosure.

Bingo and pull-tabs: Like the lottery, limited to age of majority.

VIRGIN ISLANDS—In 1995 the Virgin Islands began formal steps to legalize casinos.

Lottery: Virgin Islands Code title 32 §254 prohibits sales to anyone under the age of 18. This does not prohibit gifts by adults to minors.

VIRGINIA

Lottery: Code of Virginia §§58.1-4015 states, "No ticket shall be sold to or redeemed from any person under the age of 18 years. Any licensee who knowingly sells or offers to sell or redeem a lottery ticket or shares to or from any person under the age of 18 years is guilty of a Class 1 misdemeanor."

Pari-mutuel betting: Code of Virginia §59.1-403 prevents any person under 18 from wagering on or conducting any wagering on the outcome of a horse race.

Bingo and pull-tabs: Instant bingo is limited to players over 18. Code of Virginia §18.2-340.5.

WASHINGTON—The state has entered into compacts allowing tribes to open casinos without slot machines.

Lottery: Revised Code of Washington §67.70.120 prohibits sales to anyone under 18. This does not prohibit gifts by adults to minors.

Pari-mutuel betting: The state's racing commissioners report the minimum age as being 18. Association of Racing Commissioners International, Inc., *Pari-Mutuel Racing: 1996* at 59.

Casinos: Besides Indian casinos, Washington allows cardrooms, where poker and blackjack are played. Revised Code of Washington §9.46.0305 prevents minors from wagering.

Bingo and pull-tabs: These games may be covered by §9.46.0305, mentioned above.

WEST VIRGINIA—The West Virginia state lottery operates video lottery terminals in racetracks.

Lottery: West Virginia Code §29-22-11 prohibits sales to anyone under the age of 18. This does not prohibit gifts by adults to minors.

Pari-mutuel betting: The state's racing commissioners report the minimum age as being 18. Association of Racing Commissioners International, Inc., *Pari-Mutuel Racing: 1996* at 59.

Bingo: Bingo operators are prohibited from allowing anyone under 18 to participate in the playing of any bingo game with knowledge or reason to believe that the individual is under the age of 18. However, an individual 18 may attend the playing of a bingo game when accompanied by and under the supervision of an adult relative or a legal guardian. West Virginia Code §47-20-4

WISCONSIN

Lottery: Wisconsin has a comprehensive statutory scheme for handling minors and lottery tickets. Like many other states, the minimum age is 18, although minors may receive tickets as gifts. Wisconsin is one of the few states to specifically go after a minor's adult agent: The state makes it a crime to sell a lottery ticket not only to a minor but to an adult who is buying on behalf of the minor and not as a gift. Wisconsin Statutes §§565.17, 565.30, 565.12, and 565.10.

Pari-mutuel betting: Wisconsin Statutes §444.09 prevents any person under 18 "to be admitted to a racetrack, unless accompanied by a parent, grandparent, great-grandparent, guardian or spouse who is at least 18 years of age, or unless accompanied by another person at least 18 with the written permission of the minor's parent or guardian." Even at the track 18-year-olds may not make a wager or receive any payout on a wager and no licensee may knowingly accept a wager or pay out winnings to anyone under 18. No one under 16 may work in any pari-mutuel wagering activity.

Bingo and pull-tabs: Anyone under 18 may not play bingo, unless accompanied by that person's parent, guardian, or spouse. Wisconsin Statutes §563.51.

Casinos: The state entered into compacts allowing tribes to open full-scale, high-stake casinos—with expirations dates beginning in 1998. When the compacts came up for renewal, the state asked for more money and insisted that the age limit be raised from 18 to 21. So far, 11 of the state's 15 tribes have agreed. Wisconsin: New Compacts Guarantee State Tribal Payments, Casino Journal's National Gaming Summary at p. 12 (January 4, 1999).

WYOMING

Pari-mutuel betting: Wyoming Statutes §11-25-109 states, "No person under the age of eighteen (18) years shall place or be allowed to place a bet."

Source: I. Nelson Rose, *Gambling and the Law: Minimum Legal Age to Place A Bet*. Costa Mesa, CA: Whittier Law School, 1999. Reprinted with permission.

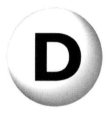

Summary of Treatment Literature

Case Studies (n of 1)

Author(s)/Year	Technique/Approach	Follow-up Period
Lindner, 1950	Psychoanalytic	not specified
Reider, 1960	Psychoanalytic	not specified
Harris, 1964	Psychoanalytic	not specified
Victor and Krug, 1967	Psychoanalytic (paradoxical intention)	not specified
Goorney, 1968	Behavioral (aversive therapy)	12 months
Kraft, 1970	Behavioral (systematic desensitization)	1 year
Cotler, 1971	Behavioral (aversive and covert sensitization)	9 months
Bannister, 1977	Cognitive (rational emotive therapy and covert sensitization)	2.5 years
Dickerson and Weeks, 1979	Behavioral (behavioral counseling)	15 months
Rankin, 1982	Behavioral (behavioral counseling)	2 years
Toneatto and Sobell, 1990	Cognitive	6 months
Hollander et al., 1992	Pharmacotreatment	not specified
Seager et al., 1992	Behavioral (marriage counseling)	not specified
Sharpe and Tarrier, 1992	Cognitive (relaxation training, imaginal and in vivo exposure, cognitive restructuring)	10 months
Haller and Hinterhuber, 1994	Pharmacotreatment (carbamazepine)	not specified

313

Noncontrolled/Descriptive Studies

Author(s)/Year	Sample Size	Technique/ Approach	Follow-up Period
Bergler, 1958	60	Psychoanalytic	not specified
Barker and Miller, 1966	5	Behavioral (aversive therapy)	several months- 2 years
Boyd and Bolen, 1970	9	Psychoanalytic (marital group therapy)	end of treatment
Seager, 1970	14	Behavioral (electrical aversion therapy)	1-3 years
Koller, 1972	20	Behavioral (aversive therapy)	6 months-2 years
Moskowitz, 1980	3	Pharmacotreatment (lithium)	not specified
Greenberg and Marks, 1982	7	Behavioral (desensitization)	6 months
Greenberg and Rankin, 1982	26	Behavioral (stimulus control exposure and covert sensitization)	9 months-5 years
Salzman, 1982	4	Behavioral (aversion)	not specified
Russo et al., 1984	60	Multimodal (group therapy, education, Gamblers Anonymous, discharge plan)	1 year
Taber et al., 1987	57	Multimodal (group therapy, education, Gamblers Anonymous, discharge plan)	6 months
Hudak et al., 1989	99 treated (26 followed- up)	Multimodal (education, individual, family and group therapy, communication skills training, specific discharge plan)	4 years
Arribas and Martinez, 1991	4	Cognitive (self-monitoring, exposure, stimulus control, response prevention, cognitive restructuring, family intervention, relapse prevention)	3 and 6 months

Author(s)/Year	Sample Size	Technique/ Approach	Follow-up Period
Schwarz and Lindner, 1992	58 treated 25 contacted at 2-year follow-up)	Multimodal (medical, group, individual, occupational and family therapy)	1 and 2 years
Sylvain and Ladouceur, 1992	3	Cognitive (education, cognitive restructuring, relapse prevention)	3 and 6 months
Bujold et al., 1994	3	Cognitive (cognitive/ behavioral)	3, 6, and 9 months
Ladouceur et al., 1994	4	Cognitive (information about gambling, cognitive restructuring, problem-solving training, social skills training, relapse prevention)	3 and 6 months
Stinchfield and Winters, 1996	274 (sample for whom discharge, 6 and 12 month data obtained)	Multimodal (individual and group psychotherapy, lectures, participation in self-help groups, family counseling)	Discharge, 6 and 12 months
Hand, 1998	68	Multimodal (motivational interviewing, behavior therapy, family counseling)	not specified

Controlled Studies (random assignment and comparison groups)			
McConaghy et al., 1983[c]	20 (imaginal desensitization = 10, aversive = 10)	Behavioral	1 year
McConaghy et al., 1988	20 (imaginal desensitization = 10, imaginal relaxation = 10)	Behavioral	1 month and 1 year

Author(s)/Year	Sample Size	Technique/ Approach	Follow-up Period
McConaghy et al., 1991	120 (imaginal desensitization = 60[a], other behavioral procedures = 60[b])	Behavioral	2-9 years
Echeburua et al., 1994	64 (individual stimulus control = 16, in vivo exposure with response prevention = 16, group cognitive restructuring = 16, waiting list = 16)	Cognitive	6 months
Sylvain et al., 1997	29 (cognitive/ behavioral = 14, control = 15)	Cognitive	6 and 12 months

[a]33 followed-up.
[b]30 followed-up.
[c]labeled as controlled, but random assignment not mentioned.

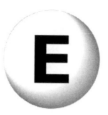

Gamblers Anonymous Meetings
by State

	1995[a]	1996[b]	1998[c]	Change from 1995 to 1998
Alabama	6	6	6	NC
Alaska	3	3	5	+2
Arizona	14	20	39	+25
Arkansas	1	1	1	NC
California	94	110	121	+27
Colorado	9	13	15	+6
Connecticut	18	20	24	+6
Delaware	3	4	6	+3
Florida	40	50	48	+8
Georgia	4	4	12	+8
Hawaii	3	1	1	−2
Idaho	2	3	4	+2
Illinois	29	34	53	+24
Indiana	12	16	16	+4
Iowa	9	21	32	+23
Kansas	4	4	7	+3
Kentucky	9	9	11	+2
Louisiana	24	34	56	+32
Maine	2	3	3	+1
Maryland	17	16	17	NC
Massachusetts	29	26	32	+3
Michigan	16	17	28	+12
Minnesota	43	56	56	+13

	1995[a]	1996[b]	1998[c]	Change from 1995 to 1998
Mississippi	13	15	16	+3
Missouri	10	11	17	+7
Montana	45	40	53	+8
Nebraska	7	11	12	+5
Nevada	63	70	101	+38
New Hampshire	4	4	5	+1
New Jersey	51	49	49	−2
New Mexico	4	7	9	+5
New York	121	112	129	+8
North Carolina	6	7	7	+1
North Dakota	5	5	6	+1
Ohio	43	44	51	+8
Oklahoma	4	4	4	NC
Oregon	25	34	44	+19
Pennsylvania	45	48	43	−2
Rhode Island	5	7	8	+3
South Carolina	20	16	27	+7
South Dakota	19	27	30	+11
Tennessee	9	14	11	+2
Texas	19	20	18	−1
Utah	3	3	2	−1
Vermont	0	0	3	+3
Virginia	5	5	7	+2
Washington	16	15	18	+2
West Virginia	4	6	3	−1
Wisconsin	25	28	40	+15
Wyoming	1	1	1	NC
Total	963		1,074	1,307

[a]Source: Gamblers Anonymous International Directory 1995, Gambler's Anonymous International Service Office. Los Angeles, CA 1995.

[b]Source: Gamblers Anonymous International Directory 1996, Gambler's Anonymous International Service Office. Los Angeles, CA 1996.

[c]Source: Gamblers Anonymous International Service Office. Los Angeles, CA, 1998. Web site visited September 16, 1998. <http://www.gamblersanonymous.org/mtgdirTOP.html>

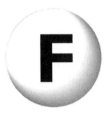

Biographical Sketches

Charles F. Wellford (*Chair*) is director of the University of Maryland Center for Applied Policy Studies and professor of criminology and criminal justice at the University of Maryland. He served as chair of the University's Department of Criminal Justice from 1981 to 1995. He serves on numerous federal and state advisory boards and commissions and is a fellow and the immediate past president of the American Society of Criminology. He currently serves as the chair of the National Research Council's Committee on Law and Justice. He has published more than 40 articles in scholarly journals and is the author of numerous reports developed for various federal agencies and the state of Maryland. He is an expert on crime and social justice issues, prosecution policies and sentencing, and civil justice. His current research interests include the determinants of sentencing and the development of comparative crime data. He received a PhD in sociology from the University of Pennsylvania in 1969.

Melissa I. Bamba (*Research Associate*) serves as a research associate to the Committee on Law and Justice for this and other studies. She previously worked as a research associate at CSR, Inc., a private research firm, on projects for the Office of National Drug Control Policy and the National Institute on Drug Abuse. She received her BA and MA degrees in criminology and criminal justice from Temple University and the University of Maryland, respectively. She is currently working on a PhD degree in criminology from the University of Maryland. Her interests lie in gender and sentencing policy analysis.

Colin F. Camerer is Axline professor of business economics (one of three chaired professors in social science) at the California Institute of Technology. He has held teaching positions at the Kellogg Graduate School of Management at Northwestern University, the Wharton School, and the University of Chicago. His research is primarily published in academic journals and he is on several of their boards, including the *Quarterly Journal of Economics, Journal of Risk and Uncertainty, Journal of Behavioral Decision Making, Strategic Management Journal*, and *Games and Economic Behavior*. His research concerns whether people make systematic mistakes in their decisions, for example in choosing among risky alternatives, engaging in competitive or strategic interactions, and trading in financial markets. He is interested in how new discoveries in neuroscience inform the basic components of economic decision making (judging probabilities, weighing the future, choosing among goods). He has an MBA in finance and a PhD in decision theory from the University of Chicago Graduate School of Business.

Linda B. Cottler is professor of epidemiology in the Department of Psychiatry at Washington University School of Medicine in St. Louis. Her contributions to the field involve risk factors for substance use, assessment of substance use and psychiatric disorders, and the consequences and prevention of substance use, particularly in connection with the human immunodeficiency virus (HIV). She has published extensively, reviews articles for numerous journals, and is on the board of College on the Problems of Drug Dependence and the American Psychopathological Association. Her latest publication (with colleague Renee M. Cunningham-Williams) focused on the epidemiology of pathological gambling among household residents in Missouri from the Epidemiologic Catchment Area (ECA) Study. She has an MPH from Boston University School of Public Health and a PhD from Washington University, St. Louis.

Sara Kiesler is professor of social and decision sciences and a faculty member in the Human Computer Interaction Institute at Carnegie Mellon University. She has a PhD in psychology from Ohio State University, with an emphasis in experimental psychology, basic research on groups, group dynamics, relationships, communication, and decision making. Her interests turned to computer networks in the early 1980s, and her current research focuses on social and behavioral aspects of computers and computer-based communications technologies. She is the author of numerous publications on such topics as flaming, electronic group dynamics, changes in decision making and employee participation, and new kinds of teamwork. With Lee Sproull she is the author of *Connections: New Ways of Working in the Networked Organization*. Most recently she edited *Culture of the Internet*.

Mark W. Lipsey is professor of public policy at Vanderbilt University's Peabody College and codirector of the Center for Evaluation Research and Methodology at the Vanderbilt Institute for Public Policy Studies. His research and teaching interests are in the areas of public policy, program evaluation research, social intervention, field research methodology, and research synthesis. The foci of his recent research have been risk and intervention for juvenile delinquency and issues of methodological quality in program evaluation research. He has published three books and more than 50 articles and technical reports in these areas and has consulted with numerous organizations and projects. He is a former editor-in-chief of *New Directions for Program Evaluation* and has served on the editorial boards of several journals. He has a BS in applied psychology from the Georgia Institute of Technology and a PhD in psychology from the Johns Hopkins University.

Eileen Luna is an assistant professor in the American Indian Studies Program, in the area of law and policy, at the University of Arizona, Tucson. She is an attorney who, for 14 years, directed government agencies that investigated and prosecuted police misconduct cases in California; she is a member of the California,

Federal, and Native American Bar Associations. She was appointed by Attorney General Janet Reno to a position on the National Citizens Advisory Panel for the Immigration and Naturalization Service and Border Patrol. She is an enrolled member of the White River Band of the Chickamauga Cherokee. She has received a grant from the National Institute of Justice to evaluate tribal government programs aimed at reducing violence against women on reservations. Luna has an MPA from the John F. Kennedy School of Government at Harvard University and a JD from Peoples College of Law, Los Angeles.

Samuel C. McQuade (*Study Director*) has over 20 years of combined criminal justice and research experience. Prior to joining the National Research Council, he managed research on behalf of the National Institute of Justice of the U.S. Department of Justice. From 1977 to 1994 he served as a law enforcement officer in the states of Arizona and Washington. He has consulted nationally on policing issues, has an MPA from the University of Washington's Graduate School of Public Affairs, and is completing doctoral studies at the Institute of Public Policy, George Mason University.

Barbara Mellers is professor of psychology at Ohio State University, specializing in psychological models of human judgment and decision making. She currently serves on the executive board of the Federation of Behavioral, Psychological, and Cognitive Sciences and is the immediate past president of the Judgment and Decision Making Society. She is the author of over 40 published papers and the editor of two books: *Decision Research from Bayesian Approaches to Normative Perspectives* and *Psychological Perspectives on Justice: Theory and Applications*. She has developed descriptive models to capture judgments that deviate from rational choice theory, either because people are influenced by context effects or response mode effects not specified by the theory, or because they process information differently, which can lead to intransitive choices or violations of dominance. Currently, she is involved in a large, observational study designed to investigate how California lottery winners expect their winnings will influence their jobs, lifestyles, risk attitudes, and personal happiness. She has a PhD from the University of Illinois, Champaign-Urbana.

Clinton V. Oster, Jr., is a professor in the School of Public and Environmental Affairs and in the School of Business (part time) at Indiana University. His current research centers on aviation safety, transportation economics, international aviation, airport and airway infrastructure, environmental and natural resource policy, and environmental remediation. He was principal investigator on a study of the economic impacts of riverboat gambling for the Indiana Gaming Commission. He is the coauthor of books on public policy, aviation safety, and various aspects of the U.S. airline industry's adaptation to deregulation. He has a BSE from Princeton University, an MS from Carnegie Mellon University, and a PhD from Harvard University.

David Rados is a professor of management at the Owen Graduate School of Management at Vanderbilt University. His research interests include the development and application of normative decision models to marketing, exploration of consumer needs for information and the value of such information, and the marketing of nonprofit goods and services. He is the author of three books on these topics, the latest of which is *Marketing for Non-Profit Organizations*. His most recent publications include "The Luck Business," published in the *Journal of Macromarketing*. He has been a referee for the *Journal of Marketing* and for *Decision Sciences*. He was the recipient of a Fulbright scholarship in 1989, and was awarded a research fellowship at Macquarie University in Australia. He has a BS in chemical engineering from the Massachusetts Institute of Technology, an MBA from the Harvard Business School, and a PhD in marketing from the Stanford Business School.

Richard J. Rosenthal is a board-certified psychiatrist who has been involved in the treatment and rehabilitation of pathological gamblers for almost 20 years. He was founder and first president of the California Council on Problem Gambling and was director of the Gambling Treatment Program at CPC Westwood Hospital. He is currently assistant clinical professor of psychiatry at the

School of Medicine, University of California, Los Angeles and on the faculty of the Los Angeles Psychoanalytic Institute. He coauthored the official diagnostic criteria for pathological gambling that appears in the American Psychiatric Association's *Diagnostic and Statistical Manual of Mental Disorders (DSM-IV)*. He was coinvestigator on the first genetic study that indicated a possible physiological predisposition for the disorder. Other contributions to the gambling literature have dealt with patterns of self-deception, transference-countertransference issues, phases of treatment, and the relationship between gambling problems and criminal behavior. He is currently on the board of directors of the National Council on Problem Gambling, the advisory board of the Institute for the Study of Gambling and Commercial Gaming, and the national advisory board of the American Academy of Health Care Providers in the Addictive Disorders. He has a BA from Cornell University and an MD from the Albert Einstein College of Medicine.

Howard J. Shaffer is associate professor at Harvard Medical School and director of the Harvard Medical School Division on Addictions. He is the founding director of the Norman E. Zinberg Center for Addiction Studies at Harvard Medical School and the Department of Psychiatry at the Cambridge Hospital. He is also founder and president of the board of trustees of the American Academy of Health Care Providers in the Addictive Disorders, the first international credentialing body for clinicians working in the addictive disorders. Recent research projects on which he has served as principal or coprincipal investigator include the Addiction Training Center of New England, the Harvard Project on Gambling and Health, and Estimating the Prevalence of Disordered Gambling in the United States and Canada, a meta-analysis of over 150 gambling prevalence studies. His major research interests include the social perception of addiction and disease, the philosophy of science, impulse control regulation and compulsive behaviors, disordered gambling, addiction treatment outcomes, and the natural history of addictive behaviors. He has a PhD in psychology from the University of Miami, Florida.

Jerome H. Skolnick came to New York University School of Law after taking early retirement from the University of California, Berkeley, where he was Claire Clements Dean's professor of law, jurisprudence, and social policy, a chair he now holds as professor emeritus. For 10 years he was director of the University of California's Center for the Study of Law and Society. At New York University Law School, Skolnick teaches seminars on police and on the regulation of vice and is co-director of the Center for Research in Crime and Justice. Among his best-known books are *Justice Without Trial*, a study of police in a democratic society; *The Politics of Protest*, written as director of the Task Force on Violent Protest and Confrontation of the National Commission on the Causes and Prevention of Violence; *House of Cards*, a study of the regulation of casino gambling; *The New Blue Line*, analyzing community-oriented policing (with David Bayley); and, most recently, *Above the Law*, a study of police use of excessive force (with James J. Fyfe). He was elected a fellow and is a past president of the American Society of Criminology (1993-1994), and recently (1997) completed a three-year term as chair of the National Research Council's Committee on Law and Justice. Skolnick has a bachelor's degree in economics and philosophy and a PhD in sociology from Yale University.

Ken Winters is director of the Center for Adolescent Substance Abuse and associate professor of psychiatry at the University of Minnesota. He also serves as senior research associate in the Department of Psychiatry at the university. He is a member of the American Psychological Association and is currently the principal investigator or coinvestigator for five projects supported by a variety of research organizations, including the National Institute on Drug Abuse (NIDA), the Walker Foundation, the National Institute on Responsible Gaming, and the Center for Substance Abuse Prevention. His research interests include the assessment and treatment of adolescent drug abuse, root causes of addiction, and problem gambling. His previous experience includes appointments as a research scientist at the State University of New York at Stony Brook and as a staff psychologist at a community mental health center. He has a BA from the University of Minnesota and a PhD in clinical psychology from the State University of New York at Stony Brook.

Index